1995 CodeLink

Otolaryngology

DISCLAIMER

1995 CodeLink

Otolaryngology

Context Software Systems Inc.

McGraw-Hill Inc.

New York St. Louis San Francisco Auckland Bogotá Caracas Lisbon
London Madrid Mexico Milan Montreal New Delhi Paris
San Juan Singapore Sydney Tokyo Toronto

A product of McGraw–Hill, Inc.

CODELINK FOR OTOLARYNGOLOGY

1 2 3 4 5 6 7 8 9 0 BKM BKM 95

ISBN 0–07–600762–6

NOTICE:

CPT is a listing of descriptive terms and five–digit numeric identifying codes and modifiers for reporting medical services performed by physicians. This presentation includes only CPT descriptive terms, numeric identifying codes and modifiers for reporting medical services and procedures that were selected by McGraw–Hill, for inclusion in this publication.

The most current CPT is available from the American Medical Association.

No fee schedules, basic unit values, relative value guides, conversion factors or scales are included in CPT. The AMA is not recommending that any specific relative values, fees, fee schedules, or related listings, be attached to CPT. Any relative listings assigned to the CPT codes are not those of the AMA and such assignment should not be construed as a recommendation for use of these relative values by the AMA.

The AMA assumes no responsibility for the consequences attributable to or related to any use or interpretation of any information contained or not contained in this Publication.

NOTICE REGARDING COPYRIGHT DATES:

The AMA CPT for 1995 is published by the AMA in calendar year 1994 and carries a 1994 copyright. These are the valid CPT codes to be used for 1995.

This book was composed and set in Helvetica using WordPerfect®, Ventura Publisher® and an IBM 4039 LaserPrinter® by Context Software Systems, Inc.

TABLE OF CONTENTS

PREFACE

The opening paragraph of the original Preface for the *CodeLink* series began with a quote attributed to Alcott: "That is a good book which is opened with expectation and closed with profit." Much to our delight, judging by the widely growing popularity of the the *CodeLink* series, it seems we have met the challange of providing a "good" book. The series began with *CodeLink* manuals for Oral & Maxillofacial Surgery, Orthopaedics, and Ophthalmology. Due to popular demand, we will be adding titles on Otolaryngology and Plastic Surgery this year, with additional titles to follow as this series continues to grow.

CodeLink was designed to provide a unique tool that will help your practice submit more accurate claims, to lift from your shoulders a bit of the burden of dealing with third party payers, and, as a result, increase your income. This manual helps guide you in the selection of proper codes by providing frequently used ICD–9–CM linkages to CPT codes used within each specialty.

This text would not have been possible without the tireless efforts of many individuals. Bill Elliott, Senior Vice President at Context, worked his computer magic on tens of millions of claims — the starting point of this text. Suzanne McGuire and Todd Winey spent endless hours checking and validating the links between CPT and ICD–9–CM codes and integrating the Medicare rules within the text. Suzanne, Denise Knaus and Leslie Garvey proofed and edited the text and worked directly with the Editorial Panel members. Leslie also designed and typeset the text. Maureen Cirnitski at McGraw–Hill spent numerous hours tying together all the loose ends to ensure the production quality of the series.

We again thank our Editorial Panel members, listed on pages ix through x of this book, for taking time away from their busy schedules to provide guidance on the contents of the text and the links between codes.

We welcome your constructive comments and suggestions on ways of making this text more usable to your practice. Please send them to my attention at the address below.

Gary M. Knaus
President
Context Software Systems, Inc.
241 South Frontage Road, Suites 38–39
Burr Ridge, Illinois 60521

EDITORIAL PANEL

The CPT to ICD–9–CM linkages found in this text are derived from claims actually submitted to third party payers. To help guarantee the quality and integrity of this information, a panel of expert otolaryngologists reviewed and validated the linkages. The following persons offered their time and expertise in this process. Their help is gratefully acknowledged.

Neal S. Beckford, M.D.

Memphis, Tennessee

Dr. Beckford, a graduate of Ohio State University, received his M.D. and postgraduate training from Howard University in Washington, DC. He has served as Chairman and Associate Professor of the Department of Otolaryngology at the University of Tennessee in Memphis, as well as on many committees for the University, hospitals, and musical foundations of Memphis. His extensive written works have been published in medical journals and books, and he has given scientific presentations for many medical, educational, and musical conferences. Dr. Beckford is in private practice in Memphis, Tennessee, specializing in voice, speech and swallowing disorders.

Roman J. Dykun, M.D.

Crystal Lake, Illinois

Dr. Dykun has been in private practice in otolaryngology–head and neck surgery in suburban Chicago, Illinois, since 1982. He is a Fellow of the American Academy of Otolaryngology–Head and Neck Surgery, and the Royal College of Surgeons of Canada. Specializing in pediatric otolaryngology and allergic naso-sinus disease, he has authored several articles and presentations on these subjects. Dr. Dykun conducts pediatric otolaryngology clinics for school children under the auspices of the University of Illinois (D.S.C.C.). He serves as Vice-Chairman of Surgery and as a member of the Board of Directors of the Northern Illinois Medical Center. Dr. Dykun received his M.D. and his residency training at the University of Toronto in Ontario, Canada.

Thomas G. Gerber, Jr., M.D.

Rice Lake, Wisconsin

Dr. Gerber is a Board Certified member of the American Board of Otolaryngology–Head and Neck Surgery. He has been in full-time private practice in Rice Lake, Wisconsin, since 1982. In addition to memberships in the Minnesota Academy of Otolaryngology–Head and Neck Surgery, the American Medical Association, and the State Medical Society of Wisconsin, he is a Fellow of the American Academy of Otolaryngology–Head and Neck Surgery, and a member of its Committee on Terminology and CPT Coding. Dr. Gerber received his B.S. from Wisconsin State University in Eau Claire, Wisconsin, and his M.D. from the Medical College of Wisconsin in Milwaukee.

Joseph Haddad, Jr., M.D.

New York, New York

Dr. Haddad is the Director of Pediatric Otolaryngology at Columbia–Presbyterian Medical Center in New York. He also serves as an Editorial Reviewer for the Annals of Otolaryngology, is the author of numerous articles, publications and abstracts, and has been the principal investigator for several significant research projects in the area of pediatric otolaryngology. He is a regular participant in the Columbia Cleft Lip and Palate Project at Tegucigalpa, Honduras, and has made many presentations at national and international medical conferences. In addition to serving on the faculty and the Curriculum Committee of the Columbia University College of Physicians and Surgeons, Dr. Haddad is a Fellow of the American College of Surgeons and the American Academy of Facial Plastic and Reconstructive Surgery. He is also a member of several other professional and scientific societies. Dr. Haddad is a member of the Committee on Terminology and CPT Coding and the Committee on Infectious Disease for the American Academy of Otolaryngology–Head and Neck Surgery. Dr. Haddad received his B.A., *cum laude*, from Wesleyan University in Middletown, Connecticut, and his M.D. from New York University School of Medicine in New York.

INTRODUCTION

To receive proper reimbursement from third party payers, otolaryngology practices are by now familiar with and using the CPT, HCPCS, and ICD–9–CM coding systems. They are also probably familiar with the guidelines regarding appropriate circumstances to use each system. However, what they may not be familiar with is the increasing scrutiny third party payers are applying to insurance claims.

Attempting to better control costs, payers are increasingly looking at the medical necessity of a procedure or service before deciding to pay for it. If it seems reasonable based on the patient's problem, it is paid. If it does not seem reasonable, it probably is not paid. This process of verifying the medical necessity is done by testing the relationships, or linkages, between the procedure and diagnosis codes submitted on the claim form. These linkages can set the stage for a paid or denied claim.

Therefore, the purpose of this text is to provide this linkage information, as well as the basic reimbursement and coding guidelines necessary to bill properly. Please be aware that this book is not to be considered a replacement for your CPT, HCPCS, or ICD–9–CM books. This manual should be used after location of the correct codes in the coding manuals to verify that your code selections make sense.

CODE LINKAGES

The code linkages in this text were derived from actual claims submitted by otolaryngologists. The linkages were statistically validated, meaning that if a linkage was infrequently reported, it was not included in this volume. The linkages were also reviewed by prominent otolaryngologists for appropriateness and completeness.

Please note that this text has limitations. While the linkages provided herein should cover the vast majority of codes reported by ENT practices, they are not intended, nor does the author or publisher purport to provide a "complete" or "all–inclusive" list. While confident of the quality and integrity of the linkages, the author and publisher make no claim that those provided are "absolute." The linkages are based on actual claims submitted to third party payers which means they are representative of the actual linkages used by ENT practices. The exclusion of a code from the linkage list does not indicate that the code may not be medically appropriate; it means only that it is infrequently reported by ENT practices. For these less–than–common linkages, you may need to submit support documentation to the third party payer to justify and explain the reasons for the procedure/service.

CPT to ICD–9–CM Linkages

The CPT to ICD–9–CM linkages provide the logically–related diagnosis code (ICD–9–CM) relationships to an individual CPT code. This information can be used to validate the diagnosis code choice when the procedure code (CPT) is already known. An example from this section of the book is provided below.

402 CODELINK for OTOLARYNGOLOGY

CPT CODE **SERVICE**

92567 Tympanometry (impedance testing)

CPT NOTES

- Diagnostic or treatment procedures usually included in a comprehensive otorhinolaryngologic evaluation or office visit, are reported as an integrated medical service, using appropriate descriptors from the 99201 series. Itemization of component procedures (e.g., otoscopy, rhinoscopy, tuning fork test) does not apply.

  Special otorhinolaryngologic services are those diagnostic and treatment services not usually included in a comprehensive otorhinolaryngologic evaluation or office visit. These services are reported separately, using descriptors from the 92500 series.

  All services include medical diagnostic evaluation. Technical procedures (which may or may not be performed by the physician personally) are often part of the service, but should not be mistaken to constitute the service itself.
- For laryngoscopy with stroboscopy, use 31579.
- For evaluation of speech, language and/or hearing problems through observation and assessment of performance, see 92506.
- This audiometric test implies the use of calibrated electronic equipment. Other hearing tests (such as whispered voice, tuning fork) are considered part of the general otorhinolaryngologic services and are not reported separately. All descriptors refer to testing both ears. Use the modifier '–52' or 09952, if a test is applied to one ear instead of to two ears. All descriptors (except 92559), apply to testing of individuals; for testing of groups, use 92559 and specify test(s) used.

ICD–9–CM

315.39	Speech/language develop disord NEC
380.32	Acquired deformity auricle/pinna
380.50	Acquired stenosis ear canal NOS
381.0x	Acute otitis media
381.10	Chron serous otitis media simp/NOS
381.19	Chronic serous otitis media NEC
381.3	Chronic nonsuppurative otitis media
381.4	Chron nonsup otitis media NOS
381.81	Dysfunction of Eustachian tube
381.9	Eustachian tube disorder NOS
382.00	Acute suppurative otitis media NOS
382.3	Chronic suppurativ otitis media NOS
384.0x	Acute myringitis
384.1	Chronic myringitis
384.82	Atrophic nonflaccid tymp membrane
384.9	Tympanic membrane disorder NOS
385.10	Adhesive middle ear disease NOS
385.2x	Other acquired abnormality ossicles
385.30	Cholesteatoma NOS
385.89	Middle Ear/Mastoid disorder NEC
387.9	Otosclerosis NOS
388.01	Presbyacusis
388.1x	Noise effects on inner ear
388.3x	Tinnitus
388.42	Hyperacusis
388.43	Impairment auditory discrimination
388.60	Otorrhea NOS
388.69	Otorrhea NEC
388.7x	Otalgia
389.08	Conductive hearing loss, comb type
389.10	Sensorineural hearing loss NOS
389.11	Sensory hearing loss
389.12	Neural hearing loss
389.18	Sensorineural hear loss comb type
389.2	Mixed hearing loss
744.02	Ext ear anomaly NEC, hearing impair
852.40	Traumatic extradural hemorrhage
951.5	Injury to acoustic nerve
V41.2	Problems with hearing
V72.1	Examination of ears/hearing

REIMBURSEMENT INFORMATION

Medicare

- Follow–up Days — global concept does not apply
- Assistant Surgeon — by report
- Supply Charges — not allowed
- Outpatient Limit — does not apply

Fifth–Digit Representation

You will note that in some cases, ICD–9–CM codes are listed as "123.4x." The "x" indicates that fifth digits apply to this code. However, in the interest of conserving space, not all fifth–digit codes are expanded, but instead are listed in this way. Be sure to check your ICD–9–CM manual for the fifth–digit code applicable to your coding situation.

HOW TO USE THIS MANUAL

This manual is arranged in sections as follows:

Coding Guidelines. This section explains the basic coding conventions and guidelines which all users of the coding systems need to know. While it is not exhaustive, it does provide an overview of topics such as the global surgical package, billing starred procedures, the basics of ICD–9–CM and CPT coding, etc.

CPT to ICD–9–CM Linkages. This section contains the "what's and why's"; that is, the logical relationships between procedures and diagnoses. A single CPT code number is listed in the left column with the logically related diagnosis (ICD–9–CM) code(s) listed in the right column. In addition, you will find general coding reminders, notes from CPT relevant to each code, and pertinent Medicare reimbursement information.

Within this section, the linkages are grouped and divided according to the sections of CPT.

To make best use of this manual, it is recommended that you become familiar with the organization of and notations used in this text. An overview of the organization was provided above. The specific notations used are discussed below.

OVERVIEW AND EXPLANATION OF NOTATIONS

Additional coding and reimbursement information is provided in the CPT to ICD–9–CM Linkages section of this manual. The example shown on the next page is representative, with an explanation of the notations provided on the following pages.

CPT CODE	SERVICE
● 31254	Nasal/sinus endoscopy, surgical; with ethmoidectomy, partial (anterior)

CPT Description

ICD-9-CM Code Number(s)/Link(s)

CPT NOTES

- A surgical sinus endoscopy always includes a sinusotomy and diagnostic endoscopy.
- Codes 31231–31294 are used to report unilateral procedures unless otherwise specified.

CPT Code Number

CPT Notes

New/Changed Code Marker

ICD-9-CM

212.0	B-Neoplasm, nasal cavity/sinus
229.8	Benign neoplasm NEC
375.56	Acquired nasolacrimal duct stenosis
461.0	Acute maxillary sinusitis
461.2	Acute ethmoidal sinusitis
461.8	Other acute sinusitis
461.9	Acute sinusitis NOS
471.0	Polyp of nasal cavity
471.1	Polypoid sinus degeneration
471.8	Nasal sinus polyp NEC
471.9	Nasal polyp NOS
473.0	Chronic maxillary sinusitis
473.2	Chronic ethmoidal sinusitis
473.8	Chronic sinusitis NEC
473.9	Chronic sinusitis NOS
478.1	Nasal and sinus disease NEC
519.8	Respiratory system disease NEC

ICD-9-CM Description(s)

REIMBURSEMENT INFORMATION

General

- New procedure, 1995 CPT.

Medicare

- Follow-up Days — 0
- Assistant Surgeon — not paid
- Supply Charges — not allowed
- Outpatient Limit — does not apply
- Minor Surgery Rules Apply

General Reimbursement Information

Medicare Reimbursement Information

CPT CODE–SERVICE

This is the code number and full description as it appears in CPT 1995.

CPT NOTES

Pertinent parenthetical or other notes found in CPT which apply specifically to the code listed are printed here for your reference. Where applicable, notes relative to an entire section of codes are reproduced as a single entry before that group of codes. For example, the notes from CPT 1995 from the Surgery/Musculoskeletal section are included as a single entry on page 83. A note in the right column under "General Information" refers you to the appropriate page of this manual which you should reference should you wish to review these notes.

ICD–9–CM

These are the logically related ICD–9–CM 1995 code numbers and shortened descriptions. Please note again that this list is not intended to be all–inclusive nor should it be construed as any kind of recommendation of "correct" medical parameters. The linkages are provided for reference. If your situation dictates that you report a code not found on the list, you may wish to add the linkage. Conversely, you may wish to delete linkages not pertinent to your practice.

REIMBURSEMENT INFORMATION

General

This notation contains general reimbursement information, such as the references to section notes, whether the code is new or the description changed in 1995, and whether certain coding rules, such as separate procedure or starred procedure rules, apply.

For the notes found at the beginning of a section of codes in CPT which are reproduced in this book, the reference in this notation says "See notes on page xx." Refer to that page in this text to find these notes. For example, the note on page 84 of this text for CPT code number 21310 instructs you to "See notes on page 83." For the instructional notes related to these repairs, you would refer to page 83 of this text for those notes. You can refer also to the section guidelines of your CPT for more complete information.

Codes for which the description changed in 1995 are noted with both the triangle (CPT's symbol for change) as well as the notation "Description changed in 1995 CPT." New codes which were added to CPT 1995 are noted with both the circle (CPT's symbol for new) as well as the notation "New procedure, 1995 CPT."

Codes for which the starred procedure billing rules or the separate procedure billing rules apply have a note under this heading which states "Starred procedure" or "Separate procedure rules apply." These notes are provided to help the coder use the codes and bill properly. These coding rules are also discussed in this text in the Coding Guidelines section. Starred procedures are discussed beginning on page 15 and separate procedures are discussed beginning on page 17.

Medicare

The notations under this heading provide information specific to Medicare. Each is explained below.

Follow–Up Days. This note indicates the number of surgical follow–up days applicable to the procedure. The numbers will be 0, 10 or 90, depending upon the procedure. If this note reads "none; included in global package of another procedure," you should interpret this to mean the procedure is actually a component of another procedure and so no follow–up days are assigned for performance of the procedure alone. A note which reads "global concept does not apply" indicates that this service is not considered surgical in nature so no follow–up days need to be assigned. A note which reads "determined by local carrier" indicates that the local carrier determines the follow–up days for this procedure on an individual basis. Typically, these are unlisted procedures.

Assistant Surgeon. This note tells you whether Medicare permits payment for an assistant surgeon for the procedure. "Paid" means Medicare may allow payment for an assistant for this procedure. "Not paid" means Medicare has determined that an assistant surgeon is not necessary for this procedure and so will not pay for one. (You are not permitted to attempt to charge the patient for the assistant.) A "by report" notation means that the individual carrier makes a determination as to whether an assistant is payable for this service.

Supply Charges. Medicare permits payment for supplies provided in the physician's office only for certain identified procedures (refer to the Coding Guidelines chapter of this manual for further information about this provision). This notation reminds you whether or not the supply of a surgical tray is payable separately. "Not allowed" means Medicare considers the tray to be part of the charge for the procedure; you cannot collect this charge from the patient. "Allowed" indicates you can charge Medicare an additional amount, using HCPCS National code A4550, for the provision of a surgical tray.

Outpatient Limit. Also called the site–of–service reduction, the outpatient limit refers to a 50 percent reduction in the practice expense component of the procedure's relative value units. The outpatient limit applies to certain identified procedures which, if provided in an outpatient department or hospital rather than the physician's office, will receive this reduction. A note which reads "applies" means that payment will be reduced if the place of service is other than the physician's office. A note which reads "does not apply" means Medicare will not adjust payment based on the place of service.

Minor or Major Procedure Rules.	Medicare's global surgical package rules can be referenced with this note. "Minor Procedure Rules" means that the minor surgical package rules apply to this procedure. "Major Procedure Rules" means the major surgical package rules apply to this procedure. For more information about Medicare's surgical package definitions, refer to the Coding Guidelines chapter of this text.

EVALUATION AND MANAGEMENT SERVICES

This section of code linkages deserves special mention. You will note an "Examples" notation folowing many of the evaluation and management (E&M) services codes. The information provided under this notation is a vignette, or illustration, of the level of care provided. These vignettes are found in the CPT code manual, either following the code or in Appendix D. They are included here for illustrative purposes.

Notes specific to a group of E&M codes are found prior to that group of codes in this manual and are referenced with the "See notes on page xx" notation. These are provided for your reference. For more complete information regarding the definitions of each component of an E&M code and other pertinent rules, refer to your CPT book.

Also, it is important to note that in some cases a limited set of ICD–9–CM linkages are provided for each level of E&M service. The author and publisher recognize that an almost unlimited set of diagnoses could be listed with each code. However, in the interest of space and to make the book easier to use, only a limited set are included. It is recommended that you add to or delete from this list as pertinent to your practice.

CODING GUIDELINES

OVERVIEW OF CODING SYSTEMS

The primary means by which ENT practices communicate to third party payers is by the use of codes. That is, codes are reported to inform the insurance carrier what was done to the patient (procedures and services) and why (diagnoses). Physicians actually use three different coding systems. Procedures and services are reported using the American Medical Association's *Current Procedural Terminology* (CPT) and the *Health Care Financing Administration's (HCFA) Common Procedure Coding System* (HCPCS). The *International Classification of Diseases, Ninth Revision, Clinical Modification* (ICD–9–CM) coding system is used to report patient diagnoses. An understanding of how to use these coding systems is essential to proper reimbursement.

PHYSICIANS' CURRENT PROCEDURAL TERMINOLOGY (CPT)

Published by the American Medical Association and updated annually in December, CPT is the most widely used procedural coding system in the United States. CPT contains codes and descriptions for more than 7,000 procedures and services rendered by doctors. Codes listed in CPT consist of two parts: a five–digit code number and the associated description. The following is an example of a CPT code and its description:

30124 Excision dermoid cyst, nose; simple, skin, subcutaneous

Most every claim submitted by ENT practices to their patients' medical insurance will contain CPT codes. Therefore, it is imperative that the reader have a grasp of the CPT system as a whole: the symbols and format utilized, modifiers, and the general rules guiding the choice and use of codes. Users of CPT need to be especially aware of the many notes contained in the coding system which provide information about how certain procedures and services are to be reported. These notes may appear before a group of codes, below a code, or at the end of a group of codes. In some cases, interpretation of these notes will vary from coder to coder, and from one third party payer to another. Experienced CPT coders have learned to accept that there is not always an absolute right way to code certain procedures and services.

Organization of the CPT Coding Manual

CPT is divided into six distinct sections of codes: Evaluation and Management (for visits and consultations); Anesthesia; Surgery (for procedures such as rhinectomy and laryngoscopy); Radiology (for X–rays); Pathology and Laboratory (for lab work such as urinalysis and cultures); and Medicine (for non-invasive services, such as injections and physical therapy). Each of the six sections are preceded by guidelines that contain rules and modifiers relevant to that section of codes.

In addition to codes, CPT also contains an introduction, four appendices, and an index. The CPT Introduction provides information about and rules related to use of the coding system and describes symbols and other important concepts. Appendix A lists all CPT modifiers and their definitions. Changes that have appeared since the previous year's volume are noted in Appendix B. (The use of symbols to indicate changes will be discussed later.) The third appendix (Appendix C) notes changes applying to those practices that use the CPT short procedure descriptions in their computer database. Appendix D contains clinical examples for E&M services. CPT's Index is located at the back of the book and is preceded by instructions related to helping the user locate codes.

Symbols

CPT utilizes three symbols that provide special information about the codes: the circle; the triangle; and the star. Each of these symbols is discussed below.

Circle (•)

A blackened circle, or bullet, is placed to the left of codes that are new to CPT. That is, these codes did not appear in the previous year's volume. Noting the circle serves two purposes. First, it allows users of CPT to quickly locate new procedures and services without having to refer back and forth between Appendix B and the code sections. Second, it reminds the coder that the procedure or service is new. This is important when billing because third party payers do not always implement new codes when they are released. Information related to patient conditions for which the procedure is appropriate, reasonable fees for the new procedures, etc., must be developed by the third party payers before the new procedure is routinely reimbursed. Therefore, when submitting new CPT codes to third party payers, it may be necessary to provide additional information that justifies both medical necessity and the charge being made. Once the third party payers begin paying for the new procedure or service on a routine basis, the supplementary support documentation may not be needed to ensure payment.

Triangle (▲)

The blackened triangle, or delta, to the left of a code signifies that the code's definition has been changed. Changes may be significant or minor, but in any case, for those codes used by the practice, a comparison of the current to the previous year's definition should be made.

The comparison is important for reimbursement and audit liability reasons. To understand why, consider a procedure for which the definition has significantly changed, but the practice is unaware of the change and continues to bill as if the code describes something which it no longer does. In such a case the physician is not reporting what was performed. Two unfortunate consequences may result. First, the physician may be inappropriately reimbursed due to the fact that what was billed was not what was actually performed. Second, if audited, this could be interpreted as fraudulent billing and might create a host of problems for the practice.

Star (*)

In the Surgery section of CPT, stars appear to the right of several code numbers. The star notes that CPT's surgical package concept does not apply to the procedure. That is, preoperative and postoperative care are to be billed separately in addition to the starred procedure, subject to a set of rules found in the Surgery section guidelines. These rules are discussed on pages 14–18 of this text.

HEALTH CARE FINANCING ADMINISTRATION'S COMMON PROCEDURE CODING SYSTEM (HCPCS)

Pronounced "hick-pix," this coding system was developed by Medicare (HCFA) and consists of the three levels of codes described below:

Level I — CPT

Level II — National Codes

Level III — Local Codes

Level I, CPT, was incorporated into HCPCS in 1984 with the permission of the American Medical Association. The Level II and III codes are created by HCFA and local Medicare carriers to supplement CPT. National Codes (Level II) contain listings of supplies and procedures not specified in CPT. These National codes may be differentiated from CPT codes in that they begin with a letter of the alphabet (A through V) followed by four numbers. An example of a National code is given below:

J2510 Injection, penicillin G procaine, aqueous, up to 600,000 units

Local codes (Level III) are created by each individual state's Medicare carrier and are for use only in that carrier's region. These codes can be distinguished from National codes in that they begin with the letter W, X, Y, or Z followed by four numbers. Local codes sometimes describe supplies, injections, and procedures that are very new, and therefore not yet listed in the CPT or National systems. In other cases, Local codes will describe variations on the services and supplies listed in the other levels. Furthermore, some states' Medicare carriers have Local codes that could be used by ENT practices while, in other states, no codes would apply.

Use of HCPCS Codes

HCPCS codes are reported in the same manner on claim forms and superbills as CPT codes. Determining which codes to use — CPT, National, or Local — is a simple process if the following rules are kept in mind:

1. Use HCPCS codes when reporting services, procedures, and supplies to Medicare, and in some states, to Medicaid.
2. Use the HCPCS code which most completely describes the procedure, service, or supply.

Although in most cases the physician will report CPT codes to Medicare and Medicaid, there are two groups of codes in the National system of interest. These are the medical and surgical supply codes (A4190–A5507) and the injection/chemotherapy codes (J0110–J9999). An example follows.

The physician treats a Medicare patient. During the visit, he/she injects 500 mg of Ampicillin intramuscularly. CPT provides an all–purpose intramuscular antibiotic injection code, 90788:

90788 Intramuscular injection of antibiotic (specify).

For non–Medicare/Medicaid patients, this CPT code could be appropriate for reporting the injection. The type of antibiotic and amount injected would be listed with the description. However, for Medicare and Medicaid patients the reporting rules differ. To report the supply of the antibiotic substance, the most specific code should be listed. The HCPCS National system contains more than 400 codes for different injectables, many of which are antibiotics. There is a code for ampicillin:

J0290 Injection, Ampicillin, up to 500 mg.

Using the second rule above, since the J0290 code more exactly describes the service it should be reported to Medicare instead of the more general CPT antibiotic injection code, 90788. As a rule, never use the CPT therapeutic injection codes (90782–90799) when reporting the supply of injectables to Medicare (or possibly Medicaid). The appropriate "J" code should be listed instead.

Note that Medicare considers the administration of the injection to be included in the service provided. Separate billing is allowed, using the appropriate HCPCS National code, for the supply of the injected material only.

Local codes can also be important to ENT practices. Their importance depends upon the specific codes used by the practice's local Medicare carrier. If the Medicare carrier has created codes for injections, supplies, procedures, and/or services, they should be reviewed for potential use by the practice. Optimal reimbursement from Medicare and Medicaid depends upon understanding the rules associated with these HCPCS National and Local codes. As such, practices need to obtain copies of both the HCPCS National and Local codes.

INTERNATIONAL CLASSIFICATION OF DISEASES, NINTH REVISION, CLINICAL MODIFICATION (ICD–9–CM)

The ICD–9–CM coding system was developed in the late 1970s by the National Center for Health Statistics as a statistical classification system. It was created to replace the older ICD–A system, and to allow for better reporting of both inpatient and outpatient conditions. Today, ICD–9–CM is used by virtually all third party payers as the coding system for describing patient conditions. ICD–9–CM is updated annually in October. It is expected that the next revision of ICD, ICD–10, will not be released until sometime after the year 2000.

Although the complete ICD–9–CM coding system consists of three volumes, physician practices need only concern themselves with Volumes 1 and 2, the Tabular List and Index, respectively. Volume 3, which contains procedures and an index to procedures, is used almost exclusively by hospitals. Volume I, the Tabular Listing, contains diagnosis codes and their descriptions. Volume 2 is the index to the codes found in the Tabular Listing. The example below was taken from Volume 1 and demonstrates an ICD–9 code:

471.0 Polyp of nasal cavity

Organization and Use of ICD–9–CM

On April 1, 1989, a law requiring that all physicians use ICD–9–CM codes when reporting patient diagnoses to Medicare took effect. Serious penalties can result from lack of compliance on claims submitted to Medicare after June 1, 1989. Penalties range from possible non-payment of assigned claims, to potential fines of $2,000 per occurrence on unassigned claims.

Although this law applies only to claims submitted to Medicare, the use of ICD–9–CM codes for reporting diagnoses to all third party payers is advisable for several reasons. First, if diagnosis codes are not used, payment may be denied or delayed. Second, when not used, the carrier's staff will locate an ICD–9–CM code based on the doctor's description of the patient's problem. This coding is usually performed by individuals with either no or very limited medical background. As a result, the codes selected by the carrier may not logically match with the procedure or service being reported, and the claim could be denied.

Finally, many third party payers have purchased or developed software programs that compare the CPT code to the ICD–9–CM code. These programs test for logical relationships. Should, for example, the procedure listed be the removal of a foreign body from the ear and the diagnosis is fracture of the nasal bones, the claim will be automatically denied for lack of medical necessity or reasonableness.

Therefore, it is becoming increasingly important that practices familiarize themselves with the ICD–9–CM coding system and its rules. To that end, discussed below is the organization of the ICD–9–CM coding manual, and the abbreviations, symbols, and notes used throughout the system. The discussion is not intended to be exhaustive.

Organization

The complete ICD–9–CM consists of three volumes. Physician practices do not need the third volume, as it contains procedure codes for hospital use. Volume 1 of ICD–9–CM, the Tabular List, contains codes and descriptions for diseases, illnesses, injuries, complaints, symptoms, etc. It is organized into 17 chapters plus two supplementary sections. These later sections are for coding patients who are not being seen for a current illness ("V" codes) or where the patient's problem is due to an external cause related to injury or poisoning ("E" codes). Volume 2 of ICD–9–CM is the index to the first volume.

Codes can be either three–digits (called categories), four–digits (called classifications), or five–digits (called sub–classifications). Many category codes are further defined by the classification and subclassification codes. The additional fourth and fifth digits typically provide additional information to the category pertinent to the body area, site, or whether the patient did or did not present complications. An example of each level of code is shown below.

385 Other Disorders of Middle Ear and Mastoid

385.1 Other Disorders of Middle Ear and Mastoid, Adhesive Middle Ear Disease; adhesive otitis, otitis media: chronic adhesive, fibrotic

385.12 Other Disorders of Middle Ear and Mastoid, Adhesive Middle Ear Disease; adhesive otitis, otitis media: chronic adhesive, fibrotic, Adhesions of Drum Head to Stapes

Symbols

Two symbols are used throughout the first volume of ICD–9–CM. The first symbol, the lozenge "□," is not relevant to physician practices. The second symbol, the section mark, "§," is important as it alerts the coder to the presence of fifth digits that need to be added to the code. In many instances, definitions for the fifth digits are found on pages preceding the code.

Abbreviations

Users of ICD–9–CM will be familiar with the two abbreviations, NEC and NOS. Each has a specific meaning and importance to coding and reimbursement.

Not Elsewhere Classifiable (NEC)

In some situations the coder will not have enough information available to determine a more specific code. This may occur in cases where highly specific codes exist. The ICD–9–CM Index provides references to specific codes when such cases arise, and uses the NEC abbreviation to help guide the coder. For example, the physician determines that a patient has an abnormality of the ear but does not provide any further information about the abnormality. The ICD–9–CM Index lists anomalies of the ear as follows:

Anomaly, anomalous (congenital) (unspecified type) 759.9
ear 744.3
causing impairment of hearing 744.00
specified type NEC 744.09
external 744.3
causing impairment of hearing 744.02
specified type NEC 744.29
inner (causing impairment of hearing) 744.05
middle, except ossicles (causing impairment of hearing) 744.03
ossicles 744.04
ossicles 744.04
prominent auricle 744.29
specified type NEC 744.29
with hearing impairment 744.09

The NEC abbreviation informs the coder that code 744.29 might be appropriate in the example cited above.

In other cases there may not be a code which completely describes the patient's condition. Not elsewhere classifiables will also be used in these situations. Referring to the previous example, suppose the physician specified the specific type of the anomaly, but that particular diagnosis is not listed in ICD–9–CM. That is, it is not one of the types mentioned (e.g., absence of ear lobe, macrotia, microtia). In this case, the Index reference to specified type NEC would apply to this coding situation. So, code 744.29 would be appropriate to use in this coding example where the anomaly is known, but the specific type of anomaly is not listed in the ICD–9–CM book.

From a reimbursement standpoint, in such cases as cited above, it may be necessary to inform the third party payer of the specific diagnosis. That is, a brief description of the patient's illness may need to be submitted to help ensure proper payment.

Not Otherwise Specified (NOS)

This abbreviation appears throughout the Tabular List and is frequently associated with the "unspecified" codes. In fact, "not otherwise specified" means the same as "unspecified." Use of codes with NOS as part of their definition will often result when the coder does not have enough information to select a more definitive diagnosis. For example, suppose a patient is seen for chronic sinusitis, but the type has not been determined. ICD–9–CM provides a code for this situation, "473.9, Chronic Sinusitis; unspecified sinusitis (chronic); NOS." NOS is listed as part of the code's definition.

When codes for unspecified conditions are reported to third party payers, special attention may need to be given to the claim if reimbursement is expected. Many carriers will often suspend for review claims that list an unspecified diagnosis code. Therefore, it may be necessary to attach a brief note to the claim explaining the patient's problem in more detail.

Notes

Users of ICD–9–CM have undoubtedly noticed the Includes and Excludes notes that appear with groups of codes as well as specific codes. These terms have specific meanings in

ICD–9–CM. Includes notes further define or give an example of the contents of a group of codes. Consider the following code from ICD–9–CM:

477. Allergic rhinitis

Includes: allergic rhinitis (nonseasonal) (seasonal)
hay fever
spasmodic rhinorrhea
temporomandibular (joint)

Patients suffering from any of these types of rhinitus could be coded using listings from the 477 series.

Excludes notes mean just the opposite of Includes notes. In ICD–9–CM, the term "Excludes:" is always surrounded by a printed box so that it is easily noticed. Coders need to be aware of conditions that are excluded from groups of codes, and therefore, should take notice of the Excludes notes. An example of an Excludes note appears on the next page:

784.1 Symptoms involving head and neck; Throat pain

Excludes: *dysphagia (787.2)*
neck pain (723.1)
sore throat (462)
chronic (472.1)

Thus, if a patient is suffering from a sore throat, codes from the 784.1 group would not be reported.

Fourth– and Fifth–Digit Codes

In many cases there will be fourth– and fifth–digit codes from which to select. If there is a fifth–digit code, it should always be used. If there are no fifth–digit codes, but there are fourth–digit codes, use a fourth–digit code. Only if there are no fourth– and fifth–digit codes may a third–digit code be used.

Fifth digits are presented in different ways in ICD–9–CM. Each fifth–digit code may be listed as is found under the series 381.6 "Obstruction of Eustachian tube." All possible fifth–digit codes are listed. Another method involves printing the fifth–digits themselves, with their definitions, prior to the fourth–digit codes to which they apply. An example of this is found for the three–digit category 015, "Tuberculosis of bones and joints" codes. The fifth–digit subclassifications for use with this category are found under the "Tuberculosis" heading before category code 010. Seven fifth–digits apply to categories 010–018, as shown below:

0 unspecified

1 bacteriological or histological examination not done

2 bacteriological or histological examination unknown (at present)

3 tubercle bacilli found (in sputum) by microscopy

4 **tubercle bacilli not found (in sputum) by microscopy, but found by bacterial culture**

5 **tubercle bacilli not found by bacteriological examination, but tuberculosis confirmed histologically**

6 **tubercle bacilli not found by bacteriological or histological examination but tuberculosis confirmed by other methods [inoculation of animals]**

These would be applied to the fourth–digit codes in the 015 series as appropriate. As an example, for a patient suffering from tuberculous mastoiditis (code 015.6) found in microscopy, the fifth–digit "3" is required to indicate the method of detection for a final code of 015.63. If the tuberculosis was confirmed by inoculation of an animal, the final code would be 015.66. Claims not listing fifth– or fourth–digit diagnoses when required may be denied.

Symptoms, Signs, and Ill–Defined Conditions

Some patients may present symptoms or signs that defy immediate diagnosis. Nonetheless, if a claim is filed, a diagnosis must be listed, and special codes can be used in such cases. Chapter 16 in ICD–9–CM serves this purpose as it provides codes for these types of conditions. For example, the physician treats a patient who has repeated nosebleeds. Until a more definitive diagnosis is established, code 784.7 for epistaxis of unknown origin can be listed.

"V" Codes

These codes appear toward the end of Volume 1 under the title "Supplementary Classification of Factors Influencing Health Status and Contact with Health Services." They are typically used when the patient is being seen for something other than a current illness or injury. A follow–up visit related to cancer that has not been present in a patient for several years would be an example.

Many physicians and staff are afraid to report "V" codes because they are aware that in most cases the patient's insurance policy will not cover services associated with "V" codes. But the problem is really not the doctors', as well meaning as they may be. Patients purchase specific coverages when they buy health insurance and few carriers today sell coverage for adult "well visits." Thus, it is the patient's responsibility to pay for non-covered services, and the physician should not feel shy about reporting "V" codes when it is appropriate to do so.

"E" Codes

The "E" codes are supplementary and are used to describe external causes of injuries and poisonings. They are never reported by themselves, and are rarely used by physicians.

EVALUATION AND MANAGEMENT (E&M) SERVICES

The 1992 CPT completely redefined both the code numbers and descriptions of all visit and consultation codes. The changes were intended to reduce the potential for differing interpretations of the codes and to increase the consistency of reporting by doctors in differing specialties. Medicare began requiring use of these codes effective for services rendered on or after January 1, 1992. Other payers phased the codes in over time.

Unlike with the old "visit" codes, it is no longer possible to make direct comparison between levels of service provided to new and established patients, or to services rendered in different locations. For example, a Level II new patient office visit is not defined in the same way as a Level II established patient office visit. General E&M coding rules and important factors associated with different types of E&M codes are covered below.

New and Established Patients

The definitions for new and established patients were changed in the 1992 CPT. New patients are those for whom the doctor has not provided professional services within the past three years. Obviously, patients provided professional services within the past three years are considered to be established. There are two key exceptions to this rule:

1. If you are on call or covering for another doctor (including locum tenens doctors, according to Medicare) and bill your services, you would report using an established patient code.
2. If you have never before provided professional services to a patient, but are a member of a group practice that bills under a group ID, and the patient received services within the last three years from a doctor of the same specialty in that group, then Medicare will consider the patient established. If the patient was seen by a practitioner of a different specialty, you may consider the patient new.

Definitions of E&M Services

Evaluation and management services (visits) are defined based upon three key components. Selection of a code requires the performance of each of the three components. Certain key words and phrases are used to define these components. The components, and their definitions, are described below.

History

The levels of E&M services recognize four types of history that are defined as follows:

- **Problem Focused.** History of the chief complaint; brief history of present illness or problem.
- **Expanded Problem Focused.** History of the chief complaint; brief history of present illness; problem pertinent system review.

- **Detailed.** History of the chief complaint; extended history of present illness; extended system review; pertinent past, family and/or social history.
- **Comprehensive.** History of the chief complaint; extended history of present illness; complete system review; complete past, family and social history.

Examination

The levels of E&M services recognize four types of examination that are defined as follows:

- **Problem Focused.** An examination that is limited to the affected body area or organ system.
- **Expanded Problem Focused.** An examination of the affected body area or organ system and other symptomatic or related organ systems.
- **Detailed.** An extended examination of the affected body area(s) and other symptomatic or related organ system(s).
- **Comprehensive.** A complete single system specialty examination or a complete multi–system examination.

Medical Decision Making

This refers to the complexity of establishing a diagnosis and/or selecting a management option as measured by:

- the number of possible diagnoses and/or the number of management options that must be considered.
- the amount and/or complexity of information (e.g., medical records, diagnostic tests, etc.) that must be obtained, reviewed and analyzed.
- the risk of significant complications, morbidity and/or mortality, as well as co-morbidities, associated with the patient's presenting problem(s), the diagnostic procedure(s), and/or the possible management options.

Four types of medical decision making are recognized: straightforward; low complexity; moderate complexity; and high complexity. For a service to qualify as involving a certain type of medical decision making, two of the three descriptions listed after each type of decision making in the table below must be met or exceeded.

Type of Decision Making	Number of Diagnoses or Management Options	Amount and/or Complexity of Data to be Reviewed	Risk of Complications and/or Morbidity or Mortality
Straightforward	Minimal	Minimal or None	Minimal
Low Complexity	Limited	Limited	Low
Moderate Complexity	Multiple	Moderate	Moderate
High Complexity	Extensive	Extensive	High

Comorbidities/underlying diseases, in and of themselves, are not considered in selecting a level of E&M service unless their presence significantly increases the complexity of the medical decision making.

Contributing Components

There are four contributory components which can affect code selection. Each of these contributory components is described below.

Nature of Presenting Problem

A presenting problem is a disease, condition, illness, injury, symptom, sign, finding, complaint, or other reason for an encounter, whether or not a diagnosis is established at the time of the encounter. Definitions for the five types of problems are found in the E&M Guidelines in your CPT.

Counseling/Coordination of Care

Counseling is a discussion with the patient and/or the family concerning one or more of the following areas:

- Diagnostic results, impressions and/or recommended diagnostic studies.
- Prognosis.
- Risks and benefits of management (treatment) options.
- Instructions for management (treatment) and/or follow–up.
- Importance of compliance with chosen management (treatment) options.
- Risk factor reduction.
- Patient and family education.

Coordination of care is not formally defined in CPT. However, it is self–explanatory.

Time

Time as an explicit factor is included to assist doctors in selecting the most appropriate level of service. It should be recognized that the specific times expressed in the visit code descriptors are averages, and therefore represent a range of times which may be higher or lower depending on actual clinical circumstances. Time is to be considered as a deciding factor in code selection only when counseling and/or coordination of care comprise more than 50 percent of the encounter.

Intra–service times are defined as face–to–face time for office and other outpatient visits and as unit/floor time for hospital and other inpatient visits. This distinction is necessary because most of the work of typical office visits takes place during the face–to–face time with the patient, while most of the work of typical hospital visits takes place during the time spent on the patient's floor or unit.

Consultations

A consultation is service provided by a physician whose opinion or advice regarding evaluation and/or management of a specific problem is requested by another physician or other appropriate source. The request for a consultation from the attending doctor or other appropriate source and the need for the consultation must be documented in the patient's medical record. The consultant's opinion and any services that were ordered or performed must also be documented in the patient's medical record and communicated to the requesting doctor or other appropriate source. "Communicated" in this sense means that a written report must be provided to the requesting doctor.

CPT provides four criteria for determining whether or not the service provided constitutes a consultation. These criteria are:

1. The opinion or advice is requested by another doctor or appropriate source.
2. During the consultation, the physician may initiate diagnostic and/or therapeutic services. (However, should the consultant continue to care for the patient, he or she should use the appropriate subsequent hospital visit or office visit codes.)
3. The request for the consultation must be documented in the patient's record.
4. The opinion and/or recommendations of the consultant must also be documented in the patient's record and communicated to the requesting doctor or other source. This means that a written report containing the consultant's opinion and/or advice should be sent to the requesting doctor.

Any specifically identifiable procedure performed on or subsequent to the date of the initial consultation should be reported separately. Additionally, any lab or other types of procedures/tests which are performed as part of the consultation should be reported separately.

CPT defines four types of consultation services:

- Office or other outpatient (office, ambulatory care facility, emergency department, etc.).
- Initial inpatient (hospital or nursing home).
- Follow-up inpatient (hospital or nursing home).
- Confirmatory (additional opinion).

A "consultation" initiated by a patient and/or the patient's family, and not requested by a doctor, is not reported using the initial consultation codes but may be reported using the codes for confirmatory consultation or office visits, as appropriate.

Office or Other Outpatient Consultations

These codes are used to report consultations provided in the office or in an outpatient or other ambulatory facility, including an emergency department.

Follow–up visits in the consultant's office or other outpatient facility that are initiated by the doctor–consultant are reported using office visit codes for established patients. If an additional request for an opinion or advice regarding the same or a new problem is received from the attending doctor and is documented in the patient's record, the office consultation codes may be used again.

Initial Inpatient Consultations

These codes are used to report consultations provided to hospital inpatients or residents of nursing facilities. Only one initial consultation should be reported by a consultant per admission. Any additional visits to the patient during the same admission, providing you have not assumed care, should be coded as follow–up consultations. In cases where the physician has assumed care of the patient's problem, use the subsequent hospital care codes. (Be aware of the possibility of concurrent care in a situation such as this.)

There are also codes for follow–up inpatient consultations and confirmatory consultations. Refer to your CPT book for further information regarding these services.

SURGICAL PROCEDURES

Billing for surgical services is complicated because the CPT definition for what is considered to be included in the surgery charge is different from the definition used by Medicare. Both the AMA's and Medicare's definitions of the global surgical package are discussed below, as are reporting starred procedures and separate procedures. Refer also to your CPT and your Medicare carrier's bulletins for more information.

Surgical Package Rules

CPT's Global Surgical Package

The CPT system provides a definition of what is called the global surgical package. Discussed in the Surgery section guidelines, it specifies those components assumed to be included in the charge for a surgery. The components are:

- The operation itself;
- Local or topical anesthetics or digital blocks (if provided); and,
- The normal, uncomplicated follow–up care related to the procedure.

The preceding three items comprise the surgical package. Since anesthetics and digital blocks are itemized, the physician should not bill separately for them; if provided, they are included in the charge for the surgery. However, questions may arise regarding follow–up care, such as what is considered normal and what is a complication. Traditionally, follow–up care is defined as the period of time after surgery during which the patient is not billed for visits, whether in the hospital or office. The amount of normal follow–up time varies by procedure. Estimates of normal follow–up days can be found in the major relative value guides, such as McGraw–Hill's *Relative Values for Physicians*. If the physician is still seeing the patient after the "normal" period of time for the procedure (perhaps due to a secondary illness affecting his recovery), consider billing for the services. The treatment of all but the most minor complications following surgery may be also billed.

Conspicuously missing from this definition is reference to preoperative care, such as consultations, office visits, and initial hospital care. This was apparently omitted because practices have historically varied with respect to charging for preoperative services; some practices always billed them separately while others did not. Due to the omission in CPT, many third party payers created their own definitions of allowable preoperative billing. These range from allowing all reasonable charges to restricting claims submitted up to two weeks prior to surgery.

It should be noted that Medicare defines the surgical package differently than CPT. The Medicare definition delineates the number of pre– and postoperative days which are included in the package as well as the types of services which are included. Medicare's definition is provided later in this section under the heading, "Medicare's Global Surgical Package."

Starred Procedures

Starred procedures are those procedures in CPT for which a star (or asterisk) appears to the right of the code number, such as the example shown below:

30020* Drainage abscess or hematoma, nasal septum

The star indicates that the surgical package as defined above does not apply to the starred procedure. A separate set of rules applies to billing these starred surgical procedures. Stars are usually given to minor procedures that typically don't have any significant associated postoperative care or where the care is so variable that the package concept won't work. The logic of the global surgical package concept is based on the predictability of an operation and its follow–up. Major differences between patients aside, the preoperative services, the operation itself, and the follow–up for any particular surgical procedure involves approximately the same level of effort from one patient to the next. Thus, each surgical procedure can have a standard charge. However, for relatively minor surgeries, this logic does not hold. One patient who is treated for acute frontal sinusitis by drainage may not require a follow-up visit where another might. Thus, there are separate rules for billing preoperative and postoperative services for these minor procedures:

1. If the patient is new to the practice and the major service rendered is a starred procedure, the physician can bill for both the procedure and a new patient visit. Usually the visit is billed with a special code, 99025, or with one of the new patient office visit codes.

2. If the patient is established and the major service rendered is a starred procedure, bill only for the procedure.

3. If in addition to the starred procedure the patient is seen and treated or evaluated for other problems, additional service charges may be made as appropriate.

4. If to perform the starred procedure the patient must be hospitalized, the physician may bill for hospital visits in addition to the starred procedure.

Note that Medicare uses a different definition of the surgical package for starred procedures. The Medicare definition is discussed below as part of Medicare's minor surgical package.

Medicare's Global Surgical Package

Medicare's definition of the global surgical package differs substantially from that found in CPT. First, according to Medicare, procedures are considered to be either major or minor. Second, Medicare defines more specifically than CPT which pre– and postoperative services are included in, and excluded from, the surgical package. Medicare's global surgical package for major surgeries includes:

- Preoperative visits. These include all preoperative visits, in or out of the hospital, by the surgeon beginning with the day before the day of surgery.
- Intra–operative services. This includes all intra–operative services that are normally a usual and necessary part of a surgical procedure.
- Complications following surgery. All additional medical or surgical services required of the surgeon providing the postoperative care within 90 days of the surgery to treat complications which do not require additional trips to the operating room are included.
- Postoperative visits. Follow–up visits within 90 days after surgery that are related to recovery from the surgery are included. These services may be provided in any setting, e.g., hospital, ambulatory surgery center, surgeon's office. Visits to a patient in an intensive care or critical care unit are also included if made by the surgeon.
- Post–surgical pain management. Pain management provided by the surgeon providing the postoperative care are included in the package.
- Supplies. Except for a surgical tray for certain procedures, all supplies are included in the package.
- Miscellaneous services. Included are items such as dressing changes; local incisional care; removal of operative pack, removal of cutaneous sutures and staples, lines, wires, tubes, drains, casts, and splints; insertion, irrigation and removal of urinary catheters, routine peripheral intravenous lines, nasogastric and rectal tubes; and changes and removal of tracheotomy tubes.

The package does not include:

- The initial evaluation or consultation of the problem by the surgeon to determine the need for surgery (even if performed the day of or the day before surgery).
- Services of other doctors except when the services included in a global package are furnished by more than one doctor.
- Visits unrelated to the diagnosis for which the surgery is performed.
- Treatment for the underlying condition or an added course of treatment which is not part of the normal recovery from surgery.
- Diagnostic tests and procedures, including radiological procedures.
- Clearly distinct surgical procedures during the postoperative period which are not re–operations or treatment for complications. (A new postoperative period begins with the subsequent procedure.) These services should be reported with modifier "–79."
- Treatment for postoperative complications which require a return trip to the operating room, including ambulatory surgery centers and hospital outpatient departments. (A reduced payment rate applies.) These services should be reported using modifier "–78." No new postoperative period begins in this case.
- The surgical tray for certain procedures performed in a physician's office.

Medicare's package for minor surgery and nonincisional procedures, which include starred procedures and diagnostic/therapeutic nonincisional endoscopic procedures, is defined the same as that for the major surgeries with two exceptions:

- The postoperative period is 10 days for some procedures. Those procedures which do not have a 90 or 10 day postoperative period have 0 days, or no postoperative period. A complete list of codes and their associated postoperative period can be obtained from your Medicare carrier. For your reference, this text provides the postoperative follow–up days for Medicare for each procedure listed.
- Visits provided on the same day as a minor surgery or endoscopy are included in the package unless a documented, separately identifiable service is furnished (generally, for a problem different from that requiring surgery). These services should be reported using modifier "–24" or "–25."

Separate Procedure Concept

About 5 percent of surgeons account for 80 percent of surgical overbillings. How do these doctors overcharge? Most do so by "fragmenting" or "unbundling" their surgical charges, for example, billing for each area viewed during a sinus endoscopy. Such "a la carte" billing results in higher charges.

Because fragmented and unbundled charging may result from ignorance, it is important to be familiar with the rule related to CPT's separate procedures. Refer to CPT codes 31231 and 31237.

31231 Nasal endoscopy, diagnostic, unilateral or bilateral (separate procedure)

31237 Nasal/sinus endoscopy, surgical; with biopsy, polypectomy or debridement (separate procedure)

The definitions for these codes contain the parenthetical note "(separate procedure)." The separate procedure notation informs the ENT practice not to bill for the procedure if it is performed as part of a larger, more global service. Using the example above, if billing for an endoscopy, separate charges would not be submitted for the each area viewed, nor would additional charges be added for these procedures.

Think of it this way: If a surgical procedure has the words "(separate procedure)" listed as part of the definition, and it is either the only procedure performed through the incision or is not related to other procedures being performed through the incision, then the physician can charge for the separate procedure code.

Rules Associated With Billing For Assistant Surgeons

A normal surgical assist is billed by reporting the appropriate CPT surgery code (i.e., the code(s) used by the primary surgeon) plus the "–80" modifier. Many payers will pay the assistant a predetermined percentage of the amount paid to the primary surgeon. Medicare will make payment to the assistant surgeon at 16 percent of the fee schedule amount allowed for the primary surgeon.

If two surgeons with different skills perform surgery for a patient at the same time, they would be considered co–surgeons rather than primary/assistant surgeons. Note that Medicare and many other payers will not make payment for a surgical assist in addition to payment for co–surgeons. In other words, it has to be one or the other (assist or co–surgeons), not both.

For those services where, on a national level, assistants are used in less than 5 percent of the cases, Medicare will not allow payment for a surgical assistant. As you may have noted in the "Overview and Explanation of Notations" section in the "Introduction" to this text, a notation is provided in the Reimbursement notes in this manual to help alert you to those instances where Medicare restricts payment for an assistant surgeon. Recall that "paid" means Medicare may allow payment for an assistant for this procedure. "Not paid" means Medicare has determined that an assistant surgeon is not necessary for this procedure and so will not pay for one. (You are not permitted to attempt to charge the patient for the assistant.) A "by report" notation means that the individual carrier makes a determination as to whether an assistant is payable for this service.

BILLING SUPPLIES

The code you will use for items supplied to the patient will be CPT code 99070. Think of it as the all–purpose, generic code for supplies. When billing a patient for supplies you need to keep the following factors in mind.

1. If you are billing for the first time for supplies that were previously included in the charge for the service, you are "unbundling" and thus might not be reimbursed by the carrier for the supply. Consider the physician who in the past always provided a surgical tray as needed when performing minor surgeries in his office. Upon discovering the supply code for a surgical tray, he decides to list a separate charge for the tray in addition to his usual charge for the minor surgery. Summed together, the two charges (tray and procedure) are greater than what he had been charging when the tray was included. This is unbundling and might be interpreted by payers as an increase in charges.

2. When billing a patient for more than one supply on the same claim, list code 99070 more than once. Next to each use of 99070, describe the supply and list the charge for each.

3. When determining whether or not to bill for supplies, consider factors related to patient satisfaction. If you feel that your patients will complain that you are "padding" your bills with charges for supplies, the patient may seek care from a different physician in the future. Use common sense when billing for supplies.

Most Medicare and Medicaid carriers reject charges for supplies when CPT code 99070 is used. Recall from the discussion of HCPCS that Medicare's HCPCS codes provide hundreds of specific codes for billing supplies. These codes should be used instead of 99070 when billing Medicare and Medicaid for supplies.

Note, however, that Medicare reimburses separately for supplies, such as surgical trays, for only a certain number of identified "facility–based" procedures which are performed in a doctor's office instead of the facility. For your reference, this text provides reference to whether Medicare will reimburse for a supply under the "Reimbursement Information" column. Be sure that the procedure for which you wish to bill the tray is identified as one for which Medicare will pay for the supply of a surgical tray. If it is not, the charge for the tray should be considered to be included as part of your charge for the procedure. You may not bill the patient for the tray, either.

CPT MODIFIERS

CPT provides two–digit modifiers which can be attached to codes. Modifiers communicate additional information to the carrier, usually that circumstances that affected the performance of a procedure or service occurred. A discussion of those modifiers relevant to ENT practices is provided below.

"–20" Microsurgery

Surgical procedures for which charges are increased due to the use of microsurgical techniques require the addition of the "–20" modifier. There are three exceptions to this rule. First, if the procedure is always performed microsurgically, use of the modifier may be considered inappropriate. Second, some procedures are described as involving microsurgical techniques. In such cases, use of the modifier would be redundant. As an example of this latter point, refer to code 31560, which is for laryngoscopy with arytenoidectomy with operating microscope. When billing code 31561 you do not need to also list the "-20" modifier because the description includes it. Finally, when reporting nerve repair by suture procedures (range 68831–64876), instead of the "–20" modifier you add an additional code, 64830, to report the use of microsurgical technique.

"–21" Prolonged Evaluation and Management Services

This modifier is for use exclusively with E&M codes. In situations where the E&M service(s) provided is prolonged or otherwise greater than that usually required for the highest level of E&M service within a given category, this modifier should be used with the highest level code to report that circumstance. A special report explaining the situation may be necessary to ensure proper payment.

"–22" Unusual Service

The unusual service modifier is primarily used to denote circumstances for which a procedure or service was significantly more difficult than usual to perform or when it required significantly more time than usual to perform. Typically, the physician also adds an additional charge for the extra time or work. This modifier is used in these circumstances. Note, however, that addition of the modifier does not guarantee increased payment. Most carriers will require support documentation for this modifier.

"–24" Unrelated Evaluation and Management Service by the Same Physician During a Postoperative Period

There are times during the follow–up period of a surgery when the physician provides E&M services for a problem unrelated to that for which the surgery was performed. To indicate that the E&M service is not part of the global surgical package, this modifier is listed next to the E&M code. Medicare requires that support documentation be submitted when this modifier is used.

"–25" Significant, Separately Identifiable Evaluation and Management Service by the Same Physician on the Day of a Procedure

Medicare and other payers do not allow separate payment for non–surgical services provided to a patient on the day of a surgery. However, for situations where the patient's condition requires that the surgeon provide E&M services above and beyond the usual pre– and post-operative care associated with the procedure, this modifier should be used. Such services may be warranted if the patient has a condition that requires E&M services for a condition unrelated to that for which surgery is being performed, for example.

"–26" Professional Component

Many procedures include both technical and professional aspects. When billing for the professional aspects, use this modifier on the appropriate CPT code.

"–32" Mandated Services

Mandated services are those requested by an insurance carrier, peer review organization, utilization review panel, HMO, PPO or other entity. Typically, the request is for a second or third opinion regarding a patient illness or treatment. When mandated services are requested, the doctor performing the service is usually required to accept assignment from the payer, and in turn, the payer reimburses the doctor 100 percent of the payer's allowable for the service. An example of a mandated service would be an extended additional opinion consultation. This would be reported as:

99272–32

The "–32" modifier is used to alert the payer's claim processors to the fact that the service was mandated and should receive special handling.

"–50" Bilateral Procedures

In 1990, all specifically listed bilateral procedure codes were deleted from CPT. Procedures are assumed to be unilateral unless they are either always performed bilaterally or are otherwise noted.

Practices are sometimes confused by the definition of bilateral. Bilateral procedures are identical procedures (i.e., use of the same CPT code) performed on the same anatomic site but on opposite sides of the body. Furthermore, each procedure should be performed through its own separate incision to qualify for bilateral.

The most commonly accepted method of reporting bilateral procedures is to list the procedure twice and add the "–50" modifier to the second procedure as shown below for meniscectomies of a patient's left and right ears:

69300	Otoplasty, protruding ear, RIGHT
69300–50	Otoplasty, protruding ear, LEFT

Note that the words "right" and "left" have been added to clarify that the procedures were indeed performed bilaterally. Also, it is common to report your full charge for each procedure and let the payer reduce the amount on the second, or bilateral, procedure.

Some payers will accept an alternative method of billing bilateral procedures. This method involves listing the procedure once and adding the "–50" modifier as shown below:

69300-50	Otoplasty, protruding ear, bilateral

If this method is used, place a "2" in the UNITS column of the claim form so that the payer is aware that two procedures are being listed on one line. The charge reported on the claim for the procedures is typically twice that of what the doctor charges for performing one of the procedures.

"–51" Multiple Procedures

This modifier has traditionally been used to identify multiple surgical procedures performed on a patient during the same operative session. For example, the repair of a simple neck wound and the closed treatment of a nasal bone fracture for a patient who had been in an automobile accident would be coded as:

21310	Treat nasal bone fracture
12005–51	Simple closure 22cm neck wound

Note that the higher charge procedure (fracture treatment in this case) is listed first and the multiple procedure modifier is added to the lesser or secondary service. If three procedures had been performed, the services would be ranked from highest to lowest charge on the claim form and the "–51" modifier would be added to all but the first (highest charge) procedure.

The definition of multiple procedures was expanded in the 1990 CPT to include not only multiple procedures performed during the same operative session, but to extend to multiple medical and/or surgical services performed for a patient on the same day.

Although it is acceptable to use the "–51" modifier when reporting multiple services and procedures, it is not known how many, if any, payers require the "–51" modifier under these circumstances. Use of the "–51" modifier is usually limited to reporting multiple surgeries performed in the same operative session. However, payer policies can change overnight and practices should keep abreast of the requirements of their major payers with regard to use of this modifier.

"–52" Reduced Services

When the physician performs only a portion of, rather than the complete or total service, this modifier can be used to denote the situation. Fees for these reduced services are invariably lowered due to the fact that only part of the service was provided.

"–54" Surgical Care Only
"–55" Postoperative Management Only
"–56" Preoperative Management Only

These three modifiers may be used, as appropriate, to report that portion(s) of surgery provided by a surgeon in situations where the surgeon does not perform all the services as defined by the surgical package. For example, if the surgeon performs preoperative and intra–operative services and a different doctor handles the patient's postoperative care, then the surgeon would list modifiers "–56" and "–54" on his claim next to the appropriate surgery code. The doctor taking responsibility for the postoperative care would list the "–55" modifier.

"–57" Decision For Surgery

Many payers, including Medicare, now bundle some or all of the surgical preoperative services as part of the global surgical package. An exception is typically allowed for the evaluation and management visit during which the decision for surgery was made. If the decision for surgery was made during the period of time normally included in the global surgical package, the evaluation and management visit may be billed by adding the "–57" modifier to the reported code. For example, a secondary tympanoplasty planned at the same time as a mastoidectomy would be considered a "staged procedure," and, therefore, use of the "–58" modifier on the tympanoplasty code would be appropriate.

"–58" Staged or Related Procedure or Service by the Same Physician During the Postoperative Period.

This modifier allows for billing of staged or related procedures that are performed by the physician during the postoperative (follow–up) period for a procedure. It is intended for use under the following circumstances:

1. If at the time of the original procedure it was known that an additional procedure(s) would be performed, add the "–58" modifier to the additional procedure(s) when reporting it (them). For example, dental implants that require more than one surgical session would be considered "staged" procedures, and therefore on the second and additional implant surgeries, the "–58" modifier would be listed.
2. If a surgery during the postoperative period was more extensive or difficult than the initial procedure, add the "–58" modifier to the postop surgical procedure code.
3. When therapeutic services are provided following diagnostic surgical procedures, add the "–58" modifier to the therapy service codes.

"–62" Two Surgeons

This modifier is reported when two surgeons are acting as co–surgeons. That is, each surgeon is acting as a "primary" surgeon performing a different aspect of a complex procedure. As an example of two surgeons acting as co–surgeons, consider procedures such as a total nerve decompression performed jointly by a neurosurgeon and an otolaryngologist. Each doctor might list the following on his/her claim:

69955–62 Fascial nerve decompression

Third party payers often allow 60 percent of the prevailing to each surgeon in such cases. Medicare allows 125 percent of its global fee for the service, dividing the payment equally between the two surgeons.

"–76" Repeat Procedure By Same Physician
"–77" Repeat Procedure By Different Physician

These two modifiers are reported to note that a procedure which was previously performed was repeated. You may find it helpful to submit an explanation with the claim to justify the need to repeat the procedure and to clarify that you are not double billing for the procedure.

"–78" Return Trip to the Operating Room for a Related Procedure During the Postoperative Period

This modifier is reported for a return trip to the operating room for a related procedure during a postoperative period. This modifier is used, for instance, for complications from surgery, to indicate that another procedure was performed during the postoperative period of a related procedure.

"–79" Unrelated Procedure By the Same Physician During the Postoperative Period

During the follow–up period for a surgery, use this modifier to indicate that the performance of a service or procedure was unrelated to the original surgery. This modifier is used only on surgical services; the "–24" modifier is used for unrelated E&M services.

"–80" Assistant Surgeon
"–81" Minimum Assistant Surgeon
"–82" Assistant Surgeon (Where Qualified Resident Not Available)

These modifiers are used to identify surgical services provided by assistants. A normal surgical assist is billed by reporting the appropriate CPT surgery code (that is, the code(s) used by the primary surgeon) plus the addition of the "–80" modifier. In cases where a second assistant surgeon is warranted, his/her surgery code(s) would also list the "–81" minimum assistant surgeon modifier. It is important to note that assistant surgeons submit their charges on claims separate from those of the primary surgeon, even if both are from the same group practice or clinic. The reason is straightforward: each doctor must submit under his/her unique identification number, and by doing so, accept responsibility for the services he/she provided.

Many hospitals have surgical residency programs that provide qualified resident assistants. In hospitals where qualified residents are available, most payers will not reimburse for the services of a non–resident assistant surgeon, arguing that the fees they pay for the patient's hospitalization, use of the surgical suite, etc., include the services of the resident assistant. With one exception, the non–resident assistant's services in such situations will usually not be covered. The exception exists when (for whatever reason) a qualified resident assistant was not available at the time of the patient's surgery. In these cases the non–resident assistant surgeon may bill for the assist by adding the "–82" modifier to the surgery code(s). However, the assistant needs to obtain a note or letter from the hospital's administration stating that a qualified resident was not available, thus necessitating the services of the non–resident assistant surgeon. A copy of the note or letter should be submitted with the claim for the assistant surgeon's services. Of course, if a hospital does not have a surgical residency program, the assistant surgeon will use the "–80" modifier.

MAJOR HCPCS NATIONAL MODIFIERS

"–LT" Left Side

This modifier is used to identify procedures performed on the left side of the body.

"–RT" Right Side

This modifier is used to identify procedures performed on the right side of the body.

EVALUATION AND MANAGEMENT

OFFICE OR OTHER OUTPATIENT SERVICES
99201—99215

These codes are used to report evaluation and management services provided in the physician's office or in an outpatient or other ambulatory facility. A patient is considered an outpatient until inpatient admission to a health care facility occurs.

To report services provided to a patient who is admitted to a hospital or nursing facility in the course of an encounter in the office or other ambulatory facility, see the notes for initial hospital inpatient care (page 41) or comprehensive nursing facility assessments (see your CPT).

For services provided by physicians in the Emergency Department, see 99281–99285.

For observation care, see 99217–99220 in your CPT.

For definitions of key components, see Evaluation and Management Services Guidelines in your CPT.

New Patient
99201–99205

Established Patient
99211–99215

For definitions of new and established patients, refer to page 1 in the Coding Guidelines section of this text.

CPT CODE	SERVICE
99201	Office or other outpatient visit for the evaluation and management of a new patient, which requires these three key components: • a problem focused history; • a problem focused examination; and • straightforward medical decision making. Counselling and/or coordination of care with other providers or agencies are provided consistent with the nature of the problem(s) and the patient's and/or family's needs. Usually, the presenting problem(s) are self limited or minor. Physicians typically spend 10 minutes face-to-face with the patient and/or family.

ICD–9–CM

380.10	Infective otitis externa NOS
380.22	Acute otitis externa NEC
380.4	Impacted cerumen
470	Deviated nasal septum

REIMBURSEMENT INFORMATION

General

- ♦ See notes on page 29.

Medicare

- ♦ Outpatient Limit — applies

CPT CODE **SERVICE**

99202 Office or other outpatient visit for the evaluation and management of a new patient, which requires these three key components:

- an expanded problem focused history;
- an expanded problem focused examination; and
- straightforward medical decision making.

Counseling and/or coordination of care with other providers or agencies are provided consistent with the nature of the problem(s) and the patient's and/or family's needs.

Usually the presenting problem(s) are of low to moderate severity. Physicians typically spend 20 minutes face-to-face with the patient and/or family.

EXAMPLES

♦ Initial office evaluation for gradual hearing loss, 58-year-old male, history and physical examination, with interpretation of complete audiogram, air bone, etc.

ICD-9-CM

380.1	Infective otitis externa
380.2	Otitis externa
380.4	Impacted cerumen
381.01	Acute serous otitis media
381.10	Chron serous otitis media simp/NOS
381.4	Chron nonsup otitis media NOS
381.81	Dysfunction of Eustachian tube
382.9	Otitis media NOS
384.20	Perforation tympanic membrane NOS
388.01	Presbyacusis
388.3	Tinnitus
388.7	Otalgia
389.0	Conductive hearing loss
389.1	Sensorineural hearing loss
389.2	Mixed hearing loss
460	Acute nasopharyngitis
461.0	Acute maxillary sinusitis
461.9	Acute sinusitis NOS
462	Acute pharyngitis
464.0	Acute laryngitis
470	Deviated nasal septum
472.0	Chronic rhinitis
472.1	Chronic pharyngitis
473.0	Chronic maxillary sinusitis
473.9	Chronic sinusitis NOS
476.0	Chronic laryngitis
477.0	Allergic rhinitis d/t pollen
477.9	Allergic rhinitis NOS
478.1	Nasal and sinus disease NEC
524.6	Temporomandibular joint disorder
527.2	Sialoadenitis
784.4	Voice disturbance
784.7	Epistaxis

REIMBURSEMENT INFORMATION

General

♦ See notes on page 29.

Medicare

♦ Outpatient Limit — applies

CPT CODE **SERVICE**

99203 Office or other outpatient visit for the evaluation and management of a new patient, which requires these three key components:

- a detailed history;
- a detailed examination; and
- medical decision making of low complexity.

Counseling and/or coordination of care with other providers or agencies are provided consistent with the nature of the problem(s) and the patient's and/or family's needs.

Usually, the presenting problems are of moderate severity. Physicians typically spend 30 minutes face-to-face with the patient and/or family.

EXAMPLES

♦ Initial office visit of an adult who presents with symptoms of an upper-respiratory infection that has progressed to unilateral purulent nasal discharge and discomfort in the right maxillary teeth.

♦ Initial office visit of a 40-year-old female with symptoms of atopic allergies including eye and sinus congestion, often associated with infections. She would like to be tested for allergies.

♦ Initial office visit of a 65-year-old with nasal stuffiness.

ICD–9–CM

381.10	Chron serous otitis media simp/NOS
381.4	Chron nonsup otitis media NOS
381.81	Dysfunction of Eustachian tube
382.9	Otitis media NOS
384.20	Perforation tympanic membrane NOS
386.11	Benign paroxysmal position vertigo
388.3	Tinnitus
389.0	Conductive hearing loss
389.1	Sensorineural hearing loss
389.2	Mixed hearing loss
461.9	Acute sinusitis NOS
464.0	Acute laryngitis
472.0	Chronic rhinitis
472.1	Chronic pharyngitis
473.0	Chronic maxillary sinusitis
477.9	Allergic rhinitis NOS
530.1	Esophagitis
780.4	Dizziness and giddiness
784.1	Throat pain
784.2	Swelling in head/neck
784.4	Voice disturbance
784.7	Epistaxis
786.2	Cough
787.2	Dysphagia

REIMBURSEMENT INFORMATION

General

♦ See notes on page 29.

Medicare

♦ Outpatient Limit — applies

CPT CODE	SERVICE
99204	Office or other outpatient visit for the evaluation and management of a new patient, which requires these three components: • a comprehensive history; • a comprehensive examination; and • medical decision making of moderate complexity. Counseling and/or coordination of care with other providers or agencies are provided consistent with the nature of the problem(s) and the patient's and/or family's needs. Usually, the presenting problem(s) are of moderate to high severity. Physicians typically spend 45 minutes face-to-face with the patient and/or family.

EXAMPLES

♦ Initial office visit of a 40-year-old with chronic draining ear, inbalance and probable cholesteatoma.

ICD–9–CM

386.1	Peripheral vertigo
386.3	Labyrinthitis
388.3	Tinnitus
389.1	Sensorineural hearing loss
472.1	Chronic pharyngitis
473.9	Chronic sinusitis NOS
478.1	Nasal and sinus disease NEC
524.6	Temporomandibular joint disorder
530.1	Esophagitis
780.4	Dizziness and giddiness
784.0	Headache
784.2	Swelling in head/neck
784.4	Voice disturbance
784.7	Epistaxis
786.2	Cough
787.2	Dysphagia

REIMBURSEMENT INFORMATION

General

♦ See notes on page 29.

Medicare

♦ Outpatient Limit — applies

CPT CODE **SERVICE**

99205 Office or other outpatient visit for the evaluation and management of a new patient, which requires these three key components:

- a comprehensive history;
- a comprehensive examination; and
- medical decision making of high complexity.

Counseling and/or coordination of care with other providers or agencies are provided consistent with the nature of the problem(s) and the patient's and/or family's needs.

Usually, the presenting problem(s) are of moderate to high severity. Physicians typically spend 60 minutes face-to-face with the patient and/or family.

ICD–9–CM

161.9	M-Neoplasm, Larynx NOS
173.3	M-Neoplasm, Skin of face NEC
386.1	Peripheral vertigo
386.5	Labyrinthine dysfunction
388.01	Presbyacusis
388.5	Acoustic nerve disorders
389.0	Conductive hearing loss
389.1	Sensorineural hearing loss
473.9	Chronic sinusitis NOS
530.1	Esophagitis
780.4	Dizziness and giddiness
784.0	Headache
784.2	Swelling in head/neck
784.4	Voice disturbance
784.7	Epistaxis
786.2	Cough
787.2	Dysphagia

REIMBURSEMENT INFORMATION

General

- ♦ See notes on page 29.

Medicare

- ♦ Outpatient Limit — applies

CPT CODE	SERVICE

99211 Office or other outpatient visit for the evaluation and management of an established patient, that may not require the presence of a physician.

Usually, the presenting problem(s) are minimal.

Typically, 5 minutes are spent performing or supervising these services.

EXAMPLES

- ♦ Office visit of a 20-year-old female established patient who receives an allergy vaccine injection and is observed for a reaction by the nurse.

ICD–9–CM

380.4	Impacted cerumen
709.9	Skin disorder NOS
995.3	Allergy, unspecified

REIMBURSEMENT INFORMATION

General

- ♦ See notes on page 29.

Medicare

- ♦ Outpatient Limit — applies

99212 Office or other outpatient visit for the evaluation and management of an established patient, which requires at least two of these three key components:

- a problem focused history;
- a problem focused examination
- straightforward medical decision making.

Counseling and/or coordination of care with other providers or agencies are provided consistent with the nature of the problem(s) and the patient's and/or family's needs.

Usually, the presenting problem(s) are self limited or minor. Physicians typically spend 10 minutes face-to-face with the patient and/or family.

EXAMPLES

- ♦ Office visit of a child established patient with chronic secretory otitis media.
- ♦ Office visit for a 21-year-old established patient who is seen in follow-up after antibiotic therapy for acute bacterial tonsillitis.
- ♦ Office visit for a 4-year-old child established patient with tympanostomy tubes, check-up.
- ♦ Office visit for an established patient who has had needle aspiration of a peritonsillar abscess.
- ♦ Follow-up office examination for evaluation and treatment of acute draining ear in a 5-year-old child with tympanotomy tubes.

380.1	Infective otitis externa
380.2	Otitis externa
380.4	Impacted cerumen
470	Deviated nasal septum

REIMBURSEMENT INFORMATION

General

- ♦ See notes on page 29.

Medicare

- ♦ Outpatient Limit — applies

CPT CODE **SERVICE**

99213 Office or other outpatient visit for the evaluation and management of an established patient, which requires at least two of these three key components:

- an expanded problem focused history;
- an expanded problem focused examination;
- medical decision making of low complexity.

Counseling and coordination of care are provided consistent with the nature of the problem(s) and the patient's and/or family's needs.

Usually, the presenting problem(s) are of low to moderate severity. Physicians typically spend 15 minutes face-to-face with the patient and/or family.

ICD–9–CM

380.1	Infective otitis externa
380.2	Otitis externa
380.4	Impacted cerumen
381.01	Acute serous otitis media
381.1	Chronic serous otitis media
381.3	Chronic nonsuppurative otitis media
381.4	Chron nonsup otitis media NOS
381.81	Dysfunction of Eustachian tube
382.9	Otitis media NOS
384.2	Perforation of tympanic membrane
388.01	Presbyacusis
388.3	Tinnitus
388.7	Otalgia
389.00	Conductive hearing loss NOS
389.1	Sensorineural hearing loss
389.2	Mixed hearing loss
389.9	Hearing loss NOS
460	Acute nasopharyngitis
462	Acute pharyngitis
464.0	Acute laryngitis
470	Deviated nasal septum
471.9	Nasal polyp NOS
472.0	Chronic rhinitis
472.1	Chronic pharyngitis
473.0	Chronic maxillary sinusitis
473.9	Chronic sinusitis NOS
476.0	Chronic laryngitis
477.0	Allergic rhinitis d/t pollen
477.9	Allergic rhinitis NOS
478.1	Nasal and sinus disease NEC
524.6	Temporomandibular joint disorder
527.2	Sialoadenitis
784.4	Voice disturbance
784.7	Epistaxis

REIMBURSEMENT INFORMATION

General

- ♦ See notes on page 29.

Medicare

- ♦ Outpatient Limit — applies

CPT CODE	SERVICE	ICD-9-CM

99214 Office or other outpatient visit for the evaluation and management of an established patient, which requires at least two of these three key components:

- a detailed history;
- a detailed examination
- medical decision making of moderate complexity.

Counseling and/or coordination of care with other providers or agencies are provided consistent with the nature of the problem(s) and the patient's and/or family's needs.

Usually, the presenting problem(s) are of moderate to high severity. Physicians typically spend 25 minutes face-to-face with the patient and/or family.

EXAMPLES

- ♦ Office visit for an adult diabetic established patient with a past history of recurrent sinusitis who presents with a one week history of double vision.

ICD-9-CM

386.1	Peripheral vertigo
386.3	Labyrinthitis
388.3	Tinnitus
389.1	Sensorineural hearing loss
472.1	Chronic pharyngitis
473.9	Chronic sinusitis NOS
476.0	Chronic laryngitis
478.1	Nasal and sinus disease NEC
524.6	Temporomandibular joint disorder
530.1	Esophagitis
780.4	Dizziness and giddiness
784.0	Headache
784.2	Swelling in head/neck
784.4	Voice disturbance
784.7	Epistaxis
786.2	Cough
787.2	Dysphagia

REIMBURSEMENT INFORMATION

General

- ♦ See notes on page 29.

Medicare

- ♦ Outpatient Limit — applies

99215 Office or other outpatient visit for the evaluation and management of an established patient, which requires at least two of these three key components:

- a comprehensive history;
- a comprehensive examination;
- medical decision making of high complexity.

Counseling and/or coordination of care with other providers or agencies are provided consistent with the nature of the problem(s) and the patient's and/or family's needs.

Usually, the presenting problem(s) are of moderate to high severity. Physicians typically spend 40 minutes face-to-face with the patient and/or family.

161.0	M-Neoplasm, Glottis
161.9	M-Neoplasm, Larynx NOS
173.3	M-Neoplasm, Skin of face NEC
386.1	Peripheral vertigo
386.5	Labyrinthine dysfunction
388.01	Presbyacusis
388.5	Acoustic nerve disorders
389.0	Conductive hearing loss
389.1	Sensorineural hearing loss
473.9	Chronic sinusitis NOS
530.1	Esophagitis
780.4	Dizziness and giddiness
784.0	Headache
784.2	Swelling in head/neck
784.4	Voice disturbance
784.7	Epistaxis
786.2	Cough
787.2	Dysphagia

REIMBURSEMENT INFORMATION

General

- ♦ See notes on page 29.

Medicare

- ♦ Outpatient Limit — applies

HOSPITAL OBSERVATION SERVICES
99217–99220

These codes are used to report evaluation and management services provided to patients designated/admitted as "observation status" in a hospital. It is not necessary that the patient be located in an observation area designated by the hospital. If such an area does exist in a hospital (as a separate unit in the hospital, in the emergency department, etc.), these codes are to be utilized if the patient is placed in such an area.

For definitions of key components and commonly used terms, please see Evaluation and Management Services Guidelines in your CPT.

Typical times have not yet been established for this category of services.

Observation Care Discharge Services
99217

Observation care discharge of a patient from "observation status" includes final examination of the patient, discussion of the hospital stay, instructions for continuing care, and preparation of discharge records.

Initial Observation Care
99218–99220

These codes are used to report the encounter(s) by the supervising physician with the patient when designated as "observation status." This refers to the initiation of observation status, supervision of the care plan for observation and performance of periodic reassessments. For observation encounters by other physicians, see Office or Other Outpatient Consultation codes (99241–99245).

To report services provided to a patient who is admitted to the hospital after receiving hospital observation care services on the same date, see the notes for initial hospital inpatient care (99221–99238). For a patient admitted to the hospital on a date subsequent to the date of observation status, the hospital admission would be reported with the appropriate Initial Hospital Care Codes (99221–99223). Do not report observation discharge in conjunction with the hospital admission.

When "observation status" is initiated in the course of an encounter in another site of service (e.g., hospital emergency department, physician's office, nursing facility) all evaluation and management services provided by the supervising physician in conjunction with initiating "observation status" are considered part of the initial observation care when performed on the same date. The observation care level of service reported by the supervising physician should include the services related to initiating "observation status" provided in the other sites of service as well as in the observation setting.

Evaluation and management services on the same date provided in sites that are not related to initiating "observation status" should NOT be reported separately.

These codes may not be utilized for post–operative recovery if the procedure is considered part of the surgical "package." This code applies to all Evaluation and Management services that are provided on the same date of initiating "observation status."

CPT CODE **SERVICE**

99217 Observation care discharge day management

CPT NOTES

♦ This code is to be utilized by the physician to report all services provided to a patient on discharge from "observation status" if the discharge is on other than the initial date of "observation status." To report services to a patient designated as "observation status" who is discharged on the same date, use only the codes for Initial Observation Services (99218–99220)).

ICD–9–CM

REIMBURSEMENT INFORMATION

General

♦ See notes on page 38.

Medicare

♦ Outpatient Limit — does not apply

99218 Initial observation care, per day, for the evaluation and management of a patient which requires these three key components:

- a detailed or comprehensive history;
- a detailed or comprehensive examination; and
- medical decision making that is straightforward or of low complexity.

Counseling and/or coordination of care with other providers or agencies are provided consistent with the nature of the problem(s) and the patient's and/or family's needs.

Usually, the problem(s) requiring admission to "observation status" are of low severity.

CPT NOTES

♦ This code is to be utilized by the physician to report all services provided to a patient on discharge from "observation status" if the discharge is on other than the initial date of "observation status." To report services to a patient designated as "observation status" who is discharged on the same date, use only the codes for Initial Observation Services (99218–99220)).

REIMBURSEMENT INFORMATION

General

♦ See notes on page 38.

Medicare

♦ Outpatient Limit — does not apply

CPT CODE	SERVICE	ICD-9-CM

99219 Initial observation care, per day, for the evaluation and management of a patient which requires these three key components:

- a detailed or comprehensive history;
- a detailed or comprehensive examination; and
- medical decision making that is straightforward or of low complexity.

Counseling and/or coordination of care with other providers or agencies are provided consistent with the nature of the problem(s) and the patient's and/or family's needs.

Usually, the problem(s) requiring admission to "observation status" are of moderate severity.

CPT NOTES

- ♦ This code is to be utilized by the physician to report all services provided to a patient on discharge from "observation status" if the discharge is on other than the initial date of "observation status." To report services to a patient designated as "observation status" who is discharged on the same date, use only the codes for Initial Observation Services (99218–99220)).

REIMBURSEMENT INFORMATION

General

- ♦ See notes on page 38.

Medicare

- ♦ Outpatient Limit — does not apply

99220 Initial observation care, per day, for the evaluation and management of a patient which requires these three key components:

- a detailed or comprehensive history;
- a detailed or comprehensive examination; and
- medical decision making that is straightforward or of low complexity.

Counseling and/or coordination of care with other providers or agencies are provided consistent with the nature of the problem(s) and the patient's and/or family's needs.

Usually, the problem(s) requiring admission to "observation status" are of high severity.

CPT NOTES

- ♦ This code is to be utilized by the physician to report all services provided to a patient on discharge from "observation status" if the discharge is on other than the initial date of "observation status." To report services to a patient designated as "observation status" who is discharged on the same date, use only the codes for Initial Observation Services (99218–99220)).

REIMBURSEMENT INFORMATION

General

- ♦ See notes on page 38.

Medicare

- ♦ Outpatient Limit — does not apply

HOSPITAL INPATIENT SERVICES
99221–99238

These codes are used to report evaluation and management services provided to hospital inpatients. Hospital inpatient services include those services provided to patients in a "partial hospital" setting. These codes are to be used to report these partial hospitalization services. See also psychiatry notes in the full text of CPT.

For definitions of key components and commonly used terms, please see Evaluation and Management Services Guidelines in your CPT. For hospital observation services, see 99218–99220.

Initial Hospital Care
New Or Established Patient
99221–99223

These codes are used to report the first hospital inpatient encounter with the patient by the admitting physician. For initial inpatient encounters by physicians other than the admitting physician, see initial inpatient consultation codes (99251–99255) or subsequent hospital care codes (99231–99233) as appropriate.

When the patient is admitted to the hospital as an inpatient in the course of an encounter in another site of service (e.g., hospital emergency department, observation status in a hospital, physician's office, nursing facility) all evaluation and management services provided by that physician in conjunction with that admission are considered part of the initial hospital care when performed on the same date as the admission. The inpatient care level of service reported by the admitting physician should include the services related to the admission he/she provided in the other sites of service as well as the inpatient setting.

Evaluation and management services on the same date provided in sites other than the hospital that are related to the admission should NOT be reported separately.

Subsequent Hospital Care
99231–99233

All levels of subsequent hospital care include reviewing the medical record and reviewing the results of diagnostic studies and changes in the patient's status (i.e., changes in history, physical condition and response to management) since the last assessment by the physician.

Hospital Discharge Services
99238

Final hospital discharge of a patient includes final examination of the patient, discussion of the hospital stay, instructions for continuing care, and preparation of discharge records.

CPT CODE **SERVICE**

99221 Initial hospital care, per day, for the evaluation and management of a patient which requires these three key components:

- a detailed or comprehensive history;
- a detailed or comprehensive examination; and
- straightforward or low complexity medical decision making.

Counseling and/or coordination of care with other providers or agencies are provided consistent with the nature of the problem(s) and the patient's and/or family's needs.

Usually, the problem(s) requiring admission are of low severity. Physicians typically spend 30 minutes at the bedside and on the patient's hospital floor or unit.

ICD–9–CM

161.9	M-Neoplasm, Larynx NOS
195.0	M-Neoplasm, Head/face/neck
210.1	B-Neoplasm, Tongue
380.4	Impacted cerumen
475	Peritonsillar abscess
682.0	Cellulitis of face
682.1	Cellulitis of neck
784.2	Swelling in head/neck
786.09	Respiratory abnormality NEC

REIMBURSEMENT INFORMATION

General

- ♦ See notes on page 41.

Medicare

- ♦ Outpatient Limit — does not apply

99222 Initial hospital care, per day, for the evaluation and management of a patient, which requires these three key components:

- a comprehensive history;
- a comprehensive examination; and
- medical decision making of moderate complexity.

Counseling and/or coordination of care with other providers or agencies are provided consistent with the nature of the problem(s) and the patient's and/or family's needs.

Usually, the problem(s) requiring admission are of moderate severity. Physicians typically spend 50 minutes at the bedside and on the patient's hospital floor or unit.

EXAMPLES

- ♦ Initial hospital visit and evaluation of a 15-year-old male admitted with peritonsillar abscess or cellulitis requiring intravenous antibiotic therapy.
- ♦ Initial hospital visit of a 15-year-old on medications for a sore throat over the last two weeks. The sore throat has worsened and now has dysphagia. The exam shows large necrotic tonsils with an adequate airway and small palpable nodes. The initial mono test was negative.
- ♦ Initial hospital evaluation of a 23-year-old allergy patient admitted with eyelid edema and pain on 5th day of oral antibiotic therapy.

198.89	M2-Neoplasm NEC
202.8	Lymphoma
276.5	Hypovolemia
380.14	Malignant otitis externa
473.9	Chronic sinusitis NOS
478.3	Paralysis of vocal cords or larynx
519.1	Trachea/bronchus disease NEC
519.8	Respiratory system disease NEC
784.2	Swelling in head/neck
784.7	Epistaxis
786.09	Respiratory abnormality NEC
787.2	Dysphagia

REIMBURSEMENT INFORMATION

General

- ♦ See notes on page 41.

Medicare

- ♦ Outpatient Limit — does not apply

CPT CODE	SERVICE
99223	Initial hospital care, per day, for the evaluation and management of a patient, which requires these three key components: • a comprehensive history; • a comprehensive examination; and • medical decision making of high complexity. Counseling and/or coordination of care with other providers or agencies are provided consistent with the nature of the problem(s) and the patient's and/or family's needs. Usually, the problem(s) requiring admission are of high severity. Physicians typically spend 70 minutes at the bedside and on the patient's hospital floor or unit.

EXAMPLES

- ♦ Initial hospital visit of a 75-year-old with progressive stridor and dysphagia with history of cancer of the larynx treated by radiation therapy in the past. Exam shows a large recurrent tumor of the glottis with a mass in the neck.
- ♦ Initial hospital visit of a 67-year-old male admitted with a large neck mass, dysphagia and history of myocardial infarction three months before.
- ♦ Initial hospital visit for a patient with suspected cerebrospinal fulid rhinorrhea which developed two weeks after head injury.
- ♦ Initial hospital exam of a pediatric patient with high fever and proptosis.

ICD–9–CM

173.4	M-Neoplasm, Scalp/skin neck
386.0	Meniere's disease
478.3	Paralysis of vocal cords or larynx
486	Pneumonia, organism NOS
780.4	Dizziness and giddiness
784.7	Epistaxis
786.09	Respiratory abnormality NEC
787.2	Dysphagia

REIMBURSEMENT INFORMATION

General

- ♦ See notes on page 41.

Medicare

- ♦ Outpatient Limit — does not apply

CPT CODE	SERVICE
99231	Subsequent hospital care, per day, for the evaluation and management of a patient, which requires at least two of these three key components:

- a problem focused interval history;
- a problem focused examination
- straightforward or low complexity medical decision making.

Counseling and/or coordination of care with other providers or agencies are provided consistent with the nature of the problem(s) and the patient's and/or family's needs.

Usually, the patient is stable, recovering or improving. Physicians typically spend 15 minutes at the bedside and on the patient's hospital floor or unit.

EXAMPLES:

- ♦ Subsequent hospital visit for a 23-year-old female with otitis externa, seen two days before in consultation, now to have otic wick removal.
- ♦ Subsequent hospital visit for a 27-year-old with acute labyrinthitis.
- ♦ Subsequent hospital visit for a patient with peritonsillar abscess.
- ♦ Subsequent hospital visit for an 18-year-old female responding to intravenous antibiotic therapy for ear or sinus infection.

ICD–9–CM

380.1	Infective otitis externa
380.4	Impacted cerumen
381.1	Chronic serous otitis media
475	Peritonsillar abscess
478.3	Paralysis of vocal cords or larynx
682.0	Cellulitis of face
682.1	Cellulitis of neck
784.4	Voice disturbance
786.1	Stridor
V55.0	Attention to tracheostomy

REIMBURSEMENT INFORMATION

General

♦ See notes on page 41.

Medicare

♦ Outpatient Limit — does not apply

CPT CODE	SERVICE
99232	Subsequent hospital care, per day, for the evaluation and management of a patient, which requires at least two of these three key components:

- an expanded problem focused interval history;
- an expanded problem focused examination;
- medical decision making of moderate complexity.

Counseling and/or coordination of care with other providers or agencies are provided consistent with the nature of the problem(s) and the patient's and/or family's needs.

Usually, the patient is responding inadequately to therapy or has developed a minor complication. Physicians typically spend 25 minutes at the bedside and on the patient's hospital floor or unit.

ICD-9-CM

161.0	M-Neoplasm, Glottis
161.9	M-Neoplasm, Larynx NOS
197.3	M2-Neoplasm, Respiratory NEC
198.89	M2-Neoplasm NEC
380.1	Infective otitis externa
382.3	Chronic suppurativ otitis media NOS
382.9	Otitis media NOS
388.01	Presbyacusis
461.0	Acute maxillary sinusitis
461.9	Acute sinusitis NOS
464.0	Acute laryngitis
464.1	Acute tracheitis
466.0	Acute bronchitis
527.2	Sialoadenitis
682.0	Cellulitis of face
682.1	Cellulitis of neck
780.4	Dizziness and giddiness
784.4	Voice disturbance
786.09	Respiratory abnormality NEC

REIMBURSEMENT INFORMATION

General

- ♦ See notes on page 41.

Medicare

- ♦ Outpatient Limit — does not apply

CPT CODE	SERVICE
99233	Subsequent hospital care, per day, for the evaluation and management of a patient, which requires at least two of these three key components:

- a detailed interval history;
- a detailed examination;
- medical decision making of high complexity.

Counseling and/or coordination of care with other providers or agencies are provided consistent with the nature of the problem(s) and the patient's and/or family's needs.

Usually, the patient is unstable or has developed a significant complication or a significant new problem. Physicians typically spend 35 minutes at the bedside and on the patient's hospital floor or unit.

EXAMPLE:

- ♦ Follow-up hospital care of a patient with parsinusitis infection complicated by a brain abscess and asthma; no response to curren treatment.
- ♦ Subsequent hospital visit for a patient with a laryngeal neoplasm who develops airway compromise, suspected metastasis.
- ♦ Follow-up hospital care of a pediatric case with stridor, laryngomalcia, established tracheostomy, complicated by multiple medical problems in PICU.

ICD–9–CM

176.8	Kaposi's sarcoma NEC
197.3	M2-Neoplasm, Respiratory NEC
231.0	CA in situ, Larynx
386.9	Vertiginous syndromes NOS
464.1	Acute tracheitis
464.2	Acute laryngotracheitis
473.2	Chronic ethmoidal sinusitis
478.7	Disease of larynx NEC
518.81	Respiratory failure
529.8	Tongue disorder NEC
780.4	Dizziness and giddiness
784.2	Swelling in head/neck
784.7	Epistaxis
786.09	Respiratory abnormality NEC
787.2	Dysphagia
802.8	Fx facial bone NEC, closed
995.1	Angioneurotic edema

REIMBURSEMENT INFORMATION

General

- ♦ See notes on page 41.

Medicare

- ♦ Outpatient Limit — does not apply

CPT CODE **SERVICE**

99238 Hospital discharge day management

CPT NOTES

- This code is to be utilized by the physician to report all services provided to a patient on the date of discharge, if other than the initial date of inpatient status. To report services to a patient who is admitted as an inpatient, and discharged on the same date use only the codes for Initial Hospital Inpatient Services, 99221–99223. To report concurrent care services provided by a physician(s) other than the attending physician, use subsequent hospital care codes (99231-99233) on the day of discharge.
- For Observation Care Discharge, use 99217.

ICD–9–CM

038.9	Septicemia NOS
173.4	M-Neoplasm, Scalp/skin neck
197.3	M2-Neoplasm, Respiratory NEC
464.1	Acute tracheitis
475	Peritonsillar abscess
486	Pneumonia, organism NOS
496	Chronic airway obstruction NEC
682.0	Cellulitis of face
784.0	Headache
784.2	Swelling in head/neck
784.7	Epistaxis

REIMBURSEMENT INFORMATION

General

- See notes on page 41.

Medicare

- Outpatient Limit — does not apply

CONSULTATIONS
99241–99275

A consultation is a type of service provided by a physician whose opinion or advice regarding evaluation and/or management of a specific problem is requested by another physician or other appropriate source.

A physician consultant may initiate diagnostic and/or therapeutic services.

The request for a consultation from the attending physician or other appropriate source and the need for consultation must be documented in the patient's medical record. The consultant's opinion and any services that were ordered or performed must also be documented in the patient's medical record and communicated to the requesting physician or other appropriate source.

A "consultation" initiated by a patient and/or family, and not requested by a physician, is not reported using the initial consultation codes but may be reported using the codes for confimatory consultation or office visits, as appropriate. If a confirmatory consultation is required, e.g., by a third party payor, the modifier –32 or 09932, mandated services, should also be reported.

Any specifically identifiable procedure (i.e., identified with a specific CPT code) performed on or subsequent to the date of the initial consultation should be reported separately.

If subsequent to the completion of a consultation, the consultant assumes responsibility for management of a portion or all of the patient's condition(s), the follow–up consultation codes should not be used. In the hospital setting, the physician receiving the patient for partial or complete transfer of care should use the appropriate inpatient hospital consultation code for the initial encounter and then subsequent hospital care codes (not follow–up consultation codes). In the office setting, the appropriate established patient code should be used.

There are four subcategories of consultations: office, initial inpatient, follow–up inpatient, and confirmatory. See each subcategory for specific reporting instructions.

For definitions of key components and commonly used terms, please see Evaluation and Management Services Guidelines in your CPT.

Office or Other Outpatient Consultations
New or Established Patient
99241–99245

These codes are used to report consultations provided in the physician's office or in an outpatient or other ambulatory facility, including hospital observation services, home services, domiciliary, rest home, custodial care, or emergency department (see above).

Follow–up visits in the consultant's office or other outpatient facility that are initiated by the physician consultant are reported using office visit codes for established patients (99211–99215). If an additional request for an opinion or advice regarding the same or a new problem is received from the attending physician and documented in the medical record, the office consultation codes may be used again.

CONSULTATIONS, cont'd.

Initial Inpatient Consultations
New or Established Patient
99251–99255

These codes are used to report physician consultations provided to hospital inpatients, residents of nursing facilities, or patients in a partial hospital setting. Only one initial consultation should be reported by a consultant per admission.

Follow–Up Inpatient Consultations
Established Patient
99261–99263

Follow–up consultations are visits to complete the initial consultation OR subsequent consultative visits requested by the attending physician. A follow–up consultation includes monitoring progress, recommending management modifications or advising on a new plan of care in response to changes in the patient's status.

If the physician consultant has initiated treatment at the initial consultation, and participates thereafter in the patient's management, the codes for subsequent hospital care should be used (99231–99233).

These codes are used to report follow–up consultations provided to hospital inpatients or nursing facility residents only. For consultative services provided in other settings, the codes for office or other outpatient consultations should be reported (99241–99245).

Confirmatory Consultations
New or Established Patient
99271–99275

These codes are used to report the evaluation and management services provided to patients when the consulting physician is aware of the confirmatory nature of the opinion sought (e.g., when a second/third opinion is requested or required on the necessity or appropriateness of a previously recommended medical treatment or surgical procedure). Confirmatory consultations may be provided in any setting.

A physician consultant providing a confirmatory consultation is expected to provide an opinion and/or advice only. Any services subsequent to the opinion are coded at the appropriate level of office visit, established patient, or subsequent hospital care. If a confirmatory consultation is required, e.g., by a third party payor, the modifier –32 or 09932, mandated services, should also be reported. (See also Consultation Notes, above.)

Typical times have not yet been established for this subcategory of services.

CPT CODE	SERVICE
99241	Office consultation for a new or established patient, which requires these three key components:

- a problem focused history;
- a problem focused examination; and
- straightforward medical decision making.

Counseling and/or coordination of care with other providers or agencies are provided consistent with the nature of the problem(s) and the patient's and/or family's needs.

Usually, the presenting problem(s) are self limited or minor. Physicians typically spend 15 minutes face-to-face with the patient and/or family.

ICD–9–CM

380.1	Infective otitis externa
380.4	Impacted cerumen
384.2	Perforation of tympanic membrane
462	Acute pharyngitis
470	Deviated nasal septum

REIMBURSEMENT INFORMATION

General

- ♦ See notes on pages 48–49.

Medicare

- ♦ Outpatient Limit — applies

CPT CODE **SERVICE**

99242 Office consultation for a new or established patient, which requires these three key components:

- an expanded problem focused history;
- an expanded problem focused examination; and
- straightforward medical decision making.

Counseling and/or coordination of care with other providers or agencies are provided consistent with the nature of the problem(s) and the patient's and/or family's needs.

Usually, the presenting problem(s) are of low severity. Physicians typically spend 30 minutes face-to-face with the patient and/or family.

ICD–9–CM

173.3	M-Neoplasm, Skin of face NEC
380.1	Infective otitis externa
381.1	Chronic serous otitis media
381.4	Chron nonsup otitis media NOS
381.8	Eustachian tube disorder
382.3	Chronic suppurativ otitis media NOS
386.1	Peripheral vertigo
388.3	Tinnitus
389.0	Conductive hearing loss
389.1	Sensorineural hearing loss
389.9	Hearing loss NOS
461.9	Acute sinusitis NOS
464.0	Acute laryngitis
472.0	Chronic rhinitis
473.9	Chronic sinusitis NOS
478.3	Paralysis of vocal cords or larynx
519.0	Tracheostomy complication
524.6	Temporomandibular joint disorder
527.2	Sialoadenitis
529.0	Glossitis
530.1	Esophagitis
784.0	Headache
784.2	Swelling in head/neck
784.4	Voice disturbance
784.7	Epistaxis
786.0	Dyspnea and respiratory abnormality
786.2	Cough
787.2	Dysphagia
802.0	Nasal bone Fx, closed
V55.0	Attention to tracheostomy

REIMBURSEMENT INFORMATION

General

- ♦ See notes on pages 48–49.

Medicare

- ♦ Outpatient Limit — applies

CPT CODE	SERVICE
99243	Office consultation for a new or established patient, which requires these three key components: • a detailed history; • a detailed examination; and • medical decision making of low complexity. Counseling and/or coordination of care with other providers or agencies are provided consistent with the nature of the problem(s) and the patient's and/or family's needs. Usually, the presenting problem(s) are of moderate severity. Physicians typically spend 40 minutes face-to-face with the patient and/or family.

ICD–9–CM

381.4	Chron noncup otitic media NOS
381.8	Eustachian tube disorder
386.1	Peripheral vertigo
388.3	Tinnitus
388.7	Otalgia
389.1	Sensorineural hearing loss
389.2	Mixed hearing loss
464.0	Acute laryngitis
472.1	Chronic pharyngitis
477.8	Allergic rhinitis NEC
478.3	Paralysis of vocal cords or larynx
519.0	Tracheostomy complication
524.6	Temporomandibular joint disorder
527.2	Sialoadenitis
530.1	Esophagitis
780.4	Dizziness and giddiness
784.0	Headache
784.2	Swelling in head/neck
784.4	Voice disturbance
784.7	Epistaxis
785.6	Enlargement of lymph nodes
786.2	Cough
787.2	Dysphagia
V55.0	Attention to tracheostomy

REIMBURSEMENT INFORMATION

General

- ♦ See notes on pages 48–49.

Medicare

- ♦ Outpatient Limit — applies

CPT CODE	SERVICE	ICD–9–CM	
99244	Office consultation for a new or established patient, which requires these three key components: • a comprehensive history; • a comprehensive examination; and • medical decision making of moderate complexity. Counseling and/or coordination of care with other providers or agencies are provided consistent with the nature of the problem(s) and the patient's and/or family's needs. Usually, the presenting problem(s) are of moderate to high severity. Physicians typically spend 60 minutes face-to-face with the patient and/or family.	210.2	B-Neoplasm, Major salivary glands
		239.0	Digestive neoplasm NOS
		351.0	Bell's palsy
		386.0	Meniere's disease
		386.1	Peripheral vertigo
		386.2	Central origin vertigo
		388.01	Presbyacusis
		389.1	Sensorineural hearing loss
		473	Chronic sinusitis
		476.0	Chronic laryngitis
		478.4	Polyp of vocal cord/larynx
		527.2	Sialoadenitis
		530.1	Esophagitis
		784.0	Headache
		784.4	Voice disturbance
		784.7	Epistaxis
		786.2	Cough
		786.3	Hemoptysis
		787.2	Dysphagia

REIMBURSEMENT INFORMATION

General

♦ See notes on pages 48–49.

Medicare

♦ Outpatient Limit — applies

CPT CODE	SERVICE	ICD–9–CM	
99245	Office consultation for a new or established patient which requires these three key components: • a comprehensive history; • a comprehensive examination; and • medical decision making of high complexity. Counseling and/or coordination of care with other providers or agencies are provided consistent with the nature of the problem(s) and the patient's and/or family's needs. Usually, the presenting problem(s) are of moderate to high severity. Physicians typically spend 80 minutes face-to-face with the patient and/or family.	235.1	UB-Neoplasm, Oral cavity/pharynx
		386.0	Meniere's disease
		386.1	Peripheral vertigo
		389.1	Sensorineural hearing loss
		784.0	Headache
		784.4	Voice disturbance
		784.7	Epistaxis
		786.2	Cough
		787.2	Dysphagia

REIMBURSEMENT INFORMATION

General

♦ See notes on pages 48–49.

Medicare

♦ Outpatient Limit — applies

CPT CODE	SERVICE
99251	Initial inpatient consultation for a new or established patient, which requires these three key components: • a problem focused history; • a problem focused examination; and • straightforward medical decision making. Counseling and/or coordination of care with other providers or agencies are provided consistent with the nature of the problem(s) and the patient's and/or family's needs. Usually, the presenting problem(s) are self limiting or minor. Physicians typically spend 20 minutes at the bedside and on the patient's hospital floor or unit.

ICD–9–CM

380.1	Infective otitis externa
380.4	Impacted cerumen
381.8	Eustachian tube disorder
382.9	Otitis media NOS
384.2	Perforation of tympanic membrane
461.0	Acute maxillary sinusitis
462	Acute pharyngitis
464.0	Acute laryngitis
478.3	Paralysis of vocal cords or larynx
478.4	Polyp of vocal cord/larynx
527.2	Sialoadenitis
682.0	Cellulitis of face
784.2	Swelling in head/neck

REIMBURSEMENT INFORMATION

General

- ♦ See notes on pages 48–49.

Medicare

- ♦ Outpatient Limit — does not apply

CPT CODE	SERVICE
99252	Initial inpatient consultation for a new or established patient, which requires these three key components: • an expanded problem focused history; • an expanded problem focused examination; and • straightforward medical decision making. Counseling and/or coordination of care with other providers or agencies are provided consistent with the nature of the problem(s) and the patient's and/or family's needs. Usually, the presenting problem(s) are of low severity. Physicians typically spend 40 minutes at the bedside and on the patient's hospital floor or unit.

381.1	Chronic serous otitis media
381.4	Chron nonsup otitis media NOS
389.1	Sensorineural hearing loss
461.0	Acute maxillary sinusitis
462	Acute pharyngitis
473.0	Chronic maxillary sinusitis
473.8	Chronic sinusitis NEC
476.0	Chronic laryngitis
478.3	Paralysis of vocal cords or larynx
784.0	Headache
784.4	Voice disturbance
786.3	Hemoptysis
802.0	Nasal bone Fx, closed

REIMBURSEMENT INFORMATION

General

- ♦ See notes on pages 48–49.

Medicare

- ♦ Outpatient Limit — does not apply

CPT CODE	SERVICE
99253	Initial inpatient consultation for a new or established patient, which requires these three key components: • a detailed history; • a detailed examination; and • medical decision making of low complexity. Counseling and/or coordination of care with other providers or agencies are provided consistent with the nature of the problem(s) and the patient's and/or family's needs. Usually, the presenting problem(s) are of moderate severity. Physicians typically spend 55 minutes at the bedside and on the patient's hospital floor or unit.

ICD–9–CM

381.1	Chronic serous otitis media
382.9	Otitis media NOS
389.0	Conductive hearing loss
389.1	Sensorineural hearing loss
389.2	Mixed hearing loss
389.9	Hearing loss NOS
461.9	Acute sinusitis NOS
464.0	Acute laryngitis
470	Deviated nasal septum
472.0	Chronic rhinitis
473.0	Chronic maxillary sinusitis
473.8	Chronic sinusitis NEC
478.1	Nasal and sinus disease NEC
518.81	Respiratory failure
519.8	Respiratory system disease NEC
527.2	Sialoadenitis
528.0	Stomatitis
682.0	Cellulitis of face
780.4	Dizziness and giddiness
784.2	Swelling in head/neck
786.09	Respiratory abnormality NEC
786.2	Cough
802.0	Nasal bone Fx, closed

REIMBURSEMENT INFORMATION

General

♦ See notes on pages 48–49.

Medicare

♦ Outpatient Limit — does not apply

CPT CODE **SERVICE**

99254 Initial inpatient consultation for a new or established patient, which requires these three key components:

- a comprehensive history;
- a comprehensive examination; and
- medical decision making of moderate complexity.

Counseling and/or coordination of care with other providers or agencies are provided consistent with the nature of the problem(s) and the patient's and/or family's needs.

Usually, the presenting problem(s) are of moderate to high severity. Physicians typically spend 80 minutes at the bedside and on the patient's hospital floor or unit.

ICD–9–CM

386.0	Meniere's disease
386.1	Peripheral vertigo
386.2	Central origin vertigo
386.3	Labyrinthitis
478.3	Paralysis of vocal cords or larynx
486	Pneumonia, organism NOS
496	Chronic airway obstruction NEC
518.81	Respiratory failure
519.8	Respiratory system disease NEC
784.2	Swelling in head/neck
784.4	Voice disturbance
784.7	Epistaxis
786.09	Respiratory abnormality NEC
786.3	Hemoptysis
787.2	Dysphagia
802.0	Nasal bone Fx, closed
959.0	Face and neck injury NOS

REIMBURSEMENT INFORMATION

General

- ♦ See notes on pages 48–49.

Medicare

- ♦ Outpatient Limit — does not apply

CPT CODE	SERVICE	ICD–9–CM

99255 Initial inpatient consultation for a new or established patient, which requires these three key components:

- a comprehensive history;
- a comprehensive examination; and
- medical decision making of high complexity.

Counseling and/or coordination of care with other providers or agencies are provided consistent with the nature of the problem(s) and the patient's and/or family's needs.

Usually, the presenting problem(s) are of moderate to high severity. Physicians typically spend 110 minutes at the bedside and on the patient's floor or unit.

161.9	M-Neoplasm, Larynx NOS
195.0	M-Neoplasm, Head/face/neck
519.8	Respiratory system disease NEC
784.7	Epistaxis
786.09	Respiratory abnormality NEC
786.3	Hemoptysis
787.2	Dysphagia
802.8	Fx facial bone NEC, closed

REIMBURSEMENT INFORMATION

General

- ♦ See notes on pages 48–49.

Medicare

- ♦ Outpatient Limit — does not apply

99261 Follow-up inpatient consultation for an established patient, which requires at least two of these three key components:

- a problem focused interval history;
- a problem focused examination;
- straightforward or low complexity medical decision making.

Counseling and/or coordination of care with other providers or agencies are provided consistent with the nature of the problem(s) and the patient's and/or family's needs.

Usually, the patient is stable, recovering or improving. Physicians typically spend 10 minutes at the bedside and on the patient's hospital floor or unit.

380.2	Otitis externa
380.4	Impacted cerumen
381.1	Chronic serous otitis media
519.8	Respiratory system disease NEC
527.2	Sialoadenitis
786.09	Respiratory abnormality NEC
786.1	Stridor

REIMBURSEMENT INFORMATION

General

- ♦ See notes on pages 48–49.

Medicare

- ♦ Outpatient Limit — does not apply

CPT CODE	SERVICE	ICD-9-CM
99262	Follow-up inpatient consultation for an established patient, which requires at least two of these three key components: • an expanded problem focused interval history; • an expanded problem focused examination; • medical decision making of moderate complexity Counseling and/or coordination of care with other providers or agencies are provided consistent with the nature of the problem(s) and the patient's and/or family's needs. Usually, the patient is responding inadequately to therapy or has developed a minor complication. Physicians typically spend 20 minutes at the bedside and on the patient's hospital floor or unit.	383.0 Acute mastoiditis 389.1 Sensorineural hearing loss 389.9 Hearing loss NOS 473 Chronic sinusitis 486 Pneumonia, organism NOS 527.2 Sialoadenitis 784.7 Epistaxis 958.3 Posttraumatic wound infection NEC **REIMBURSEMENT INFORMATION** General ♦ See notes on pages 48–49. Medicare ♦ Outpatient Limit — does not apply
99263	Follow-up inpatient consultation for an established patient, which requires at least two of these three key components: • a detailed interval history; • a detailed examination; • medical decision making of high complexity. Counseling and/or coordination of care with other providers or agencies are provided consistent with the nature of the problem(s) and the patient's and/or family's needs. Usually, the patient is unstable or has developed a significant complication or a significant new problem. Physicians typically spend 30 minutes at the bedside and on the patient's hospital floor or unit.	682.0 Cellulitis of face 682.1 Cellulitis of neck 784.7 Epistaxis 786.09 Respiratory abnormality NEC 787.2 Dysphagia 802.8 Fx facial bone NEC, closed 802.9 Fx facial bone NEC, open **REIMBURSEMENT INFORMATION** General ♦ See notes on pages 48–49.

CPT CODE	SERVICE	ICD-9-CM
99271	Confirmatory consultation for a new or established patient, which requires these three key components: • a problem focused history; • a problem focused examination; and • straightforward medical decision making. Counseling and/or coordination of care with other providers or agencies are provided consistent with the nature of the problem(s) and the patient's and/or family's needs. Usually, the presenting problem(s) are self limited or minor.	380.4 Impacted cerumen 692.9 Dermatitis NOS 784.49 Voice disturbance NEC **REIMBURSEMENT INFORMATION** General ♦ See notes on pages 48–49. Medicare ♦ Outpatient Limit — applies
99272	Confirmatory consultation for a new or established patient, which requires these three key components: • an expanded problem focused history; • an expanded problem focused examination; and • straightforward medical decision making. Counseling and/or coordination of care with other providers or agencies are provided consistent with the nature of the problem(s) and the patient's and/or family's needs. Usually the presenting problem(s) are of low severity.	381.1 Chronic serous otitis media 461 Acute sinusitis 462 Acute pharyngitis 472.0 Chronic rhinitis 473 Chronic sinusitis 477 Allergic rhinitis **REIMBURSEMENT INFORMATION** General ♦ See notes on pages 48–49. Medicare ♦ Outpatient Limit — applies

CPT CODE	SERVICE
99273	Confirmatory consultation for a new or established patient, which requires these three key components: • a detailed history; • a detailed examination; and • medical decision making of low complexity Counseling and/or coordination of care with other providers or agencies are provided consistent with the nature of the problem(s) and the patient's and/or family's needs. Usually, the presenting problem(s) are of moderate severity.

ICD–9–CM

381.0	Acute nonsuppurative otitis media
381.8	Eustachian tube disorder
388.3	Tinnitus
389.1	Sensorineural hearing loss
461.9	Acute sinusitis NOS
470	Deviated nasal septum
472.0	Chronic rhinitis
473	Chronic sinusitis
474.0	Chronic tonsillitis
478.29	Disease of pharynx NEC
478.4	Polyp of vocal cord/larynx
527.2	Sialoadenitis

REIMBURSEMENT INFORMATION

General

- See notes on pages 48–49.

Medicare

- Outpatient Limit — applies

CPT CODE	SERVICE
99274	Confirmatory consultation for a patient, which requires these three key components: • a comprehensive history; • a comprehensive examination; and • medical decision making of moderate complexity. Counseling and/or coordination of care with other providers or agencies are provided consistent with the nature of the problem(s) and the patient's and/or family's needs. Usually, the presenting problem(s) are of moderate to high severity.

ICD–9–CM

202.8	Lymphoma
240.9	Goiter NOS
346.9	Migraine NOS
351.0	Bell's palsy
383.0	Acute mastoiditis
386.5	Labyrinthine dysfunction
389.1	Sensorineural hearing loss
464.2	Acute laryngotracheitis
478.3	Paralysis of vocal cords or larynx
780.4	Dizziness and giddiness
780.5	Sleep disturbance
784.2	Swelling in head/neck
784.4	Voice disturbance
784.7	Epistaxis
786.1	Stridor

REIMBURSEMENT INFORMATION

General

- ♦ See notes on pages 48–49.

Medicare

- ♦ Outpatient Limit — applies

CPT CODE	SERVICE
99275	Confirmatory consultation for a patient, which requires these three key components: • a comprehensive history; • a comprehensive examination; and • medical decision making of high complexity. Counseling and/or coordination of care with other providers or agencies are provided consistent with the nature of the problem(s) and the patient's and/or family's needs. Usually, the presenting problem(s) are of moderate to high severity.

ICD–9–CM

161.9	M-Neoplasm, Larynx NOS
230.0	CA in situ, Oral cavity/pharynx
235.1	UB-Neoplasm, Oral cavity/pharynx
351.8	Facial nerve disorder NEC
386.0	Meniere's disease
388.0	Degenerative/vascular ear disorder
389.11	Sensory hearing loss
530.6	Acquired esophageal diverticulum

REIMBURSEMENT INFORMATION

General

- ♦ See notes on pages 48–49.

Medicare

- ♦ Outpatient Limit — applies

EMERGENCY DEPARTMENT SERVICES
99281–99288

New or Established Patient
99281–99285

These codes are used to report evaluation and management services provided in the Emergency Department. No distinction is made between new and established patients in the Emergency Department.

An Emergency Department is defined as an organized hospital–based facility for the provision of unscheduled episodic services to patients who present for immediate medical attention. The facility must be available 24 hours a day.

For critical care services provided in the Emergency Department, see Critical Care notes and 99291, 99292 in your CPT.

For evaluation and management services provided to a patient in an observation area of a hospital, see 99217–99220 in your CPT.

For definitions of key components and commonly used terms, see Evaluation and Management Services Guidelines in your CPT.

CPT CODE	SERVICE	ICD–9–CM
99281	Emergency department visit for the evaluation and management of a patient, which requires these three key components: • a problem focused history; • a problem focused examination; and • straightforward medical decision making. Counseling and/or coordination of care with other providers or agencies are provided consistent with the nature of the problem(s) and the patient's and/or family's needs. Usually, the presenting problem(s) are self limited or minor.	380.1 Infective otitis externa 384.2 Perforation of tympanic membrane 388.6 Otorrhea 872.61 Open wound of eardrum **REIMBURSEMENT INFORMATION** General ♦ See notes on page 62. Medicare ♦ Outpatient Limit — does not apply
99282	Emergency department visit for the evaluation and management of a patient, which requires these three key components: • an expanded problem focused history; • an expanded problem focused examination; and • medical decision making of low complexity. Counseling and/or coordination of care with other providers or agencies are provided consistent with the nature of the problem(s) and the patient's and/or family's needs. Usually, the presenting problem(s) are of low to moderate severity.	210.2 B-Neoplasm, Major salivary glands 380.2 Otitis externa 380.4 Impacted cerumen 381.0 Acute nonsuppurative otitis media 382.0 Acute suppurative otitis media 462 Acute pharyngitis 478.2 Diseases of pharynx NEC 519.0 Tracheostomy complication 527.2 Sialoadenitis 738.0 Acquired nose deformity 872.9 Open wound of ear NOS, complicated 919.0 Abrasion NEC 920 Contusion face/scalp/neck V55.0 Attention to tracheostomy **REIMBURSEMENT INFORMATION** General ♦ See notes on page 62. Medicare ♦ Outpatient Limit — does not apply

CPT CODE **SERVICE**

99283 Emergency department visit for the evaluation and management of a patient, which requires these three key components:

- an expanded problem focused history;
- an expanded problem focused examination; and
- medical decision making of moderate complexity.

Counseling and/or coordination of care with other providers or agencies are provided consistent with the nature of the problem(s) and the patient's and/or family's needs.

Usually, the presenting problem(s) are of moderate severity.

ICD–9–CM

235.1	UB Neoplasm, Oral cavity/pharynx
462	Acute pharyngitis
475	Peritonsillar abscess
490	Bronchitis NOS
496	Chronic airway obstruction NEC
524.6	Temporomandibular joint disorder
682.0	Cellulitis of face
780.4	Dizziness and giddiness
784.0	Headache
784.41	Aphonia
784.7	Epistaxis
787.2	Dysphagia
802.0	Nasal bone Fx, closed
873.42	Open wound of forehead
874.9	Open wound of neck NEC, complicated
933.0	Foreign body in pharynx
935.1	Foreign body in esophagus
959.0	Face and neck injury NOS
995.2	Adverse effect med/biol substnc NOS

REIMBURSEMENT INFORMATION

General

- ♦ See notes on page 62.

Medicare

- ♦ Outpatient Limit — does not apply

99284 Emergency department visit for the evaluation and management of a patient, which requires these three key components:

- a detailed history;
- a detailed examination; and
- medical decision making of moderate complexity.

Counseling and/or coordination of care with other providers or agencies are provided consistent with the nature of the problem(s) and the patient's and/or family's needs.

Usually, the presenting problem(s) are of high severity, and require urgent evaluation by the physician but do not pose an immediate significant threat to life or physiologic function.

478.3	Paralysis of vocal cords or larynx
486	Pneumonia, organism NOS
496	Chronic airway obstruction NEC
519.8	Respiratory system disease NEC
780.6	Pyrexia of unknown origin
784.2	Swelling in head/neck
784.7	Epistaxis
786.09	Respiratory abnormality NEC
787.2	Dysphagia
933.0	Foreign body in pharynx

REIMBURSEMENT INFORMATION

General

- ♦ See notes on page 62.

Medicare

- ♦ Outpatient Limit — does not apply

CPT CODE	SERVICE
99285	Emergency department visit for the evaluation and management of a patient, which requires these three key components within the constraints imposed by the urgency of the patient's clinical condition and mental status: • a comprehensive history; • a comprehensive examination; and • medical decision making of high complexity. Counseling and/or coordination of care with other providers or agencies are provided consistent with the nature of the problem(s) and the patient's and/or family's needs. Usually, the presenting problem(s) are of high severity and pose an immediate significant threat to life of physiologic function.

ICD–9–CM

145.2	M-Neoplasm, Hard palate
195.0	M-Neoplasm, Head/face/neck
351.0	Bell's palsy
478.74	Stenosis of larynx
519.0	Tracheostomy complication
807.5	Fracture larynx/trachea-closed
933.0	Foreign body in pharynx
933.1	Foreign body in larynx
934.0	Foreign body, trachea
935.1	Foreign body in esophagus
995.1	Angioneurotic edema

REIMBURSEMENT INFORMATION

General

- ♦ See notes on page 62.

Medicare

- ♦ Outpatient Limit — does not apply

CRITICAL CARE SERVICES
99291 99292

Critical care includes the care of critically ill or injured patients in a variety of medical emergencies that requires the constant attendance of the physician (e.g., cardiac arrest, shock, bleeding, respiratory failure, postoperative complications). Critical care is usually, but not always, given in a critical care area, such as the coronary care unit, intensive care unit, respiratory care unit, or the emergency care facility.

Services for a patient who is not critically ill but happens to be in a critical care unit are reported using subsequent hospital care codes (see 99231–99233) or hospital consultation codes (see 99251–99263) as appropriate.

The following services are included in reporting critical care when performed during the critical period by the physician providing critical care: the interpretation of cardiac output measurements (93561, 93562), chest X–rays (71010, 71020), blood gases, and information data stored in computers (e.g., ECGs, blood pressures, hematologic data (99090)); gastric intubation (91105); temporary transcutaneous pacing (92953); ventilator management (94656, 94657, 94660, 94662); and, vascular access procedures (36000, 36410, 36415, 36600). Any services performed which are not listed above should be reported separately.

The critical care codes are used to report the total duration of time spent by a physician providing constant attention to a critically ill or injured patient, even if the time spent by the physician providing critical care services on that date is not continuous. Code 99291 is used to report the first hour of critical care on a given date. It should be used only once per date even if the time spent by the physician is not continuous on that date. Critical care of less than 30 minutes total duration on a given date should be reported with the appropriate E/M code. Code 99292 is used to report each additional 30 minutes beyond the first hour. It also may be used to report the final 15-30 minutes of critical care on a given date. Critical care of less than 15 minutes beyond the first hour or less than 15 minutes beyond the final 30 minutes is not reported separately.

The following examples illustrate the correct reporting of critical care services:

Total Duration of Critical Care	Codes
a. less than 30 minutes (less than 1/2 hour)	99232 or 99233
b. 30–74 minutes (1/2 hr. – 1 hr. 14 min.)	99291 x 1
c. 75–104 minutes (1 hr. 15 min. – 2 hr. 14 min.)	99291 x 1 AND 99292 x 1
d. 105–134 minutes (1 hr. 45 min. – 2 hr. 14 min.)	99291 x 1 AND 99292 x 2
e. 135–164 minutes (2 hr. 15 min. – 2 hr. 44 min.)	99291 x 1 AND 99292 x 3
f. 165–194 minutes (2 hr. 45 min. – 3 hr. 14 min.)	99291 x 1 AND 99292 x 4

CPT CODE	SERVICE	ICD–9–CM
99291	Critical care, evaluation and management of the critically ill or critically injured patient, requiring the constant attendance of the physician; first hour	464.1 Acute tracheitis 464.3 Acute epiglottitis 478.75 Laryngeal spasm 518.5 Post traum pulmonary insufficiency 518.81 Respiratory failure 784.2 Swelling in head/neck 784.7 Epistaxis 786.09 Respiratory abnormality NEC 874.9 Open wound of neck NEC, complicated 995.1 Angioneurotic edema **REIMBURSEMENT INFORMATION** General ♦ See notes on page 66. Medicare ♦ Outpatient Limit — does not apply
99292	Critical care, evaluation and management of the critically ill or critically injured patient, requiring the constant attendance of the physician; each additional 30 minues	464.1 Acute tracheitis 464.3 Acute epiglottitis 478.75 Laryngeal spasm 518.5 Post traum pulmonary insufficiency 518.81 Respiratory failure 784.2 Swelling in head/neck 784.7 Epistaxis 786.09 Respiratory abnormality NEC 874.9 Open wound of neck NEC, complicated 995.1 Angioneurotic edema **REIMBURSEMENT INFORMATION** General ♦ See notes on page 66. Medicare ♦ Outpatient Limit — does not apply

NURSING FACILITY SERVICES
99301–99313

The following codes are used to report evaluation and management services to patients in Nursing Facilities (formerly called Skilled Nursing Facilities (SNFs), Intermediate Care Facilities (ICFs) or Long Term Care Facilities (LTCFs)).

These codes should also be used to report evaluation and management services provided to a patient in a psychiatric residential treatment center (a facility or a distinct part of a facility for psychiatric care, which provides a 24 hour therapeutically planned and professionally staffed group living and learning environment). If procedures such as medical psychotherapy are provided in addition to evaluation and management services, these should be reported in addition to the evaluation and management services provided.

Nursing facilities that provide convalescent, rehabilitative, or long term care are required to conduct comprehensive, accurate, standardized, and reproducible assessments of each resident's functional capacity using a Resident Assessment Instrument (RAI). All RAIs include the Minimum Data Set (MDS), Resident Assessment Protocols (RAPs) and utilization guidelines. The MDS is the primary screening and assessment tool; the RAPs trigger the identification of potential problems and provide guidelines for follow–up assessments.

Physicians have a central role in assuring that all residents receive thorough assessments and that medical plans of care are instituted or revised to enhance or maintain the residents' physical and psychosocial functioning.

Two subcategories of nursing facility services are recognized: Comprehensive Nursing Facility Assessments and Subsequent Nursing Facility Care. Both subcategories apply to new or established patients. Comprehensive Assessments may be performed at one or more sites in the assessment process: the hospital, office, nursing facility, domiciliary/non–nursing facility or patient's home.

For definitions of key components and commonly used terms, please see Evaulation and Management Services Guidelines in your CPT.

Comprehensive Nursing Facility Assessments
New or Established Patient
99301–99303

When the patient is admitted to the nursing facility in the course of an encounter in another site of service (e.g., hospital emergency department, physician's office), all evaluation and management services provided by that physician in conjunction with that admission are considered part of the initial nursing facility care when performed as part of the admission. The nursing facility care level of service reported by the admitting physician should include the services related to the admission he/she provided in the other sites of service as well as in the nursing facility setting. With the exception of hospital discharge services, evaluation and management services on the same date provided in sites other than the nursing facility that are related to the admission should NOT be reported separately. Hospital discharge services may be reported separately.

More than one comprehensive assessment may be necessary during an inpatient confinement.

NURSING FACILITY SERVICES (Cont'd.)

Subsequent Nursing Facility Care
New or Established Patient
99311–99312

These codes are used to report the services provided to residents of nursing facilities who do not require a comprehensive assessment, and/or who have not had a major, permanent change of status.

All levels include reviewing the medical record, noting changes in the resident's status since the last visit, and reviewing and signing orders.

CPT CODE	SERVICE	ICD–9–CM

99301 Evaluation and management of a new or established patient involving an annual nursing facility assessment which requires these three key components:

- a detailed interval history
- a comprehensive examination and
- straightforward or low complexity medical decision making.

Counseling and/or coordination of care with other providers or agencies are provided consistent with the nature of the problem(s) and the patient's and/or family's needs.

Usually, the patient is stable, recovering or improving. The review and affirmation of the medical plan of care is required. Physicians typically spend 30 minutes at the bedside and on the patient's facility floor or unit.

ICD–9–CM:

519.0	Tracheostomy complication
787.2	Dysphagia

REIMBURSEMENT INFORMATION

General

- ♦ See notes on pages 68–69.

Medicare

- ♦ Outpatient Limit — does not apply

99302 Evaluation and management of a new or established patient involving a nursing facility assessment which requires these three key components:

- a detailed interval history
- a comprehensive examination and
- medical decision making of moderate to high complexity.

Counseling and/or coordination of care with other providers or agencies are provided consistent with the nature of the problem(s) and the patient's and/or family's needs.

Usually, the patient has developed a significant complication or a significant new problem and has had a major permanent change in status.

The creation of a new medical plan of care is required. Physicians typically spend 40 minutes at the bedside and on the patient's facility floor or unit.

ICD–9–CM:

388.31	Subjective tinnitus
529.0	Glossitis
784.2	Swelling in head/neck
787.2	Dysphagia

REIMBURSEMENT INFORMATION

General

- ♦ See notes on pages 68–69.

Medicare

- ♦ Outpatient Limit — does not apply

CPT CODE	SERVICE	ICD–9–CM
99303	Evaluation and management of a new or established patient involving a nursing facility assessment at the time of initial admission to the facility, which requires these three key components: • a comprehensive history • a comprehensive examination and • medical decision making of moderate to high complexity. Counseling and/or coordination of care with other providers or agencies are provided consistent with the nature of the problem(s) and the patient's and/or family's needs. The creation of a medical plan of care is required. Physicians typically spend 50 minutes at the bedside and on the patient's facility floor or unit.	V44.0 Tracheostomy status **REIMBURSEMENT INFORMATION** General ♦ See notes on pages 68–69. Medicare ♦ Outpatient Limit — does not apply
99311	Subsequent nursing facility care, per day, for the evaluation and management of a new or established patient, which requires at least TWO of these three key components: • a problem focused interval history • a problem focused examination • straightforward or low complexity medical decision making. Counseling and/or coordination of care with other providers or agencies are provided consistent with the nature of the problem(s) and the patient's and/or family's needs. Usually, the patient is stable, recovering or improving. Physicians typically spend 15 minutes at the bedside and on the patient's facility floor or unit.	380.4 Impacted cerumen 380.5 Stenosis of external ear canal **REIMBURSEMENT INFORMATION** General ♦ See notes on pages 68–69. Medicare ♦ Outpatient Limit — does not apply

CPT CODE	SERVICE
99312	Subsequent nursing facility care, per day, for the evaluation and management of a new or established patient, which requires at least TWO of these three key components:

- an expanded problem focused interval history
- an expanded problem focused examination
- medical decision making of moderate complexity.

Counseling and/or coordination of care with other providers or agencies are provided consistent with the nature of the problem(s) and the patient's and/or family's needs.

Usually, the patient is responding inadequately to therapy or has developed a minor complication. Physicians typically spend 25 minutes at the bedside and on the patient's facility floor or unit.

ICD–9–CM

000 Hearing loss
518.81 Respiratory failure

REIMBURSEMENT INFORMATION

General

- ♦ See notes on pages 68–69.

Medicare

- ♦ Outpatient Limit — does not apply

99313 Subsequent nursing facility care, per day, for the evaluation and management of a new or established patient, which requires at least TWO of these three components:

- a detailed interval history
- a detailed examination
- medical decision making of moderate to high complexity.

Counseling and/or coordination of care with other providers or agencies are provided consistent with the nature of the problem(s) and the patient's and/or family's needs.

Usually, the patient has developed a significant complication or a significant new problem. Physicians typically spend 35 minutes at the bedside and on the patient's facility floor or unit.

389.1 Sensorineural hearing loss
478.4 Polyp of vocal cord/larynx

REIMBURSEMENT INFORMATION

General

- ♦ See notes on pages 68–69.

Medicare

- ♦ Outpatient Limit — does not apply

DOMICILIARY, REST HOME (e.g., Boarding Home), or CUSTODIAL CARE SERVICES

New Patient
99321–99323

Established Patient
99331–99333

These codes are used to report evaluation and management services in a facility which provides room, board and other personal assistance services, generally on a long–term basis. The facility's services do not include a medical component.

For definitions of key components and commonly used terms, please see Evaluation and Management Services Guidelines in your CPT.

Typical times have not yet been established for this category of services.

CPT CODE	SERVICE	ICD–9–CM
99321	Domiciliary or rest home visit for the evaluation and management of a new patient, which requires these three key components: • a problem focused history; • a problem focused examination; and • straightforward or low complexity medical decision making. Counseling and/or coordination of care with other providers or agencies are provided consistent with the nature of the problem(s) and the patient's and/or family's needs. Usually, the presenting problem(s) are of low severity.	380.4 Impacted cerumen 477.9 Allergic rhinitis NOS 780.4 Dizziness and giddiness **REIMBURSEMENT INFORMATION** General ♦ See notes on page 73. Medicare ♦ Outpatient Limit — does not apply
99322	Domiciliary or rest home visit for the evaluation and management of a new patient, which requires these three key components: • an expanded problem focused history; • an expanded problem focused examination; and • medical decision making of moderate complexity. Counseling and/or coordination of care with other providers or agencies are provided consistent with the nature of the problem(s) and the patient's and/or family's needs. Usually, the presenting problem(s) are of moderate severity.	380.4 Impacted cerumen 389.2 Mixed hearing loss **REIMBURSEMENT INFORMATION** General ♦ See notes on page 73. Medicare ♦ Outpatient Limit — does not apply
99323	Domiciliary or rest home visit for the evaluation and management of a new patient, which requires these three key components: • a detailed history; • an detailed examination; and • medical decision making of high complexity. Counseling and/or coordination of care with other providers or agencies are provided consistent with the nature of the problem(s) and the patient's and/or family's needs. Usually, the presenting problem(s) are of high complexity.	380.4 Impacted cerumen 388.01 Presbyacusis **REIMBURSEMENT INFORMATION** General ♦ See notes on page 73. Medicare ♦ Outpatient Limit — does not apply

CPT CODE **SERVICE**

99331 Domiciliary or rest home visit for the evaluation and management of an established patient, which requires at least two of these three key components:

- an problem focused interval history;
- an problem focused examination;
- straightforward or low complexity medical decision making.

Counseling and/or coordination of care with other providers or agencies are provided consistent with the nature of the problem(s) and the patient's and/or family's needs.

Usually, the patient is responding inadequately to therapy or has developed a minor complication.

ICD–9–CM

380.4 Impacted cerumen
388.31 Subjective tinnitus

REIMBURSEMENT INFORMATION

General

- ♦ See notes on page 73.

Medicare

- ♦ Outpatient Limit — does not apply

99332 Domiciliary or rest home visit for the evaluation and management of an established patient, which requires at least two of these three key components:

- an expanded problem focused interval history;
- an expanded problem focused examination;
- medical decision making of moderate complexity.

Counseling and/or coordination of care with other providers or agencies are provided consistent with the nature of the problem(s) and the patient's and/or family's needs.

Usually, the patient is responding inadequately to therapy or has developed a minor complication.

388.01 Presbyacusis
470 Deviated nasal septum

REIMBURSEMENT INFORMATION

General

- ♦ See notes on page 73.

Medicare

- ♦ Outpatient Limit — does not apply

CPT CODE	SERVICE
99333	Domiciliary or rest home visit for the evaluation and management of an established patient, which requires at least two of these three key components:

- a detailed interval history;
- a detailed examination;
- medical decision making of high complexity.

Counseling and/or coordination of care with other providers or agencies are provided consistent with the nature of the problem(s) and the patient's and/or family's needs.

Usually, the patient is unstable or has developed a significant complication or a signifiant new problem.

ICD–9–CM

161.9	M-Neoplasm, Larynx NOS
195.0	M-Neoplasm, Head/face/neck

REIMBURSEMENT INFORMATION

General

- ♦ See notes on page 73.

Medicare

- ♦ Outpatient Limit — does not apply

HOME SERVICES

New Patient
99341–99343

Established Patient
99351–99353

These codes are used to report evaluation and management services provided in a private residence.

For definitions of key components and commonly used terms, please see Evaluation and Management Services Guidelines in your CPT. Typical times have not yet been established for this category of services.

CPT CODE **SERVICE** | **ICD–9–CM**

99341 Home visit for the evaluation and management of a new patient, which requires these three key components:

- a problem focused history;
- a problem focused examination; and
- straightforward or low complexity medical decision making.

Counseling and/or coordination of care with other providers or agencies are provided consistent with the nature of the problem(s) and the patient's and/or family's needs.

Usually, the presenting problem(s) are of low severity.

346.0 Classical migraine
380.4 Impacted cerumen

REIMBURSEMENT INFORMATION

General

- ♦ See notes on page 77.

Medicare

- ♦ Outpatient Limit — does not apply

99342 Home visit for the evaluation and management of a new patient, which requires these three key components:

- an expanded problem focused history;
- an expanded problem focused examination; and
- medical decision making of moderate complexity.

Counseling and/or coordination of care with other providers or agencies are provided consistent with the nature of the problem(s) and the patient's and or family's needs.

Usually, the presenting problem(s) are of moderate severity.

380.1 Infective otitis externa
470 Deviated nasal septum
490 Bronchitis NOS
506.4 Fume/vapor chronic respiratory cond

REIMBURSEMENT INFORMATION

General

- ♦ See notes on page 77.

Medicare

- ♦ Outpatient Limit — does not apply

99343 Home visit for the evaluation and management of a new patient, which requires these three key components:

- a detailed history;
- a detailed examination; and
- medical decision making of high complexity.

Counseling and/or coordination of care with other providers or agencies are provided consistent with the nature of the problem(s) and the patient's and or family's needs.

Usually, the presenting problem(s) are of high severity.

161.9 M-Neoplasm, Larynx NOS
195.0 M-Neoplasm, Head/face/neck

REIMBURSEMENT INFORMATION

General

- ♦ See notes on page 77.

Medicare

- ♦ Outpatient Limit — does not apply

CPT CODE	SERVICE	ICD–9–CM

99351 Home visit for the evaluation and management of an established patient, which requires at least two of these three key components:

- a problem focused history;
- a problem focused examination;
- medical decision making that is straightforward and of low complexity.

Counseling and/or coordination of care with other providers or agencies are provided consistent with the nature of the problem(s) and the patient's and or family's needs.

Usually, the patient is stable, recovering or improving.

380.4 Impacted cerumen
780.4 Dizziness and giddiness
784.7 Epistaxis

REIMBURSEMENT INFORMATION

General

- ♦ See notes on page 77.

Medicare

- ♦ Outpatient Limit — does not apply

99352 Home visit for the evaluation and management of an established patient, which requires at least two of these three key components:

- an expanded problem focused history;
- an expanded problem focused examination;
- medical decision making of moderate complexity.

Counseling and/or coordination of care with other providers or agencies are provided consistent with the nature of the problem(s) and the patient's and or family's needs.

Usually, the patient is responding inadequately to therapy or has developed a minor complicaton.

346.0 Classical migraine
380.4 Impacted cerumen
381.1 Chronic serous otitis media
389.1 Sensorineural hearing loss
478.5 Vocal cord disease NEC

REIMBURSEMENT INFORMATION

General

- ♦ See notes on page 77.

Medicare

- ♦ Outpatient Limit — does not apply

99353 Home visit for the evaluation and management of an established patient, which requires at least two of these three key components:

- a detailed interval history;
- a detailed examination;
- medical decision making of high complexity.

Counseling and/or coordination of care with other providers or agencies are provided consistent with the nature of the problem(s) and the patient's and or family's needs.

Usually, the patient is unstable or has developed a significant complication or a significant new problem.

161.9 M-Neoplasm, Larynx NOS
195.0 M-Neoplasm, Head/face/neck

REIMBURSEMENT INFORMATION

General

- ♦ See notes on page 77.

Medicare

- ♦ Outpatient Limit — does not apply

SURGERY

MUSCULOSKELETAL SYSTEM

Cast and strapping procedures appear at the end of this section. The services listed include the application and removal of the first cast or traction device only. Subsequent replacement of cast and/or traction device may require an additional listing.

The terms "closed treatment," "open treatment" and "percutaneous skeletal fixation" have been carefully chosen to accurately reflect current orthopedic procedural treatments.

Definitions

The terms "closed treatment, "open treament," and "percutaneous skeletal fixation" have been carefully chosen to accurately reflect current orthopaedic procedural treatments.

Closed Treatment. "Closed treatment" specifically means that the fracture site is not surgically opened (exposed to the external environment and directly visualized). This terminology is used to describe procedures that treat fractures by three methods: 1) without manipulation. 2) with manipulation. 3) with or without traction.

Open Treatment. "Open treatment" is used when the fracture is surgically opened (exposed to the external environment). In this instance, the fracture (bone ends) is visualized and internal fixation may be used.

Percutaneous Skeletal Fixation. "Percutaneous skeletal fixation" describes fracture treatment which is neither open nor closed. In this procedure, the fracture fragments are not visualized, but fixation (e.g., pins) is placed across the fracture site, usually under X–ray imaging.

The type of fracture (e.g., open, compound, closed) does not have any coding correlation with the type of treatment (e.g., closed, open or percutaneous) provided.

The codes for treatment of fractures and joint injuries (dislocations) are categorized by the type of manipulation (reduction) and stabilization (fixation or immobilization). These codes can apply to either open (compound) or closed fractures or joint injuries.

Skeletal traction is the application of a force (distracting or traction force) to a limb segment through a wire, pin, screw or clamp that is attached (e.g., penetrates) to bone.

Skin traction is the application of a force (longitudinal) to a limb using felt or strapping applied directly to skin only.

External fixation is the usage of skeletal pins plus an attaching mechanism/device used for temporary or definitive treatment of acute or chronic bony deformity.

Codes for obtaining autogenous bone grafts, cartilage, tendon fascia lata grafts or other tissues, through separate incisions are to be used only when the graft is not already listed as part of the basic procedure.

Re–reduction of a fracture and/or dislocation performed by the primary physician may be identified by either the addition of the modifier "–76" to the usual procedure number or by use of modifier code 09976 to indicate "Repeat Procedure by Same Physician." (See Surgery Guidelines in your CPT.)

Codes for external fixation are to be used only when external fixation is not already listed as part of the basic procedure.

All codes for suction irrigation have been deleted. To report, list only the primary surgical procedure performed (e.g., sequestrectomy, deep incision).

Manipulation. The term manipulation is used throughout the musculoskeletal fracture and dislocation subsections to specifically mean the attempted reduction or restoration of a fracture or joint dislocation to its normal anatomic alignment by the application of manually applied forces.

CPT CODE | **SERVICE** | **ICD–9–CM**

21310 Closed treatment of nasal bone fracture without manipulation

802.0 Nasal bone Fx, closed
802.1 Nasal bone Fx, open

REIMBURSEMENT INFORMATION

General

- See notes on pages 83.

Medicare

- Follow–up Days — 0
- Assistant Surgeon — not paid
- Supply Charges — not allowed
- Outpatient Limit — does not apply
- Minor Surgery Rules Apply

21315* Closed treatment, nasal bone fracture; without stabilization

802.0 Nasal bone Fx, closed
802.1 Nasal bone Fx, open

REIMBURSEMENT INFORMATION

General

- See notes on pages 83.
- Starred procedure.

Medicare

- Follow–up Days — 10
- Assistant Surgeon — not paid
- Supply Charges — not allowed
- Outpatient Limit — does not apply
- Minor Surgery Rules Apply

21345 Closed treatment of nasomaxillary complex fracture (LeFort II type), with interdental wire fixation or fixation of denture or splint

802.0 Nasal bone Fx, closed
802.1 Nasal bone Fx, open
802.4 Fx malar/maxillary, closed
802.5 Fx malar/maxillary, open

REIMBURSEMENT INFORMATION

General

- See notes on pages 83.

Medicare

- Follow–up Days — 90
- Assistant Surgeon — by report
- Supply Charges — not allowed
- Outpatient Limit — does not apply
- Major Surgery Rules Apply

CPT CODE	SERVICE	ICD–9–CM
21346	Open treatment of nasomaxillary complex fracture (LeFort II type); with wiring and/or local fixation	802.0 Nasal bone Fx, closed 802.1 Nasal bone Fx, open 802.4 Fx malar/maxillary, closed 802.5 Fx malar/maxillary, open **REIMBURSEMENT INFORMATION** General ♦ See notes on pages 83. Medicare ♦ Follow–up Days — 90 ♦ Assistant Surgeon — paid ♦ Supply Charges — not allowed ♦ Outpatient Limit — does not apply ♦ Major Surgery Rules Apply
21347	Open treatment of nasomaxillary complex fracture (LeFort II type); requiring multiple open approaches	802.0 Nasal bone Fx, closed 802.1 Nasal bone Fx, open 802.4 Fx malar/maxillary, closed 802.5 Fx malar/maxillary, open **REIMBURSEMENT INFORMATION** General ♦ See notes on pages 83. Medicare ♦ Follow–up Days — 90 ♦ Assistant Surgeon — paid ♦ Supply Charges — not allowed ♦ Outpatient Limit — does not apply ♦ Major Surgery Rules Apply
21348	Open treatment of nasomaxillary complex fracture (LeFort II type); with bone grafting (includes obtaining graft)	802.0 Nasal bone Fx, closed 802.1 Nasal bone Fx, open 802.4 Fx malar/maxillary, closed 802.5 Fx malar/maxillary, open **REIMBURSEMENT INFORMATION** General ♦ See notes on pages 83. Medicare ♦ Follow–up Days — 90 ♦ Assistant Surgeon — paid ♦ Supply Charges — not allowed ♦ Outpatient Limit — does not apply ♦ Major Surgery Rules Apply

CPT CODE	SERVICE	ICD-9-CM
21365	Open treatment of complicated, (eg, comminuted or involving cranial nerve foramina) fracture(s) of malar area, including zygomatic arch and malar tripod; with internal fixation and multiple surgical approaches	802.4 Fx malar/maxillary, closed 802.5 Fx malar/maxillary, open 802.6 Fx orbital floor, closed

REIMBURSEMENT INFORMATION

General

- See notes on pages 83.

Medicare

- Follow–up Days — 90
- Assistant Surgeon — paid
- Supply Charges — not allowed
- Outpatient Limit — does not apply
- Major Surgery Rules Apply

CPT CODE	SERVICE	ICD-9-CM
21366	Open treatment of complicated (eg, comminuted or involving cranial nerve foramina) fracture(s) of malar area, including zygomatic arch and malar tripod; with bone grafting (includes obtaining graft)	802.4 Fx malar/maxillary, closed 802.5 Fx malar/maxillary, open 802.6 Fx orbital floor, closed

REIMBURSEMENT INFORMATION

General

- See notes on pages 83.

Medicare

- Follow–up Days — 90
- Assistant Surgeon — paid
- Supply Charges — not allowed
- Outpatient Limit — does not apply
- Major Surgery Rules Apply

CPT CODE	SERVICE	ICD-9-CM
21385	Open treatment of orbital floor "blowout" fracture; transantral approach (Caldwell-Luc type operation)	802.4 Fx malar/maxillary, closed 802.5 Fx malar/maxillary, open 802.6 Fx orbital floor, closed 802.7 Fx orbital floor, open

REIMBURSEMENT INFORMATION

General

- See notes on pages 83.

Medicare

- Follow–up Days — 90
- Assistant Surgeon — paid
- Supply Charges — not allowed
- Outpatient Limit — does not apply
- Major Surgery Rules Apply

CPT CODE	SERVICE	ICD–9–CM
21386	Open treatment of orbital floor "blowout" fracture; periorbital approach	802.4 Fx malar/maxillary, closed 802.5 Fx malar/maxillary, open 802.6 Fx orbital floor, closed 802.7 Fx orbital floor, open **REIMBURSEMENT INFORMATION** General ♦ See notes on pages 83. Medicare ♦ Follow–up Days — 90 ♦ Assistant Surgeon — paid ♦ Supply Charges — not allowed ♦ Outpatient Limit — does not apply ♦ Major Surgery Rules Apply
21387	Open treatment of orbital floor "blowout" fracture; combined approach	802.4 Fx malar/maxillary, closed 802.5 Fx malar/maxillary, open 802.6 Fx orbital floor, closed 802.7 Fx orbital floor, open **REIMBURSEMENT INFORMATION** General ♦ See notes on pages 83. Medicare ♦ Follow–up Days — 90 ♦ Assistant Surgeon — paid ♦ Supply Charges — not allowed ♦ Outpatient Limit — does not apply ♦ Major Surgery Rules Apply
21390	Open treatment of orbital floor "blowout" fracture; periorbital approach, with alloplastic or other implant	802.4 Fx malar/maxillary, closed 802.5 Fx malar/maxillary, open 802.6 Fx orbital floor, closed 802.7 Fx orbital floor, open **REIMBURSEMENT INFORMATION** General ♦ See notes on pages 83. Medicare ♦ Follow–up Days — 90 ♦ Assistant Surgeon — paid ♦ Supply Charges — not allowed ♦ Outpatient Limit — does not apply ♦ Major Surgery Rules Apply

CPT CODE	SERVICE	ICD-9-CM

21395 Open treatment of orbital floor "blowout" fracture; periorbital approach with bone graft (includes obtaining graft)

802.4	Fx malar/maxillary, closed
802.5	Fx malar/maxillary, open
802.6	Fx orbital floor, closed
802.7	Fx orbital floor, open

REIMBURSEMENT INFORMATION

General

- ♦ See notes on pages 83.

Medicare

- ♦ Follow–up Days — 90
- ♦ Assistant Surgeon — paid
- ♦ Supply Charges — not allowed
- ♦ Outpatient Limit — does not apply
- ♦ Major Surgery Rules Apply

21408 Open treatment of fracture of orbit, except "blowout"; with bone grafting (includes obtaining graft)

802.4	Fx malar/maxillary, closed
802.5	Fx malar/maxillary, open
802.6	Fx orbital floor, closed

REIMBURSEMENT INFORMATION

General

- ♦ See notes on pages 83.

Medicare

- ♦ Follow–up Days — 90
- ♦ Assistant Surgeon — paid
- ♦ Supply Charges — not allowed
- ♦ Outpatient Limit — does not apply
- ♦ Major Surgery Rules Apply

21497 Interdental wiring, for condition other than fracture

170.0	M-Neoplasm, Skull/Face bone
213.0	B-Neoplasm, Skull/Face bone
213.1	B-Neoplasm, Lower jaw bone
239.2	Bone/Skin neoplasm NOS
526.0	Developmental odontogenic cysts

REIMBURSEMENT INFORMATION

General

- ♦ See notes on pages 83.

Medicare

- ♦ Follow–up Days — 90
- ♦ Assistant Surgeon — by report
- ♦ Supply Charges — not allowed
- ♦ Outpatient Limit — does not apply
- ♦ Major Surgery Rules Apply

CPT CODE	SERVICE	ICD-9-CM

21501 Incision and drainage, deep abscess or hematoma, soft tissues of neck or thorax

CPT NOTES

- For incision and drainage of abscess or hematoma, superficial, see 10060, 10140.

478.1	Nasal and sinus disease NEC
682.1	Cellulitis of neck
682.2	Cellulitis of trunk
744.42	Branchial cleft cyst
759.2	Endocrine gland anomaly NEC
906.3	Late effect of contusion
906.4	Late effect of crushing
909.3	Late effect of surg/med complic
920	Contusion face/scalp/neck
922.1	Contusion of chest wall
925	Crushing injury, face/scalp/neck
926.19	Crushing injury, trunk NEC

REIMBURSEMENT INFORMATION

General

- See notes on pages 83.

Medicare

- Follow-up Days — 90
- Assistant Surgeon — not paid
- Supply Charges — not allowed
- Outpatient Limit — does not apply
- Major Surgery Rules Apply

21550 Biopsy, soft tissue of neck or thorax

CPT NOTES

- For bone biopsy, see 20220–20251.
- For needle biopsy of soft tissue, see 20206.

171.0	M-Neoplasm, Soft tissue, head
171.4	M-Neoplasm, Soft tissue, thorax
171.8	M-Neoplasm, Soft tissue NEC
195.0	M-Neoplasm, Head/face/neck
195.1	M-Neoplasm, Thorax
215.0	B-Neoplasm, Soft tissue, head
215.4	B-Neoplasm, Soft tissue, thorax
229.0	B-Neoplasm, Lymph nodes
229.8	Benign neoplasm NEC
229.9	Benign neoplasm NOS
238.1	UB-Neoplasm, Soft tissue
239.2	Bone/Skin neoplasm NOS
241.0	Nontoxic uninodular goiter
784.2	Swelling in head/neck

REIMBURSEMENT INFORMATION

General

- See notes on pages 83.

Medicare

- Follow-up Days — 10
- Assistant Surgeon — not paid
- Supply Charges — not allowed
- Outpatient Limit — does not apply
- Minor Surgery Rules Apply

CPT CODE	**SERVICE**
21555	Excision tumor, soft tissue of neck or thorax; subcutaneous

CPT NOTES

- For bone biopsy, see 20220–20251.

ICD–9–CM

171.4	M-Neoplasm, Soft tissue, thorax
171.8	M-Neoplasm, Soft tissue NEC
195.0	M-Neoplasm, Head/face/neck
195.1	M-Neoplasm, Thorax
214.0	Lipoma, Skin of face
215.0	B-Neoplasm, Soft tissue, head
215.4	B-Neoplasm, Soft tissue, thorax
229.0	B-Neoplasm, Lymph nodes
229.8	Benign neoplasm NEC
229.9	Benign neoplasm NOS
238.1	UB-Neoplasm, Soft tissue
239.2	Bone/Skin neoplasm NOS
528.4	Oral soft tissue cyst
784.2	Swelling in head/neck

REIMBURSEMENT INFORMATION

General

- See notes on pages 83.

Medicare

- Follow–up Days — 90
- Assistant Surgeon — not paid
- Supply Charges — not allowed
- Outpatient Limit — does not apply
- Major Surgery Rules Apply

CPT CODE SERVICE	ICD–9–CM
21556 Excision tumor, soft tissue of neck or thorax; deep, subfascial, intramuscular **CPT NOTES** ♦ For bone biopsy, see 20220–20251.	171.4 M-Neoplasm, Soft tissue, thorax 171.8 M-Neoplasm, Soft tissue NEC 195.0 M-Neoplasm, Head/face/neck 195.1 M-Neoplasm, Thorax 214.0 Lipoma, Skin of face 215.0 B-Neoplasm, Soft tissue, head 215.4 B-Neoplasm, Soft tissue, thorax 229.0 B-Neoplasm, Lymph nodes 229.8 Benign neoplasm NEC 229.9 Benign neoplasm NOS 238.1 UB-Neoplasm, Soft tissue 239.2 Bone/Skin neoplasm NOS 528.4 Oral soft tissue cyst 706.2 Sebaceous cyst 784.2 Swelling in head/neck **REIMBURSEMENT INFORMATION** General ♦ See notes on pages 83. Medicare ♦ Follow–up Days — 90 ♦ Assistant Surgeon — not paid ♦ Supply Charges — not allowed ♦ Outpatient Limit — does not apply ♦ Major Surgery Rules Apply
21557 Radical resection of tumor (eg, malignant neoplasm), soft tissue of neck or thorax **CPT NOTES** ♦ For bone biopsy, see 20220–20251.	171.4 M-Neoplasm, Soft tissue, thorax 171.8 M-Neoplasm, Soft tissue NEC 195.0 M-Neoplasm, Head/face/neck 195.1 M-Neoplasm, Thorax 238.1 UB-Neoplasm, Soft tissue 239.2 Bone/Skin neoplasm NOS **REIMBURSEMENT INFORMATION** General ♦ See notes on pages 83. Medicare ♦ Follow–up Days — 90 ♦ Assistant Surgeon — paid ♦ Supply Charges — not allowed ♦ Outpatient Limit — does not apply ♦ Major Surgery Rules Apply

CPT CODE	SERVICE	ICD–9–CM
30000*	Drainage abscess or hematoma, nasal, internal approach	473.0 Chronic sinusitis NEC 478.1 Nasal and sinus disease NEC 682.0 Cellulitis of face 920 Contusion face/scalp/neck 959.0 Face and neck injury NOS

CPT NOTES

- For external approach, see 10060, 10140.

REIMBURSEMENT INFORMATION

General

- Starred procedure.

Medicare

- Follow–up Days — 10
- Assistant Surgeon — not paid
- Supply Charges — not allowed
- Outpatient Limit — does not apply
- Minor Surgery Rules Apply

CPT CODE	SERVICE	ICD–9–CM
30020*	Drainage abscess or hematoma, nasal septum	478.1 Nasal and sinus disease NEC 738.0 Acquired nose deformity 802.0 Nasal bone Fx, closed 802.1 Nasal bone Fx, open 920 Contusion face/scalp/neck 959.0 Face and neck injury NOS

CPT NOTES

- For lateral rhinotomy, see specific application (e.g., 30118, 30320).

REIMBURSEMENT INFORMATION

General

- Starred procedure.

Medicare

- Follow–up Days — 10
- Assistant Surgeon — not paid
- Supply Charges — not allowed
- Outpatient Limit — does not apply
- Minor Surgery Rules Apply

CPT CODE SERVICE	ICD–9–CM
30100 Biopsy, intranasal **CPT NOTES** ♦ For biopsy skin of nose, see 11100, 11101.	160.0 M-Neoplasm, Nasal cavities 160.2 M-Neoplasm, Maxillary sinus 160.3 M-Neoplasm, Ethmoidal sinus 160.4 M-Neoplasm, Frontal sinus 160.5 M-Neoplasm, Sphenoidal sinus 212.0 B-Neoplasm, Nasal cavity/sinus 235.9 UB-Neoplasm, Respiratory system NOS 239.1 Respiratory system neoplasm NOS 471.0 Polyp of nasal cavity 471.8 Nasal sinus polyp NEC 478.1 Nasal and sinus disease NEC **REIMBURSEMENT INFORMATION** Medicare ♦ Follow–up Days — 0 ♦ Assistant Surgeon — not paid ♦ Supply Charges — not allowed ♦ Outpatient Limit — applies ♦ Minor Surgery Rules Apply
30110 Excision, nasal polyp(s), simple **CPT NOTES** ♦ Would normally be completed in an office setting.	471.0 Polyp of nasal cavity 471.8 Nasal sinus polyp NEC **REIMBURSEMENT INFORMATION** Medicare ♦ Follow–up Days — 10 ♦ Assistant Surgeon — not paid ♦ Supply Charges — not allowed ♦ Outpatient Limit — applies ♦ Minor Surgery Rules Apply
30115 Excision, nasal polyp(s), extensive **CPT NOTES** ♦ Would normally require the facilities available in a hospital setting.	471.0 Polyp of nasal cavity 471.8 Nasal sinus polyp NEC 471.9 Nasal polyp NOS 478.1 Nasal and sinus disease NEC **REIMBURSEMENT INFORMATION** Medicare ♦ Follow–up Days — 90 ♦ Assistant Surgeon — not paid ♦ Supply Charges — not allowed ♦ Outpatient Limit — does not apply ♦ Major Surgery Rules Apply

CPT CODE **SERVICE** | **ICD–9–CM**

30117 Excision or destruction, any method (including laser), intranasal lesion; internal approach

160.0 M-Neoplasm, Nasal cavities
210.7 B-Neoplasm, Nasopharynx
212.0 B-Neoplasm, Nasal cavity/sinus
478.1 Nasal and sinus disease NEC

REIMBURSEMENT INFORMATION

Medicare

- Follow–up Days — 90
- Assistant Surgeon — not paid
- Supply Charges — not allowed
- Outpatient Limit — does not apply
- Major Surgery Rules Apply

30118 Excision or destruction, any method (including laser), intranasal lesion; external approach (lateral rhinotomy)

160.0 M-Neoplasm, Nasal cavities
210.7 B-Neoplasm, Nasopharynx
212.0 B-Neoplasm, Nasal cavity/sinus
478.1 Nasal and sinus disease NEC

REIMBURSEMENT INFORMATION

Medicare

- Follow–up Days — 90
- Assistant Surgeon — paid
- Supply Charges — not allowed
- Outpatient Limit — does not apply
- Major Surgery Rules Apply

30120 Excision or surgical planing of skin of nose for rhinophyma

695.3 Rosacea

REIMBURSEMENT INFORMATION

Medicare

- Follow–up Days — 90
- Assistant Surgeon — not paid
- Supply Charges — not allowed
- Outpatient Limit — does not apply
- Major Surgery Rules Apply

CPT CODE	SERVICE	ICD–9–CM
30124	Excision dermoid cyst, nose; simple, skin, subcutaneous	212.0 B-Neoplasm, Nasal cavity/sinus 528.4 Oral soft tissue cyst 709.8 Skin disorders NEC **REIMBURSEMENT INFORMATION** Medicare ♦ Follow–up Days — 90 ♦ Assistant Surgeon — not paid ♦ Supply Charges — not allowed ♦ Outpatient Limit — does not apply ♦ Major Surgery Rules Apply
30125	Excision dermoid cyst, nose; complex, under bone or cartilage	212.0 B-Neoplasm, Nasal cavity/sinus 528.4 Oral soft tissue cyst **REIMBURSEMENT INFORMATION** Medicare ♦ Follow–up Days — 90 ♦ Assistant Surgeon — paid ♦ Supply Charges — not allowed ♦ Outpatient Limit — does not apply ♦ Major Surgery Rules Apply
30130	Excision turbinate, partial or complete	170.0 M-Neoplasm, Skull/Face bone 213.0 B-Neoplasm, Skull/Face bone 375.56 Acquired nasolacrimal duct stenosis 470 Deviated nasal septum 473.0 Chronic maxillary sinusitis 473.1 Chronic frontal sinusitis 473.2 Chronic ethmoidal sinusitis 473.3 Chronic sphenoidal sinusitis 473.8 Chronic sinusitis NEC 477.0 Allergic rhinitis d/t pollen 477.8 Allergic rhinitis NEC 477.9 Allergic rhinitis NOS 478.0 Hypertrophy of nasal turbinates 478.1 Nasal and sinus disease NEC 738.0 Acquired nose deformity **REIMBURSEMENT INFORMATION** Medicare ♦ Follow–up Days — 90 ♦ Assistant Surgeon — not paid ♦ Supply Charges — not allowed ♦ Outpatient Limit — does not apply ♦ Major Surgery Rules Apply

CPT CODE SERVICE	ICD–9–CM

30140 Submucous resection turbinate, partial or complete

CPT NOTES

- For submucous resection of nasal septum, use 30520.
- For reduction of turbinates, use 30140 with modifier -52.

170.0 M-Neoplasm, Skull/Face bone
213.0 B-Neoplasm, Skull/Face bone
470 Deviated nasal septum
473.0 Chronic maxillary sinusitis
473.1 Chronic frontal sinusitis
473.2 Chronic ethmoidal sinusitis
473.3 Chronic sphenoidal sinusitis
473.8 Chronic sinusitis NEC
478.0 Hypertrophy of nasal turbinates
478.1 Nasal and sinus disease NEC
738.0 Acquired nose deformity

REIMBURSEMENT INFORMATION

Medicare

- Follow–up Days —90
- Assistant Surgeon — not paid
- Supply Charges — not allowed
- Outpatient Limit — does not apply
- Major Surgery Rules Apply

30150 Rhinectomy; partial

CPT NOTES

- For closure and/or reconstruction, primary or delayed, see Integumentary System, 13150–13152, 14060–14300, 15120, 15121, 15260, 15261, 15760, 20900–20912.

160.0 M-Neoplasm, Nasal cavities
195.0 M-Neoplasm, Head/face/neck

REIMBURSEMENT INFORMATION

Medicare

- Follow–up Days — 90
- Assistant Surgeon — paid
- Supply Charges — not allowed
- Outpatient Limit — does not apply
- Major Surgery Rules Apply

30160 Rhinectomy; total

CPT NOTES

- For closure and/or reconstruction, primary or delayed, see Integumentary System, 13150–13152, 14060–14300, 15120, 15121, 15260, 15261, 15760, 20900–20912.

160.0 M-Neoplasm, Nasal cavities
195.0 M-Neoplasm, Head/face/neck

REIMBURSEMENT INFORMATION

Medicare

- Follow–up Days — 90
- Assistant Surgeon — paid
- Supply Charges — not allowed
- Outpatient Limit — does not apply
- Major Surgery Rules Apply

CPT CODE	SERVICE	ICD-9-CM	
30200*	Injection into turbinate(s), therapeutic	461.0	Acute maxillary sinusitis
		461.1	Acute frontal sinusitis
		461.2	Acute ethmoidal sinusitis
		461.3	Acute sphenoidal sinusitis
		461.8	Other acute sinusitis
		470	Deviated nasal septum
		477.0	Allergic rhinitis d/t pollen
		477.8	Allergic rhinitis NEC
		477.9	Allergic rhinitis NOS
		478.0	Hypertrophy of nasal turbinates
		478.1	Nasal and sinus disease NEC
		784.0	Headache

REIMBURSEMENT INFORMATION

General

- Starred procedure.

Medicare

- Follow-up Days — 0
- Assistant Surgeon — not paid
- Supply Charges — not allowed
- Outpatient Limit — applies
- Minor Surgery Rules Apply

CPT CODE	SERVICE	ICD-9-CM	
30210*	Displacement therapy (Proetz type)	381.3	Chronic nonsuppurative otitis media
		381.4	Chron nonsup otitis media NOS
		381.81	Dysfunction of Eustachian tube
		460	Acute nasopharyngitis
		461.0	Acute maxillary sinusitis
		478.1	Nasal and sinus disease NEC

REIMBURSEMENT INFORMATION

General

- Starred procedure.

Medicare

- Follow-up Days — 10
- Assistant Surgeon — not paid
- Supply Charges — not allowed
- Outpatient Limit — applies
- Minor Surgery Rules Apply

CPT CODE	SERVICE	ICD-9-CM
30220	Insertion, nasal septal prosthesis (button)	470.1 Nasal and sinus disease NEC 748.1 Congenital nose anomaly NEC **REIMBURSEMENT INFORMATION** Medicare ♦ Follow-up Days — 10 ♦ Assistant Surgeon — not paid ♦ Supply Charges — not allowed ♦ Outpatient Limit — does not apply ♦ Minor Surgery Rules Apply
30300*	Removal foreign body, intranasal; office type procedure	932 Foreign body in nose **REIMBURSEMENT INFORMATION** General ♦ Starred procedure. Medicare ♦ Follow-up Days — 10 ♦ Assistant Surgeon — not paid ♦ Supply Charges — not allowed ♦ Outpatient Limit — does not apply ♦ Minor Surgery Rules Apply
30310	Removal foreign body, intranasal; requiring general anesthesia	932 Foreign body in nose **REIMBURSEMENT INFORMATION** Medicare ♦ Follow-up Days — 10 ♦ Assistant Surgeon — by report ♦ Supply Charges — not allowed ♦ Outpatient Limit — does not apply ♦ Minor Surgery Rules Apply
30320	Removal foreign body, intranasal; by lateral rhinotomy	932 Foreign body in nose **REIMBURSEMENT INFORMATION** Medicare ♦ Follow-up Days — 90 ♦ Assistant Surgeon — by report ♦ Supply Charges — not allowed ♦ Outpatient Limit — does not apply ♦ Major Surgery Rules Apply

CPT CODE	SERVICE	ICD–9–CM
30400	Rhinoplasty, primary; lateral and alar cartilages and/or elevation of nasal tip	470 Deviated nasal septum 478.1 Nasal and sinus disease NEC 738.0 Acquired nose deformity 748.1 Congenital nose anomaly NEC
30410	Rhinoplasty, primary; complete, external parts including bony pyramid, lateral and alar cartilages, and/or elevation of nasal tip	470 Deviated nasal septum 738.0 Acquired nose deformity 754.0 Congen skull/face/jaw deformity
30420	Rhinoplasty, primary; including major septal repair	195.0 M-Neoplasm, Head/face/neck 470 Deviated nasal septum 478.1 Nasal and sinus disease NEC 738.0 Acquired nose deformity 748.1 Congenital nose anomaly NEC 754.0 Congen skull/face/jaw deformity 802.0 Nasal bone Fx, closed 802.6 Fx orbital floor, closed 905.0 Late effect, skull/face fracture

30400

CPT NOTES

- For obtaining tissues for graft, see 20900-20926, 21210.
- For columellar reconstruction, see 13150, et seq.

REIMBURSEMENT INFORMATION

Medicare

- Follow–up Days — 90
- Assistant Surgeon — not paid
- Supply Charges — not allowed
- Outpatient Limit — does not apply
- Major Surgery Rules Apply

30410

CPT NOTES

- For obtaining tissues for graft, see 20900-20926, 21210.

REIMBURSEMENT INFORMATION

Medicare

- Follow–up Days — 90
- Assistant Surgeon — paid
- Supply Charges — not allowed
- Outpatient Limit — does not apply
- Major Surgery Rules Apply

30420

CPT NOTES

- For obtaining tissues for graft, see 20900-20926, 21210.

REIMBURSEMENT INFORMATION

Medicare

- Follow–up Days — 90
- Assistant Surgeon — not paid
- Supply Charges — not allowed
- Outpatient Limit — does not apply
- Major Surgery Rules Apply

CPT CODE	SERVICE	ICD–9–CM

30430 Rhinoplasty, secondary; minor revision (small amount of nasal tip work)

CPT NOTES

- For obtaining tissues for graft, see 20900-20926, 21210.

160.0	M-Neoplasm, Nasal cavities
212.0	B-Neoplasm, Nasal cavity/sinus
216.3	B-Neoplasm, Skin of face NEC
470	Deviated nasal septum
738.0	Acquired nose deformity
748.1	Congenital nose anomaly NEC

REIMBURSEMENT INFORMATION

Medicare

- Follow–up Days — 90
- Assistant Surgeon — paid
- Supply Charges — not allowed
- Outpatient Limit — does not apply
- Major Surgery Rules Apply

30435 Rhinoplasty, secondary; intermediate revision (bony work with osteotomies)

CPT NOTES

- For obtaining tissues for graft, see 20900-20926, 21210.

160.0	M-Neoplasm, Nasal cavities
212.0	B-Neoplasm, Nasal cavity/sinus
478.1	Nasal and sinus disease NEC
716.08	Kaschin-Beck disease NEC
738.0	Acquired nose deformity
905.0	Late effect, skull/face fracture

REIMBURSEMENT INFORMATION

Medicare

- Follow–up Days — 90
- Assistant Surgeon — paid
- Supply Charges — not allowed
- Outpatient Limit — does not apply
- Major Surgery Rules Apply

30450 Rhinoplasty, secondary; major revision (nasal tip work and osteotomies)

CPT NOTES

- For obtaining tissues for graft, see 20900-20926, 21210.

160.0	M-Neoplasm, Nasal cavities
173.3	M-Neoplasm, Skin of face NEC
212.0	B-Neoplasm, Nasal cavity/sinus
216.3	B-Neoplasm, Skin of face NEC
478.1	Nasal and sinus disease NEC
716.08	Kaschin-Beck disease NEC
905.0	Late effect, skull/face fracture

REIMBURSEMENT INFORMATION

Medicare

- Follow–up Days — 90
- Assistant Surgeon — paid
- Supply Charges — not allowed
- Outpatient Limit — does not apply
- Major Surgery Rules Apply

CPT CODE	SERVICE	ICD-9-CM
30460	Rhinoplasty for nasal deformity secondary to congenital cleft lip and/or palate, including columellar lengthening; tip only	748.1 Congenital nose anomaly NEC 749.00 Cleft palate NOS 749.01 Unilateral cleft palate, complete 749.02 Unilateral cleft palate, incomplete 749.03 Bilateral cleft palate, complete 749.04 Bilateral cleft palate, incomplete 749.10 Cleft lip NOS 749.11 Unilateral cleft lip, complete 749.12 Unilateral cleft lip, incomplete 749.13 Bilateral cleft lip, complete 749.14 Bilateral cleft lip, incomplete 749.21 Unilat cleft palate/lip, complete 749.22 Unilat cleft palate/lip, incomplete 749.23 Bilat cleft palate/lip, complete 749.24 Bilat cleft palate/lip, incomplete 749.25 Cleft palate w/cleft lip NEC

CPT NOTES

- For obtaining tissues for graft, see 20900-20926, 21210.

REIMBURSEMENT INFORMATION

Medicare

- Follow–up Days — 90
- Assistant Surgeon — paid
- Supply Charges — not allowed
- Outpatient Limit — does not apply
- Major Surgery Rules Apply

CPT CODE	SERVICE	ICD-9-CM
30462	Rhinoplasty for nasal deformity secondary to congenital cleft lip and/or palate, including columellar lengthening; tip, septum, osteotomies	748.1 Congenital nose anomaly NEC 749.00 Cleft palate NOS 749.01 Unilateral cleft palate, complete 749.02 Unilateral cleft palate, incomplete 749.03 Bilateral cleft palate, complete 749.04 Bilateral cleft palate, incomplete 749.10 Cleft lip NOS 749.11 Unilateral cleft lip, complete 749.12 Unilateral cleft lip, incomplete 749.13 Bilateral cleft lip, complete 749.14 Bilateral cleft lip, incomplete 749.21 Unilat cleft palate/lip, complete 749.22 Unilat cleft palate/lip, incomplete 749.23 Bilat cleft palate/lip, complete 749.24 Bilat cleft palate/lip, incomplete 749.25 Cleft palate w/cleft lip NEC

CPT NOTES

- For obtaining tissues for graft, see 20900-20926, 21210.

REIMBURSEMENT INFORMATION

Medicare

- Follow–up Days — 90
- Assistant Surgeon — paid
- Supply Charges — not allowed
- Outpatient Limit — does not apply
- Major Surgery Rules Apply

CPT CODE **SERVICE**

ICD–9–CM

30520 Septoplasty or submucous resection, with or without cartilage scoring, contouring or replacement with graft

CPT NOTES

- For obtaining tissues for graft, see 20900-20926, 21210.
- For submucous resection of turbinates, use 30140.

461.0	Acute maxillary sinusitis
461.8	Other acute sinusitis
470	Deviated nasal septum
473.0	Chronic maxillary sinusitis
473.2	Chronic ethmoidal sinusitis
473.8	Chronic sinusitis NEC
477.9	Allergic rhinitis NOS
478.0	Hypertrophy of nasal turbinates
478.1	Nasal and sinus disease NEC
738.0	Acquired nose deformity
748.1	Congenital nose anomaly NEC
754.0	Congen skull/face/jaw deformity
802.0	Nasal bone Fx, closed
802.1	Nasal bone Fx, open

REIMBURSEMENT INFORMATION

Medicare

- Follow–up Days — 90
- Assistant Surgeon — not paid
- Supply Charges — not allowed
- Outpatient Limit — does not apply
- Major Surgery Rules Apply

30540 Repair choanal atresia; intranasal

CPT NOTES

- For obtaining tissues for graft, see 20900-20926, 21210.

478.1	Nasal and sinus disease NEC
748.0	Congenital choanal atresia

REIMBURSEMENT INFORMATION

Medicare

- Follow–up Days — 90
- Assistant Surgeon — paid
- Supply Charges — not allowed
- Outpatient Limit — does not apply
- Major Surgery Rules Apply

30545 Repair choanal atresia; transpalatine

CPT NOTES

- For obtaining tissues for graft, see 20900-20926, 21210.

478.1	Nasal and sinus disease NEC
748.0	Congenital choanal atresia

REIMBURSEMENT INFORMATION

Medicare

- Follow–up Days — 90
- Assistant Surgeon — paid
- Supply Charges — not allowed
- Outpatient Limit — does not apply
- Major Surgery Rules Apply

CPT CODE **SERVICE**

30560* Lysis intranasal synechia

CPT NOTES

- For obtaining tissues for graft, see 20900-20926, 21210.

ICD–9–CM

461.0	Acute maxillary sinusitis
470	Deviated nasal septum
471.0	Polyp of nasal cavity
471.8	Nasal sinus polyp NEC
473.2	Chronic ethmoidal sinusitis
473.3	Chronic sphenoidal sinusitis
473.8	Chronic sinusitis NEC
478.1	Nasal and sinus disease NEC
519.8	Respiratory system disease NEC
784.7	Epistaxis
959.0	Face and neck injury NOS

REIMBURSEMENT INFORMATION

General

- Starred procedure.

Medicare

- Follow–up Days — 10
- Assistant Surgeon — not paid
- Supply Charges — not allowed
- Outpatient Limit — does not apply
- Minor Surgery Rules Apply

30580 Repair fistula; oromaxillary (combine with 31030 if antrotomy is included)

CPT NOTES

- For obtaining tissues for graft, see 20900-20926, 21210.

461.0	Acute maxillary sinusitis
473.0	Chronic maxillary sinusitis
522.7	Periapical abscess w/sinus
524.3	Tooth position anomaly
526.0	Developmental odontogenic cysts
526.4	Inflammation of jaw
526.5	Alveolitis of jaw
528.3	Cellulitis/abscess of mouth
959.0	Face and neck injury NOS

REIMBURSEMENT INFORMATION

Medicare

- Follow–up Days — 90
- Assistant Surgeon — not paid
- Supply Charges — not allowed
- Outpatient Limit — does not apply
- Major Surgery Rules Apply

CPT CODE **SERVICE**

30600 Repair fistula, oronasal

CPT NOTES

- For obtaining tissues for graft, see 20900-20926, 21210.

ICD–9–CM

473.0	Chronic maxillary sinusitis
524.3	Tooth position anomaly
526.0	Developmental odontogenic cysts
526.4	Inflammation of jaw
528.3	Cellulitis/abscess of mouth
749.00	Cleft palate NOS
749.01	Unilateral cleft palate, complete
749.02	Unilateral cleft palate, incomplete
749.03	Bilateral cleft palate, complete
749.04	Bilateral cleft palate, incomplete
749.2	Cleft palate w/cleft lip
959.0	Face and neck injury NOS

REIMBURSEMENT INFORMATION

<u>Medicare</u>

- Follow–up Days — 90
- Assistant Surgeon — not paid
- Supply Charges — not allowed
- Outpatient Limit — does not apply
- Major Surgery Rules Apply

30620 Septal or other intranasal dermatoplasty (does not include obtaining graft)

CPT NOTES

- For obtaining tissues for graft, see 20900-20926, 21210.

448.0	Heredit hemorrhagic telangiectasia
459.0	Hemorrhage NOS
459.89	Circulatory disease NEC
461.0	Acute maxillary sinusitis
470	Deviated nasal septum
471.0	Polyp of nasal cavity
471.8	Nasal sinus polyp NEC
473.8	Chronic sinusitis NEC
478.1	Nasal and sinus disease NEC
738.0	Acquired nose deformity
754.0	Congen skull/face/jaw deformity
784.7	Epistaxis
802.0	Nasal bone Fx, closed
802.1	Nasal bone Fx, open
959.0	Face and neck injury NOS

REIMBURSEMENT INFORMATION

<u>Medicare</u>

- Follow–up Days — 90
- Assistant Surgeon — not paid
- Supply Charges — not allowed
- Outpatient Limit — does not apply
- Major Surgery Rules Apply

CPT CODE **SERVICE**

30630 Repair nasal septal perforations

CPT NOTES

- For obtaining tissues for graft, see 20900-20926, 21210.

ICD–9–CM

470	Deviated nasal septum
478.1	Nasal and sinus disease NEC
748.1	Congenital nose anomaly NEC
802.1	Nasal bone Fx, open

REIMBURSEMENT INFORMATION

Medicare

- Follow–up Days — 90
- Assistant Surgeon — not paid
- Supply Charges — not allowed
- Outpatient Limit — does not apply
- Major Surgery Rules Apply

30801* Cauterization and/or ablation, mucosa of turbinates, unilateral or bilateral, any method, (separate procedure); superficial

473.2	Chronic ethmoidal sinusitis
473.8	Chronic sinusitis NEC
473.9	Chronic sinusitis NOS
477.0	Allergic rhinitis d/t pollen
477.8	Allergic rhinitis NEC
477.9	Allergic rhinitis NOS
478.0	Hypertrophy of nasal turbinates
478.1	Nasal and sinus disease NEC
519.8	Respiratory system disease NEC
784.0	Headache
784.7	Epistaxis

REIMBURSEMENT INFORMATION

General

- Starred procedures.
- Separate procedure rules apply.

Medicare

- Follow–up Days — 10
- Assistant Surgeon — not paid
- Supply Charges — not allowed
- Outpatient Limit — does not apply
- Minor Surgery Rules Apply

CPT CODE	SERVICE
30802*	Cauterization and/or ablation, mucosa of turbinates, unilateral or bilateral, any method, (separate procedure); intramural

ICD–9–CM

473.2	Chronic ethmoidal sinusitis
473.8	Chronic sinusitis NEC
473.9	Chronic sinusitis NOS
477.0	Allergic rhinitis d/t pollen
477.8	Allergic rhinitis NEC
477.9	Allergic rhinitis NOS
478.0	Hypertrophy of nasal turbinates
478.1	Nasal and sinus disease NEC
519.8	Respiratory system disease NEC
784.0	Headache
784.7	Epistaxis

REIMBURSEMENT INFORMATION

General

- ♦ Starred procedures.
- ♦ Separate procedure rules apply.

Medicare

- ♦ Follow–up Days — 10
- ♦ Assistant Surgeon — not paid
- ♦ Supply Charges — not allowed
- ♦ Outpatient Limit — does not apply
- ♦ Minor Surgery Rules Apply

CPT CODE	SERVICE
30901*	Control nasal hemorrhage, anterior, simple (limited cautery and/or packing) any method

160.0	M-Neoplasm, Nasal cavities
212.0	B-Neoplasm, Nasal cavity/sinus
401.9	Essential hypertension NOS
784.7	Epistaxis
932	Foreign body in nose
959.0	Face and neck injury NOS
998.1	Hemorrhage complicating a procedure

REIMBURSEMENT INFORMATION

General

- ♦ Starred procedures.

Medicare

- ♦ Follow–up Days — 0
- ♦ Assistant Surgeon — not paid
- ♦ Supply Charges — not allowed
- ♦ Outpatient Limit — applies
- ♦ Minor Surgery Rules Apply

CPT CODE	SERVICE	ICD–9–CM
30903*	Control nasal hemorrhage, anterior, complex (extensive cautery and/or packing) any method	160.0 M-Neoplasm, Nasal cavities 212.0 B-Neoplasm, Nasal cavity/sinus 375.56 Acquired nasolacrimal duct stenosis 784.7 Epistaxis 802.0 Nasal bone Fx, closed 959.0 Face and neck injury NOS 998.1 Hemorrhage complicating a procedure **REIMBURSEMENT INFORMATION** General ♦ Starred procedure Medicare ♦ Follow–up Days — 0 ♦ Assistant Surgeon — not paid ♦ Supply Charges — not allowed ♦ Outpatient Limit — does not apply ♦ Minor Surgery Rules Apply
30905*	Control nasal hemorrhage, posterior, with posterior nasal packs and/or cauterization, any method; initial	147.9 M-Neoplasm, Nasopharynx NOS 160.0 M-Neoplasm, Nasal cavities 210.7 B-Neoplasm, Nasopharynx 212.0 B-Neoplasm, Nasal cavity/sinus 478.1 Nasal and sinus disease NEC 784.7 Epistaxis 959.0 Face and neck injury NOS 998.1 Hemorrhage complicating a procedure **REIMBURSEMENT INFORMATION** General ♦ Starred procedure Medicare ♦ Follow–up Days — 0 ♦ Assistant Surgeon — not paid ♦ Supply Charges — not allowed ♦ Outpatient Limit — does not apply ♦ Minor Surgery Rules Apply

CPT CODE	SERVICE	ICD–9–CM

30906* Control nasal hemorrhage, posterior, with posterior nasal packs and/or cauterization, any method; subsequent

478.1 Nasal and sinus disease NEC
784.7 Epistaxis
959.0 Face and neck injury NOS
998.1 Hemorrhage complicating a procedure

REIMBURSEMENT INFORMATION

General

- Starred procedure

Medicare

- Follow–up Days — 0
- Assistant Surgeon — not paid
- Supply Charges — not allowed
- Outpatient Limit — does not apply
- Minor Surgery Rules Apply

30915 Ligation arteries; ethmoidal

CPT NOTES

- For ligation external carotid artery, see 37600.

170.0 M-Neoplasm, Skull/Face bone
195.0 M-Neoplasm, Head/face/neck
213.0 B-Neoplasm, Skull/Face bone
229.8 Benign neoplasm NEC
473.2 Chronic ethmoidal sinusitis
784.7 Epistaxis

REIMBURSEMENT INFORMATION

Medicare

- Follow–up Days — 90
- Assistant Surgeon — not paid
- Supply Charges — not allowed
- Outpatient Limit — does not apply
- Major Surgery Rules Apply

30920 Ligation arteries; internal maxillary artery, transantral

CPT NOTES

- For ligation external carotid artery, see 37600.

170.0 M-Neoplasm, Skull/Face bone
195.0 M-Neoplasm, Head/face/neck
213.0 B-Neoplasm, Skull/Face bone
229.8 Benign neoplasm NEC
784.7 Epistaxis

REIMBURSEMENT INFORMATION

Medicare

- Follow–up Days — 90
- Assistant Surgeon — not paid
- Supply Charges — not allowed
- Outpatient Limit — does not apply
- Major Surgery Rules Apply

CPT CODE	SERVICE	ICD–9–CM
30930	Fracture nasal turbinate(s), therapeutic	375.55 Neonatal nasolacrimal obstruction 471.0 Polyp of nasal cavity 472.0 Chronic rhinitis 473.3 Chronic sphenoidal sinusitis 473.8 Chronic sinusitis NEC 477.0 Allergic rhinitis d/t pollen 477.8 Allergic rhinitis NEC 477.9 Allergic rhinitis NOS 478.1 Nasal and sinus disease NEC 738.0 Acquired nose deformity 959.0 Face and neck injury NOS **REIMBURSEMENT INFORMATION** Medicare ♦ Follow–up Days — 10 ♦ Assistant Surgeon — not paid ♦ Supply Charges — not allowed ♦ Outpatient Limit — does not apply ♦ Minor Surgery Rules Apply
30999	Unlisted procedure, nose	231.8 CA in situ, Respiratory system NEC 461.0 Acute maxillary sinusitis 470 Deviated nasal septum 473.9 Chronic sinusitis NOS 474.10 Hypertrophy of tonsils/adenoids 478.0 Hypertrophy of nasal turbinates 478.1 Nasal and sinus disease NEC 738.0 Acquired nose deformity 784.7 Epistaxis 802.0 Nasal bone Fx, closed 932 Foreign body in nose 959.0 Face and neck injury NOS **REIMBURSEMENT INFORMATION** Medicare ♦ Follow–up Days — determined by local carrier ♦ Assistant Surgeon — determined by local carrier ♦ Supply Charges — determined by local carrier ♦ Outpatient Limit — determined by local carrier

CPT CODE	SERVICE	ICD–9–CM
31000*	Lavage by cannulation; maxillary sinus (antrum puncture or natural ostium)	461.0 Acute maxillary sinusitis 461.8 Other acute sinusitis 461.9 Acute sinusitis NOS 471.8 Nasal sinus polyp NEC 473.0 Chronic maxillary sinusitis 473.2 Chronic ethmoidal sinusitis 473.8 Chronic sinusitis NEC 473.9 Chronic sinusitis NOS

REIMBURSEMENT INFORMATION

General

- Starred procedure.

Medicare

- Follow–up Days — 10
- Assistant Surgeon — not paid
- Supply Charges — not allowed
- Outpatient Limit — applies
- Minor Surgery Rules Apply

CPT CODE	SERVICE	ICD–9–CM
31002*	Lavage by cannulation; sphenoid sinus	461.3 Acute sphenoidal sinusitis 473.3 Chronic sphenoidal sinusitis

REIMBURSEMENT INFORMATION

General

- Starred procedure.

Medicare

- Follow–up Days — 10
- Assistant Surgeon — by report
- Supply Charges — not allowed
- Outpatient Limit — does not apply
- Minor Surgery Rules Apply

CPT CODE	SERVICE	ICD–9–CM
31020	Sinusotomy, maxillary (antrotomy); intranasal	461.0 Acute maxillary sinusitis 461.8 Other acute sinusitis 473.0 Chronic maxillary sinusitis 473.8 Chronic sinusitis NEC 473.9 Chronic sinusitis NOS 754.0 Congen skull/face/jaw deformity 932 Foreign body in nose **REIMBURSEMENT INFORMATION** Medicare ♦ Follow–up Days — 90 ♦ Assistant Surgeon — not paid ♦ Supply Charges — not allowed ♦ Outpatient Limit — does not apply ♦ Major Surgery Rules Apply
31030	Sinusotomy, maxillary (antrotomy); radical (Caldwell-Luc) without removal of antrochoanal polyps	461.0 Acute maxillary sinusitis 461.8 Other acute sinusitis 473.0 Chronic maxillary sinusitis 473.8 Chronic sinusitis NEC 478.1 Nasal and sinus disease NEC 754.0 Congen skull/face/jaw deformity 802.6 Fx orbital floor, closed 802.7 Fx orbital floor, open **REIMBURSEMENT INFORMATION** Medicare ♦ Follow–up Days — 90 ♦ Assistant Surgeon — not paid ♦ Supply Charges — not allowed ♦ Outpatient Limit — does not apply ♦ Major Surgery Rules Apply
31032	Sinusotomy, maxillary (antrotomy); radical (Caldwell-Luc) with removal of antrochoanal polyps	461.0 Acute maxillary sinusitis 471.0 Polyp of nasal cavity 471.8 Nasal sinus polyp NEC 473.0 Chronic maxillary sinusitis **REIMBURSEMENT INFORMATION** Medicare ♦ Follow–up Days — 90 ♦ Assistant Surgeon — not paid ♦ Supply Charges — not allowed ♦ Outpatient Limit — does not apply ♦ Major Surgery Rules Apply

CPT CODE	SERVICE	ICD–9–CM

31040 Pterygomaxillary fossa surgery, any approach

CPT NOTES

- For transantral ligation of internal maxillary artery, see 30920.

195.0 M-Neoplasm, Head/face/neck
784.7 Epistaxis

REIMBURSEMENT INFORMATION

Medicare

- Follow–up Days — 90
- Assistant Surgeon — not paid
- Supply Charges — not allowed
- Outpatient Limit — does not apply
- Major Surgery Rules Apply

31050 Sinusotomy, sphenoid, with or without biopsy

160.5 M-Neoplasm, Sphenoidal sinus
170.0 M-Neoplasm, Skull/Face bone
194.3 M-Neoplasm, Pituitary gland
212.0 B-Neoplasm, Nasal cavity/sinus
227.3 B-Neoplasm, Pituitary gland
461.3 Acute sphenoidal sinusitis
461.8 Other acute sinusitis
473.3 Chronic sphenoidal sinusitis
473.8 Chronic sinusitis NEC
473.9 Chronic sinusitis NOS

REIMBURSEMENT INFORMATION

Medicare

- Follow–up Days — 90
- Assistant Surgeon — not paid
- Supply Charges — not allowed
- Outpatient Limit — does not apply
- Major Surgery Rules Apply

31051 Sinusotomy, sphenoid, with or without biopsy; with mucosal stripping or removal of polyp(s)

160.5 M-Neoplasm, Sphenoidal sinus
212.0 B-Neoplasm, Nasal cavity/sinus
461.3 Acute sphenoidal sinusitis
461.8 Other acute sinusitis
473.3 Chronic sphenoidal sinusitis
473.8 Chronic sinusitis NEC
473.9 Chronic sinusitis NOS

REIMBURSEMENT INFORMATION

Medicare

- Follow–up Days — 90
- Assistant Surgeon — not paid
- Supply Charges — not allowed
- Outpatient Limit — does not apply
- Major Surgery Rules Apply

CPT CODE	SERVICE	ICD-9-CM
31070	Sinusotomy frontal; external, simple (trephine operation)	461.1 Acute frontal sinusitis 461.8 Other acute sinusitis 473.1 Chronic frontal sinusitis 473.8 Chronic sinusitis NEC **REIMBURSEMENT INFORMATION** Medicare ♦ Follow-up Days — 90 ♦ Assistant Surgeon — not paid ♦ Supply Charges — not allowed ♦ Outpatient Limit — does not apply ♦ Major Surgery Rules Apply
31075	Sinusotomy frontal; transorbital, unilateral (for mucocele or osteoma, Lynch type)	461.1 Acute frontal sinusitis 461.8 Other acute sinusitis 473.1 Chronic frontal sinusitis 473.8 Chronic sinusitis NEC **REIMBURSEMENT INFORMATION** Medicare ♦ Follow-up Days — 90 ♦ Assistant Surgeon — paid ♦ Supply Charges — not allowed ♦ Outpatient Limit — does not apply ♦ Major Surgery Rules Apply
31080	Sinusotomy frontal; obliterative without osteoplastic flap, brow incision (includes ablation)	213.0 B-Neoplasm, Skull/Face bone 473.1 Chronic frontal sinusitis 802.0 Nasal bone Fx, closed 802.1 Nasal bone Fx, open 802.8 Fx facial bone NEC, closed 802.9 Fx facial bone NEC, open **REIMBURSEMENT INFORMATION** Medicare ♦ Follow-up Days — 90 ♦ Assistant Surgeon — paid ♦ Supply Charges — not allowed ♦ Outpatient Limit — does not apply ♦ Major Surgery Rules Apply

CPT CODE	SERVICE	ICD-9-CM

31081 Sinusotomy frontal; obliterative without osteoplastic flap, coronal incision (includes ablation)

213.0	B-Neoplasm, Skull/Face bone
473.1	Chronic frontal sinusitis
802.0	Nasal bone Fx, closed
802.1	Nasal bone Fx, open
802.8	Fx facial bone NEC, closed
802.9	Fx facial bone NEC, open

REIMBURSEMENT INFORMATION

Medicare

- Follow-up Days — 90
- Assistant Surgeon — paid
- Supply Charges — not allowed
- Outpatient Limit — does not apply
- Major Surgery Rules Apply

31084 Sinusotomy frontal; obliterative, with osteoplastic flap, brow incision

213.0	B-Neoplasm, Skull/Face bone
473.1	Chronic frontal sinusitis
738.0	Acquired nose deformity

REIMBURSEMENT INFORMATION

Medicare

- Follow-up Days — 90
- Assistant Surgeon — paid
- Supply Charges — not allowed
- Outpatient Limit — does not apply
- Major Surgery Rules Apply

31085 Sinusotomy frontal; obliterative, with osteoplastic flap, coronal incision

213.0	B-Neoplasm, Skull/Face bone
473.1	Chronic frontal sinusitis
738.0	Acquired nose deformity

REIMBURSEMENT INFORMATION

Medicare

- Follow-up Days — 90
- Assistant Surgeon — paid
- Supply Charges — not allowed
- Outpatient Limit — does not apply
- Major Surgery Rules Apply

CPT CODE	SERVICE	ICD–9–CM
31086	Sinusotomy frontal; nonobliterative, with osteoplastic flap, brow incision	473.1 Chronic frontal sinusitis 473.8 Chronic sinusitis NEC 473.9 Chronic sinusitis NOS **REIMBURSEMENT INFORMATION** Medicare ♦ Follow–up Days — 90 ♦ Assistant Surgeon — paid ♦ Supply Charges — not allowed ♦ Outpatient Limit — does not apply ♦ Major Surgery Rules Apply
31087	Sinusotomy frontal; nonobliterative, with osteoplastic flap, coronal incision	473.1 Chronic frontal sinusitis 473.8 Chronic sinusitis NEC 473.9 Chronic sinusitis NOS **REIMBURSEMENT INFORMATION** Medicare ♦ Follow–up Days — 90 ♦ Assistant Surgeon — paid ♦ Supply Charges — not allowed ♦ Outpatient Limit — does not apply ♦ Major Surgery Rules Apply

CPT CODE	SERVICE	ICD–9–CM
31090	Sinusotomy combined, three or more sinuses	160.2 M-Neoplasm, Maxillary sinus 160.3 M-Neoplasm, Ethmoidal sinus 160.4 M-Neoplasm, Frontal sinus 160.5 M-Neoplasm, Sphenoidal sinus 160.8 M-Neoplasm, Accessory sinuses NEC 160.9 M-Neoplasm, Accessory sinus NOS 212.0 B-Neoplasm, Nasal cavity/sinus 461.0 Acute maxillary sinusitis 461.1 Acute frontal sinusitis 461.2 Acute ethmoidal sinusitis 461.3 Acute sphenoidal sinusitis 461.8 Other acute sinusitis 461.9 Acute sinusitis NOS 473.0 Chronic maxillary sinusitis 473.1 Chronic frontal sinusitis 473.2 Chronic ethmoidal sinusitis 473.3 Chronic sphenoidal sinusitis 473.8 Chronic sinusitis NEC 473.9 Chronic sinusitis NOS **REIMBURSEMENT INFORMATION** <u>Medicare</u> ♦ Follow–up Days — 90 ♦ Assistant Surgeon — not paid ♦ Supply Charges — not allowed ♦ Outpatient Limit — does not apply ♦ Major Surgery Rules Apply
31200	Ethmoidectomy; intranasal, anterior	160.0 M-Neoplasm, Nasal cavities 160.2 M-Neoplasm, Maxillary sinus 160.3 M-Neoplasm, Ethmoidal sinus 160.4 M-Neoplasm, Frontal sinus 160.5 M-Neoplasm, Sphenoidal sinus 160.8 M-Neoplasm, Accessory sinuses NEC 160.9 M-Neoplasm, Accessory sinus NOS 212.0 B-Neoplasm, Nasal cavity/sinus 375.56 Acquired nasolacrimal duct stenosis 461.2 Acute ethmoidal sinusitis 461.8 Other acute sinusitis 471.1 Polypoid sinus degeneration 473.2 Chronic ethmoidal sinusitis 473.8 Chronic sinusitis NEC **REIMBURSEMENT INFORMATION** <u>Medicare</u> ♦ Follow–up Days — 90 ♦ Assistant Surgeon — not paid ♦ Supply Charges — not allowed ♦ Outpatient Limit — does not apply ♦ Major Surgery Rules Apply

CPT CODE	SERVICE	ICD-9-CM
31201	Ethmoidectomy; intranasal, total	160.0 M-Neoplasm, Nasal cavities 160.2 M-Neoplasm, Maxillary sinus 160.3 M-Neoplasm, Ethmoidal sinus 160.4 M-Neoplasm, Frontal sinus 160.5 M-Neoplasm, Sphenoidal sinus 160.8 M-Neoplasm, Accessory sinuses NEC 160.9 M-Neoplasm, Accessory sinus NOS 212.0 B-Neoplasm, Nasal cavity/sinus 461.2 Acute ethmoidal sinusitis 461.8 Other acute sinusitis 473.2 Chronic ethmoidal sinusitis 473.8 Chronic sinusitis NEC **REIMBURSEMENT INFORMATION** Medicare ♦ Follow–up Days — 90 ♦ Assistant Surgeon — not paid ♦ Supply Charges — not allowed ♦ Outpatient Limit — does not apply ♦ Major Surgery Rules Apply
31205	Ethmoidectomy; extranasal, total	160.0 M-Neoplasm, Nasal cavities 160.2 M-Neoplasm, Maxillary sinus 160.3 M-Neoplasm, Ethmoidal sinus 160.4 M-Neoplasm, Frontal sinus 160.5 M-Neoplasm, Sphenoidal sinus 160.8 M-Neoplasm, Accessory sinuses NEC 160.9 M-Neoplasm, Accessory sinus NOS 212.0 B-Neoplasm, Nasal cavity/sinus 375.56 Acquired nasolacrimal duct stenosis 461.2 Acute ethmoidal sinusitis 461.8 Other acute sinusitis 473.2 Chronic ethmoidal sinusitis 473.8 Chronic sinusitis NEC **REIMBURSEMENT INFORMATION** Medicare ♦ Follow–up Days — 90 ♦ Assistant Surgeon — paid ♦ Supply Charges — not allowed ♦ Outpatient Limit — does not apply ♦ Major Surgery Rules Apply

CPT CODE	SERVICE	ICD–9–CM
31225	Maxillectomy; without orbital exenteration	160.2 M-Neoplasm, Maxillary sinus 170.0 M-Neoplasm, Skull/Face bone 195.0 M-Neoplasm, Head/face/neck 200.81 Mixed lymphosarcoma, head/neck/face 235.1 UB-Neoplasm, Oral cavity/pharynx 238.0 UB-Neoplasm, Bone 239.2 Bone/Skin neoplasm NOS

CPT NOTES

- For orbital exenteration only, see 65110 et seq.
- For skin grafts, see 15120 et seq.

REIMBURSEMENT INFORMATION

Medicare

- Follow–up Days — 90
- Assistant Surgeon — paid
- Supply Charges — not allowed
- Outpatient Limit — does not apply
- Major Surgery Rules Apply

CPT CODE	SERVICE	ICD–9–CM
31230	Maxillectomy; with orbital exenteration (en bloc)	170.0 M-Neoplasm, Skull/Face bone 195.0 M-Neoplasm, Head/face/neck 200.81 Mixed lymphosarcoma, head/neck/face 235.1 UB-Neoplasm, Oral cavity/pharynx 238.0 UB-Neoplasm, Bone 239.2 Bone/Skin neoplasm NOS

CPT NOTES

- For orbital exenteration only, see 65110 et seq.
- For skin grafts, see 15120 et seq.

REIMBURSEMENT INFORMATION

Medicare

- Follow–up Days — 90
- Assistant Surgeon — paid
- Supply Charges — not allowed
- Outpatient Limit — does not apply
- Major Surgery Rules Apply

CPT CODE **SERVICE**

31231 Nasal endoscopy, diagnostic, unilateral or bilateral (separate procedure)

CPT NOTES

- A surgical sinus endoscopy always includes a sinusotomy and diagnostic endoscopy.
- Codes 31231–31294 are used to report unilateral procedures unless otherwise specified.
- The codes 31231–31235 for diagnostic evaluation refer to employing a nasal/sinus endoscope to inspect the interior of the nasal cavity and the middle and superior meatus, the turbinates, and the spheno–ethmoid recess. Any time a diagnostic evaluation is performed all these areas would be inspected and a separate code is not reported for each area.

ICD–9–CM

160.0	M-Neoplasm, Nasal cavities
212.0	B-Neoplasm, Nasal cavity/sinus
229.8	Benign neoplasm NEC
231.8	CA in situ, Respiratory system NEC
375.56	Acquired nasolacrimal duct stenosis
381.81	Dysfunction of Eustachian tube
461.0	Acute maxillary sinusitis
461.1	Acute frontal sinusitis
461.2	Acute ethmoidal sinusitis
461.3	Acute sphenoidal sinusitis
461.8	Other acute sinusitis
461.9	Acute sinusitis NOS
470	Deviated nasal septum
471.0	Polyp of nasal cavity
471.1	Polypoid sinus degeneration
471.8	Nasal sinus polyp NEC
472.0	Chronic rhinitis
472.1	Chronic pharyngitis
472.2	Chronic nasopharyngitis
473.0	Chronic maxillary sinusitis
473.1	Chronic frontal sinusitis
473.2	Chronic ethmoidal sinusitis
473.3	Chronic sphenoidal sinusitis
473.8	Chronic sinusitis NEC
473.9	Chronic sinusitis NOS
477.0	Allergic rhinitis d/t pollen
478.0	Hypertrophy of nasal turbinates
478.1	Nasal and sinus disease NEC
738.0	Acquired nose deformity
748.1	Congenital nose anomaly NEC
781.1	Smell/taste sensation disturbance
784.7	Epistaxis
932	Foreign body in nose
941.05	Burn NOS, nose

REIMBURSEMENT INFORMATION

General

- Separate procedure rules apply.

Medicare

- Follow–up Days — 0
- Assistant Surgeon — not paid
- Supply Charges — not allowed
- Outpatient Limit — does not apply
- Minor Surgery Rules Apply

CPT CODE **SERVICE**

31233 Nasal/sinus endoscopy, diagnostic with maxillary sinusoscopy (via inferior meatus or canine fossa puncture)

CPT NOTES

- A surgical sinus endoscopy always includes a sinusotomy and diagnostic endoscopy.
- Codes 31231–31294 are used to report unilateral procedures unless otherwise specified.
- The codes 31231–31235 for diagnostic evaluation refer to employing a nasal/sinus endoscope to inspect the interior of the nasal cavity and the middle and superior meatus, the turbinates, and the spheno–ethmoid recess. Any time a diagnostic evaluation is performed all these areas would be inspected and a separate code is not reported for each area.

ICD–9–CM

160.0	M-Neoplasm, Nasal cavities
212.0	B-Neoplasm, Nasal cavity/sinus
229.8	Benign neoplasm NEC
231.8	CA in situ, Respiratory system NEC
375.56	Acquired nasolacrimal duct stenosis
381.81	Dysfunction of Eustachian tube
461.0	Acute maxillary sinusitis
461.1	Acute frontal sinusitis
461.2	Acute ethmoidal sinusitis
461.3	Acute sphenoidal sinusitis
461.8	Other acute sinusitis
461.9	Acute sinusitis NOS
470	Deviated nasal septum
471.0	Polyp of nasal cavity
471.1	Polypoid sinus degeneration
471.8	Nasal sinus polyp NEC
472.0	Chronic rhinitis
472.1	Chronic pharyngitis
472.2	Chronic nasopharyngitis
473.0	Chronic maxillary sinusitis
473.1	Chronic frontal sinusitis
473.2	Chronic ethmoidal sinusitis
473.3	Chronic sphenoidal sinusitis
473.8	Chronic sinusitis NEC
473.9	Chronic sinusitis NOS
477.0	Allergic rhinitis d/t pollen
478.0	Hypertrophy of nasal turbinates
478.1	Nasal and sinus disease NEC
738.0	Acquired nose deformity
748.1	Congenital nose anomaly NEC
781.1	Smell/taste sensation disturbance
784.7	Epistaxis
941.05	Burn NOS, nose

REIMBURSEMENT INFORMATION

Medicare

- Follow–up Days — 0
- Assistant Surgeon — not paid
- Supply Charges — not allowed
- Outpatient Limit — does not apply
- Minor Surgery Rules Apply

CPT CODE **SERVICE**

31235 Nasal/sinus endoscopy, diagnostic with sphenoid sinusoscopy (via puncture of sphenoidal face or cannulation of osteum)

CPT NOTES

- A surgical sinus endoscopy always includes a sinusotomy and diagnostic endoscopy.
- Codes 31231–31294 are used to report unilateral procedures unless otherwise specified.
- The codes 31231–31235 for diagnostic evaluation refer to employing a nasal/sinus endoscope to inspect the interior of the nasal cavity and the middle and superior meatus, the turbinates, and the spheno–ethmoid recess. Any time a diagnostic evaluation is performed all these areas would be inspected and a separate code is not reported for each area.

ICD–9–CM

160.0	M-Neoplasm, Nasal cavities
212.0	B-Neoplasm, Nasal cavity/sinus
229.8	Benign neoplasm NEC
231.8	CA in situ, Respiratory system NEC
375.56	Acquired nasolacrimal duct stenosis
381.81	Dysfunction of Eustachian tube
461.0	Acute maxillary sinusitis
461.1	Acute frontal sinusitis
461.2	Acute ethmoidal sinusitis
461.3	Acute sphenoidal sinusitis
461.8	Other acute sinusitis
461.9	Acute sinusitis NOS
470	Deviated nasal septum
471.0	Polyp of nasal cavity
471.1	Polypoid sinus degeneration
471.8	Nasal sinus polyp NEC
472.0	Chronic rhinitis
472.1	Chronic pharyngitis
472.2	Chronic nasopharyngitis
473.0	Chronic maxillary sinusitis
473.1	Chronic frontal sinusitis
473.2	Chronic ethmoidal sinusitis
473.3	Chronic sphenoidal sinusitis
473.8	Chronic sinusitis NEC
473.9	Chronic sinusitis NOS
477.0	Allergic rhinitis d/t pollen
478.0	Hypertrophy of nasal turbinates
478.1	Nasal and sinus disease NEC
738.0	Acquired nose deformity
748.1	Congenital nose anomaly NEC
781.1	Smell/taste sensation disturbance
784.7	Epistaxis
941.05	Burn NOS, nose

REIMBURSEMENT INFORMATION

Medicare

- Follow–up Days — 0
- Assistant Surgeon — not paid
- Supply Charges — not allowed
- Outpatient Limit — does not apply
- Minor Surgery Rules Apply

CPT CODE **SERVICE**

31237 Nasal/sinus endoscopy, surgical, with biopsy, polypectomy or debridement (separate procedure)

CPT NOTES

- A surgical sinus endoscopy always includes a sinusotomy and diagnostic endoscopy.
- Codes 31231–31294 are used to report unilateral procedures unless otherwise specified.

ICD–9–CM

471.0	Polyp of nasal cavity
471.1	Polypoid sinus degeneration
471.8	Nasal sinus polyp NEC
471.9	Nasal polyp NOS
478.1	Nasal and sinus disease NEC
932	Foreign body in nose

REIMBURSEMENT INFORMATION

General

- Separate procedure rules apply.

Medicare

- Follow–up Days — 0
- Assistant Surgeon — not paid
- Supply Charges — not allowed
- Outpatient Limit — does not apply
- Minor Surgery Rules Apply

31238 Nasal/sinus endoscopy, surgical; with control of epistaxis

CPT NOTES

- A surgical sinus endoscopy always includes a sinusotomy and diagnostic endoscopy.
- Codes 31231–31294 are used to report unilateral procedures unless otherwise specified.

160.0	M-Neoplasm, Nasal cavities
160.2	M-Neoplasm, Maxillary sinus
160.3	M-Neoplasm, Ethmoidal sinus
160.4	M-Neoplasm, Frontal sinus
160.5	M-Neoplasm, Sphenoidal sinus
160.8	M-Neoplasm, Accessory sinuses NEC
160.9	M-Neoplasm, Accessory sinus NOS
212.0	B-Neoplasm, Nasal cavity/sinus
471.0	Polyp of nasal cavity
471.1	Polypoid sinus degeneration
471.8	Nasal sinus polyp NEC
471.9	Nasal polyp NOS
478.1	Nasal and sinus disease NEC
784.7	Epistaxis

REIMBURSEMENT INFORMATION

Medicare

- Follow–up Days — 0
- Assistant Surgeon — by report
- Supply Charges — not allowed
- Outpatient Limit — does not apply
- Minor Surgery Rules Apply

CPT CODE	SERVICE	ICD–9–CM

31239 Nasal/sinus endoscopy, surgical; with dacryocystorhinostomy

CPT NOTES

- A surgical sinus endoscopy always includes a sinusotomy and diagnostic endoscopy.
- Codes 31231–31294 are used to report unilateral procedures unless otherwise specified.

ICD–9–CM

375.20	Epiphora NOS
375.21	Epiphora d/t excess lacrimation
375.22	Epiphora d/t insufficient drainage
375.56	Acquired nasolacrimal duct stenosis
471.0	Polyp of nasal cavity
471.1	Polypoid sinus degeneration
471.8	Nasal sinus polyp NEC
471.9	Nasal polyp NOS
478.1	Nasal and sinus disease NEC

REIMBURSEMENT INFORMATION

Medicare

- Follow–up Days — 0
- Assistant Surgeon — by report
- Supply Charges — not allowed
- Outpatient Limit — does not apply
- Minor Surgery Rules Apply

31240 Nasal/sinus endoscopy, surgical; with concha bullosa resection

CPT NOTES

- A surgical sinus endoscopy always includes a sinusotomy and diagnostic endoscopy.
- Codes 31231–31294 are used to report unilateral procedures unless otherwise specified.

471.0	Polyp of nasal cavity
471.1	Polypoid sinus degeneration
471.8	Nasal sinus polyp NEC
471.9	Nasal polyp NOS
473.0	Chronic maxillary sinusitis
473.2	Chronic ethmoidal sinusitis
478.1	Nasal and sinus disease NEC
784.0	Headache

REIMBURSEMENT INFORMATION

Medicare

- Follow–up Days — 0
- Assistant Surgeon — by report
- Supply Charges — not allowed
- Outpatient Limit — does not apply
- Minor Surgery Rules Apply

CPT CODE **SERVICE**

● **31254** Nasal/sinus endoscopy, surgical, with ethmoidectomy, partial (anterior)

CPT NOTES

- A surgical sinus endoscopy always includes a sinusotomy and diagnostic endoscopy.
- Codes 31231–31294 are used to report unilateral procedures unless otherwise specified.

ICD–9–CM

212.0	B-Neoplasm, Nasal cavity/sinus
229.8	Benign neoplasm NEC
375.56	Acquired nasolacrimal duct stenosis
461.0	Acute maxillary sinusitis
461.2	Acute ethmoidal sinusitis
461.8	Other acute sinusitis
461.9	Acute sinusitis NOS
471.0	Polyp of nasal cavity
471.1	Polypoid sinus degeneration
471.8	Nasal sinus polyp NEC
471.9	Nasal polyp NOS
473.0	Chronic maxillary sinusitis
473.2	Chronic ethmoidal sinusitis
473.8	Chronic sinusitis NEC
473.9	Chronic sinusitis NOS
478.1	Nasal and sinus disease NEC
519.8	Respiratory system disease NEC

REIMBURSEMENT INFORMATION

General

- New procedure, 1995 CPT.

Medicare

- Follow–up Days — 0
- Assistant Surgeon — not paid
- Supply Charges — not allowed
- Outpatient Limit — does not apply
- Minor Surgery Rules Apply

CPT CODE **SERVICE**

● **31255** Nasal/sinus endoscopy, surgical; with ethmoidectomy, total (anterior and posterior)

CPT NOTES

- A surgical sinus endoscopy always includes a sinusotomy and diagnostic endoscopy.
- Codes 31231–31294 are used to report unilateral procedures unless otherwise specified.

ICD–9–CM

212.0	B-Neoplasm, Nasal cavity/sinus
229.8	Benign neoplasm NEC
375.56	Acquired nasolacrimal duct stenosis
461.0	Acute maxillary sinusitis
461.2	Acute ethmoidal sinusitis
461.8	Other acute sinusitis
461.9	Acute sinusitis NOS
471.0	Polyp of nasal cavity
471.1	Polypoid sinus degeneration
471.8	Nasal sinus polyp NEC
471.9	Nasal polyp NOS
473.0	Chronic maxillary sinusitis
473.2	Chronic ethmoidal sinusitis
473.8	Chronic sinusitis NEC
473.9	Chronic sinusitis NOS
478.1	Nasal and sinus disease NEC
519.8	Respiratory system disease NEC

REIMBURSEMENT INFORMATION

General

- New procedure, 1995 CPT.

Medicare

- Follow–up Days — 0
- Assistant Surgeon — not paid
- Supply Charges — not allowed
- Outpatient Limit — does not apply

CPT CODE	SERVICE
● 31256	Nasal/sinus endoscopy, surgical with maxillary antrostomy

CPT NOTES

- A surgical sinus endoscopy always includes a sinusotomy and diagnostic endoscopy.
- Codes 31231–31294 are used to report unilateral procedures unless otherwise specified.

ICD–9–CM

212.0	D-Neoplasm, Nasal cavity/sinus
229.8	Benign neoplasm NEC
235.9	UB-Neoplasm, Respiratory system NOS
461.0	Acute maxillary sinusitis
461.1	Acute frontal sinusitis
461.8	Other acute sinusitis
461.9	Acute sinusitis NOS
471.0	Polyp of nasal cavity
471.1	Polypoid sinus degeneration
471.8	Nasal sinus polyp NEC
471.9	Nasal polyp NOS
473.0	Chronic maxillary sinusitis
473.2	Chronic ethmoidal sinusitis
473.8	Chronic sinusitis NEC
473.9	Chronic sinusitis NOS
478.1	Nasal and sinus disease NEC
519.8	Respiratory system disease NEC

REIMBURSEMENT INFORMATION

General

- New procedure, 1995 CPT.

Medicare

- Follow–up Days — 0
- Assistant Surgeon — not paid
- Supply Charges — not allowed
- Outpatient Limit — does not apply

CPT CODE	SERVICE	ICD–9–CM

● **31267** Nasal/sinus endoscopy, surgical; with removal of tissue from maxillary sinus

CPT NOTES

- A surgical sinus endoscopy always includes a sinusotomy and diagnostic endoscopy.
- Codes 31231–31294 are used to report unilateral procedures unless otherwise specified.

212.0	B-Neoplasm, Nasal cavity/sinus
229.8	Benign neoplasm NEC
235.9	UB-Neoplasm, Respiratory system NOS
461.0	Acute maxillary sinusitis
461.2	Acute ethmoidal sinusitis
461.8	Other acute sinusitis
461.9	Acute sinusitis NOS
471.0	Polyp of nasal cavity
471.1	Polypoid sinus degeneration
471.8	Nasal sinus polyp NEC
471.9	Nasal polyp NOS
473.0	Chronic maxillary sinusitis
473.2	Chronic ethmoidal sinusitis
473.8	Chronic sinusitis NEC
473.9	Chronic sinusitis NOS
478.1	Nasal and sinus disease NEC
519.8	Respiratory system disease NEC

REIMBURSEMENT INFORMATION

General

- New procedure, 1995 CPT.

Medicare

- Follow–up Days — 0
- Assistant Surgeon — not paid
- Supply Charges — not allowed
- Outpatient Limit — does not apply

● **31276** Nasal/sinus endoscopy, surgical with frontal sinus exploration, with or without removal of tissue from frontal sinus

CPT NOTES

- A surgical sinus endoscopy always includes a sinusotomy and diagnostic endoscopy.
- Codes 31231–31294 are used to report unilateral procedures unless otherwise specified.

212.0	B-Neoplasm, Nasal cavity/sinus
461.1	Acute frontal sinusitis
461.2	Acute ethmoidal sinusitis
461.8	Other acute sinusitis
471.8	Nasal sinus polyp NEC
471.9	Nasal polyp NOS
473.1	Chronic frontal sinusitis
473.2	Chronic ethmoidal sinusitis
473.8	Chronic sinusitis NEC
478.1	Nasal and sinus disease NEC

REIMBURSEMENT INFORMATION

General

- New procedure, 1995 CPT.

Medicare

- Follow–up Days — 0
- Assistant Surgeon — not paid
- Supply Charges — not allowed
- Outpatient Limit — does not apply

CPT CODE **SERVICE** | **ICD–9–CM**

31287 Nasal/sinus endoscopy, surgical, with sphenoidotomy

CPT NOTES

- A surgical sinus endoscopy always includes a sinusotomy and diagnostic endoscopy.
- Codes 31231–31294 are used to report unilateral procedures unless otherwise specified.

160.0	M-Neoplasm, Nasal cavities
160.2	M-Neoplasm, Maxillary sinus
160.3	M-Neoplasm, Ethmoidal sinus
160.4	M-Neoplasm, Frontal sinus
160.5	M-Neoplasm, Sphenoidal sinus
160.8	M-Neoplasm, Accessory sinuses NEC
160.9	M-Neoplasm, Accessory sinus NOS
194.3	M-Neoplasm, Pituitary gland
212.0	B-Neoplasm, Nasal cavity/sinus
227.3	B-Neoplasm, Pituitary gland
461.3	Acute sphenoidal sinusitis
461.8	Other acute sinusitis
470	Deviated nasal septum
473.3	Chronic sphenoidal sinusitis
473.8	Chronic sinusitis NEC

REIMBURSEMENT INFORMATION

Medicare

- Follow–up Days — 0
- Assistant Surgeon — not paid
- Supply Charges — not allowed
- Outpatient Limit — does not apply
- Minor Surgery Rules Apply

31288 Nasal/sinus endoscopy, surgical, with sphenoidotomy; with removal of tissue from the sphenoid sinus

CPT NOTES

- A surgical sinus endoscopy always includes a sinusotomy and diagnostic endoscopy.
- Codes 31231–31294 are used to report unilateral procedures unless otherwise specified.

160.0	M-Neoplasm, Nasal cavities
160.2	M-Neoplasm, Maxillary sinus
160.3	M-Neoplasm, Ethmoidal sinus
160.4	M-Neoplasm, Frontal sinus
160.5	M-Neoplasm, Sphenoidal sinus
160.8	M-Neoplasm, Accessory sinuses NEC
160.9	M-Neoplasm, Accessory sinus NOS
194.3	M-Neoplasm, Pituitary gland
212.0	B-Neoplasm, Nasal cavity/sinus
227.3	B-Neoplasm, Pituitary gland
461.3	Acute sphenoidal sinusitis
461.8	Other acute sinusitis
470	Deviated nasal septum
473.3	Chronic sphenoidal sinusitis
473.8	Chronic sinusitis NEC

REIMBURSEMENT INFORMATION

Medicare

- Follow–up Days — 0
- Assistant Surgeon — not paid
- Supply Charges — not allowed
- Outpatient Limit — does not apply
- Minor Surgery Rules Apply

CPT CODE	SERVICE	ICD–9–CM

31290 Nasal/sinus endoscopy, surgical, with repair of cerebrospinal fluid leak; ethmoid region

CPT NOTES

- A surgical sinus endoscopy always includes a sinusotomy and diagnostic endoscopy.
- Codes 31231–31294 are used to report unilateral procedures unless otherwise specified.

349.81 Cerebrospinal fluid rhinorrhea

REIMBURSEMENT INFORMATION

Medicare

- Follow–up Days — 10
- Assistant Surgeon — by report
- Supply Charges — not allowed
- Outpatient Limit — does not apply
- Minor Surgery Rules Apply

31291 Nasal/sinus endoscopy, surgical, with repair of cerebrospinal fluid leak; sphenoid region

CPT NOTES

- A surgical sinus endoscopy always includes a sinusotomy and diagnostic endoscopy.
- Codes 31231–31294 are used to report unilateral procedures unless otherwise specified.

349.81 Cerebrospinal fluid rhinorrhea

REIMBURSEMENT INFORMATION

Medicare

- Follow–up Days — 10
- Assistant Surgeon — by report
- Supply Charges — not allowed
- Outpatient Limit — does not apply
- Minor Surgery Rules Apply

31292 Nasal/sinus endoscopy, surgical; with medial or inferior orbital wall decompression

CPT NOTES

- A surgical sinus endoscopy always includes a sinusotomy and diagnostic endoscopy.
- Codes 31231–31294 are used to report unilateral procedures unless otherwise specified.

376.01 Orbital cellulitis
376.33 Orbital edema
461.2 Acute ethmoidal sinusitis
473.2 Chronic ethmoidal sinusitis
921.9 Contusion of eye NOS

REIMBURSEMENT INFORMATION

Medicare

- Follow–up Days — 10
- Assistant Surgeon — by report
- Supply Charges — not allowed
- Outpatient Limit — does not apply
- Minor Surgery Rules Apply

CPT CODE	SERVICE	ICD-9-CM
31293	Nasal/sinus endoscopy, surgical; with medial orbital wall and inferior orbital wall decompression	

376.01 Orbital cellulitis
376.33 Orbital edema
461.2 Acute ethmoidal sinusitis
473.2 Chronic ethmoidal sinusitis
921.9 Contusion of eye NOS

CPT NOTES

- A surgical sinus endoscopy always includes a sinusotomy and diagnostic endoscopy.
- Codes 31231–31294 are used to report unilateral procedures unless otherwise specified.

REIMBURSEMENT INFORMATION

Medicare

- Follow–up Days — 10
- Assistant Surgeon — by report
- Supply Charges — not allowed
- Outpatient Limit — does not apply
- Minor Surgery Rules Apply

31294 Nasal/sinus endoscopy, surgical; with optic nerve decompression

377.49 Optic nerve disorder NEC
461.2 Acute ethmoidal sinusitis
473.2 Chronic ethmoidal sinusitis
950.0 Optic nerve injury

CPT NOTES

- A surgical sinus endoscopy always includes a sinusotomy and diagnostic endoscopy.
- Codes 31231–31294 are used to report unilateral procedures unless otherwise specified.

REIMBURSEMENT INFORMATION

Medicare

- Follow–up Days — 10
- Assistant Surgeon — by report
- Supply Charges — not allowed
- Outpatient Limit — does not apply
- Minor Surgery Rules Apply

CPT CODE	SERVICE	ICD–9–CM
31299	Unlisted procedure, accessory sinuses **CPT NOTES** ♦ For hypophysectomy, transantral or transeptal approach, see 61548. ♦ For transcranial hypophysectomy, see 61546.	375.56 Acquired nasolacrimal duct stenosis 461.0 Acute maxillary sinusitis 461.1 Acute frontal sinusitis 461.8 Other acute sinusitis 461.9 Acute sinusitis NOS 471.8 Nasal sinus polyp NEC 471.9 Nasal polyp NOS 473.0 Chronic maxillary sinusitis 473.2 Chronic ethmoidal sinusitis 473.8 Chronic sinusitis NEC 478.0 Hypertrophy of nasal turbinates 478.1 Nasal and sinus disease NEC 519.8 Respiratory system disease NEC 738.0 Acquired nose deformity 784.0 Headache **REIMBURSEMENT INFORMATION** Medicare ♦ Follow–up Days — determined by local carrier ♦ Assistant Surgeon — determined by local carrier ♦ Supply Charges — determined by local carrier ♦ Outpatient Limit — determined by local carrier
31300	Laryngotomy (thyrotomy, laryngofissure); with removal of tumor or laryngocele, cordectomy	161.0 M-Neoplasm, Glottis 161.1 M-Neoplasm, Supraglottis 161.2 M-Neoplasm, Subglottis 161.3 M-Neoplasm, Laryngeal cartilages 161.8 M-Neoplasm, Larynx NEC 161.9 M-Neoplasm, Larynx NOS 212.1 B-Neoplasm, Larynx 784.49 Voice disturbance NEC **REIMBURSEMENT INFORMATION** Medicare ♦ Follow–up Days — 90 ♦ Assistant Surgeon — paid ♦ Supply Charges — not allowed ♦ Outpatient Limit — does not apply ♦ Major Surgery Rules Apply

CPT CODE	SERVICE	ICD-9-CM
31320	Laryngotomy (thyrotomy, laryngofissure); diagnostic	161.0 M-Neoplasm, Glottis 161.1 M-Neoplasm, Supraglottis 161.2 M-Neoplasm, Subglottis 161.3 M-Neoplasm, Laryngeal cartilages 161.8 M-Neoplasm, Larynx NEC 161.9 M-Neoplasm, Larynx NOS 212.1 B-Neoplasm, Larynx 496 Chronic airway obstruction NEC 519.8 Respiratory system disease NEC 784.49 Voice disturbance NEC

REIMBURSEMENT INFORMATION

Medicare

- Follow–up Days — 90
- Assistant Surgeon — by report
- Supply Charges — not allowed
- Outpatient Limit — does not apply
- Major Surgery Rules Apply

CPT CODE	SERVICE	ICD-9-CM
31360	Laryngectomy; total, without radical neck dissection	146.8 M-Neoplasm, Oropharynx NEC 148.8 M-Neoplasm, Hypopharynx NEC 161.0 M-Neoplasm, Glottis 161.1 M-Neoplasm, Supraglottis 161.2 M-Neoplasm, Subglottis 161.3 M-Neoplasm, Laryngeal cartilages 161.8 M-Neoplasm, Larynx NEC 161.9 M-Neoplasm, Larynx NOS 195.0 M-Neoplasm, Head/face/neck 197.3 M2-Neoplasm, Respiratory NEC 730.18 Chronic osteomyelitis NEC

REIMBURSEMENT INFORMATION

Medicare

- Follow–up Days — 90
- Assistant Surgeon — paid
- Supply Charges — not allowed
- Outpatient Limit — does not apply
- Major Surgery Rules Apply

CPT CODE	SERVICE	ICD–9–CM
31365	Laryngectomy; total, with radical neck dissection	146.8 M-Neoplasm, Oropharynx NEC 148.8 M-Neoplasm, Hypopharynx NEC 161.0 M-Neoplasm, Glottis 161.1 M-Neoplasm, Supraglottis 161.2 M-Neoplasm, Subglottis 161.3 M-Neoplasm, Laryngeal cartilages 161.8 M-Neoplasm, Larynx NEC 161.9 M-Neoplasm, Larynx NOS 197.3 M2-Neoplasm, Respiratory NEC 231.0 CA in situ, Larynx **REIMBURSEMENT INFORMATION** Medicare ♦ Follow–up Days — 90 ♦ Assistant Surgeon — paid ♦ Supply Charges — not allowed ♦ Outpatient Limit — does not apply ♦ Major Surgery Rules Apply
31367	Laryngectomy; subtotal supraglottic, without radical neck dissection	161.1 M-Neoplasm, Supraglottis 161.8 M-Neoplasm, Larynx NEC 231.0 CA in situ, Larynx **REIMBURSEMENT INFORMATION** Medicare ♦ Follow–up Days — 90 ♦ Assistant Surgeon — paid ♦ Supply Charges — not allowed ♦ Outpatient Limit — does not apply ♦ Major Surgery Rules Apply
31368	Laryngectomy; subtotal supraglottic, with radical neck dissection	161.1 M-Neoplasm, Supraglottis 161.8 M-Neoplasm, Larynx NEC 197.3 M2-Neoplasm, Respiratory NEC 231.0 CA in situ, Larynx **REIMBURSEMENT INFORMATION** Medicare ♦ Follow–up Days — 90 ♦ Assistant Surgeon — paid ♦ Supply Charges — not allowed ♦ Outpatient Limit — does not apply ♦ Major Surgery Rules Apply

CPT CODE	SERVICE	ICD-9-CM
31370	Partial laryngectomy (hemilaryngectomy), horizontal	161.0 M-Neoplasm, Glottis 161.1 M-Neoplasm, Supraglottis 161.2 M-Neoplasm, Subglottis 161.3 M-Neoplasm, Laryngeal cartilages 161.8 M-Neoplasm, Larynx NEC 231.0 CA in situ, Larynx **REIMBURSEMENT INFORMATION** Medicare ♦ Follow–up Days — 90 ♦ Assistant Surgeon — paid ♦ Supply Charges — not allowed ♦ Outpatient Limit — does not apply ♦ Major Surgery Rules Apply
31375	Partial laryngectomy (hemilaryngectomy); laterovertical	161.0 M-Neoplasm, Glottis 161.1 M-Neoplasm, Supraglottis 161.2 M-Neoplasm, Subglottis 161.3 M-Neoplasm, Laryngeal cartilages 161.8 M-Neoplasm, Larynx NEC 231.0 CA in situ, Larynx **REIMBURSEMENT INFORMATION** Medicare ♦ Follow–up Days — 90 ♦ Assistant Surgeon — paid ♦ Supply Charges — not allowed ♦ Outpatient Limit — does not apply ♦ Major Surgery Rules Apply
31380	Partial laryngectomy (hemilaryngectomy); anterovertical	161.0 M-Neoplasm, Glottis 161.1 M-Neoplasm, Supraglottis 161.2 M-Neoplasm, Subglottis 161.3 M-Neoplasm, Laryngeal cartilages 161.8 M-Neoplasm, Larynx NEC 231.0 CA in situ, Larynx **REIMBURSEMENT INFORMATION** Medicare ♦ Follow–up Days — 90 ♦ Assistant Surgeon — paid ♦ Supply Charges — not allowed ♦ Outpatient Limit — does not apply ♦ Major Surgery Rules Apply

CPT CODE	SERVICE	ICD–9–CM
31382	Partial laryngectomy (hemilaryngectomy); antero-latero-vertical	161.0 M-Neoplasm, Glottis 161.1 M-Neoplasm, Supraglottis 161.2 M-Neoplasm, Subglottis 161.3 M-Neoplasm, Laryngeal cartilages 161.8 M-Neoplasm, Larynx NEC 231.0 CA in situ, Larynx **REIMBURSEMENT INFORMATION** Medicare ♦ Follow–up Days — 90 ♦ Assistant Surgeon — paid ♦ Supply Charges — not allowed ♦ Outpatient Limit — does not apply ♦ Major Surgery Rules Apply
31390	Pharyngolaryngectomy, with radical neck dissection; without reconstruction	148.8 M-Neoplasm, Hypopharynx NEC 161.0 M-Neoplasm, Glottis 161.1 M-Neoplasm, Supraglottis 161.2 M-Neoplasm, Subglottis 161.3 M-Neoplasm, Laryngeal cartilages 161.8 M-Neoplasm, Larynx NEC 231.0 CA in situ, Larynx **REIMBURSEMENT INFORMATION** Medicare ♦ Follow–up Days — 90 ♦ Assistant Surgeon — paid ♦ Supply Charges — not allowed ♦ Outpatient Limit — does not apply ♦ Major Surgery Rules Apply
31395	Pharyngolaryngectomy, with radical neck dissection; with reconstruction	148.8 M-Neoplasm, Hypopharynx NEC 161.0 M-Neoplasm, Glottis 161.1 M-Neoplasm, Supraglottis 161.2 M-Neoplasm, Subglottis 161.3 M-Neoplasm, Laryngeal cartilages 161.8 M-Neoplasm, Larynx NEC 231.0 CA in situ, Larynx **REIMBURSEMENT INFORMATION** Medicare ♦ Follow–up Days — 90 ♦ Assistant Surgeon — paid ♦ Supply Charges — not allowed ♦ Outpatient Limit — does not apply ♦ Major Surgery Rules Apply

CPT CODE	SERVICE	ICD–9–CM
31400	Arytenoidectomy or arytenoidopexy, external approach	478.30 Vocal cord/larynx paralysis NOS 478.74 Stenosis of larynx 478.79 Disease of larynx NEC 959.0 Face and neck injury NOS

CPT NOTES

- For endoscopic arytenoidectomy, see 31560.

REIMBURSEMENT INFORMATION

Medicare

- Follow–up Days — 90
- Assistant Surgeon — paid
- Supply Charges — not allowed
- Outpatient Limit — does not apply
- Major Surgery Rules Apply

CPT CODE	SERVICE	ICD–9–CM
31420	Epiglottidectomy	161.1 M-Neoplasm, Supraglottis 161.8 M-Neoplasm, Larynx NEC 212.1 B-Neoplasm, Larynx

REIMBURSEMENT INFORMATION

Medicare

- Follow–up Days — 90
- Assistant Surgeon — paid
- Supply Charges — not allowed
- Outpatient Limit — does not apply
- Major Surgery Rules Apply

CPT CODE	SERVICE	ICD-9-CM

31500 Intubation, endotracheal, emergency procedure

CPT NOTES

- For injection procedure for bronchography, see 31656, 31708, 31710.

ICD-9-CM

427.5 Cardiac arrest
478.6 Edema of larynx
482.1 Pseudomonal pneumonia
518.5 Post traum pulmonary insufficiency
518.81 Respiratory failure
518.82 Other pulmonary insufficiency
519.8 Respiratory system disease NEC
748.3 Congenital laryngotrach anomaly NEC
770.0 NB Congenital pneumonia
770.1 NB meconium aspiration syndrome
770.2 NB interstitial emphysema
770.6 NB transitory tachypnea
770.8 Post-birth resp problem NEC
770.9 NB respiratory condition NOS
799.1 Respiratory arrest

REIMBURSEMENT INFORMATION

Medicare

- Follow-up Days — 0
- Assistant Surgeon — not paid
- Supply Charges — not allowed
- Outpatient Limit — does not apply
- Minor Surgery Rules Apply

31502 Tracheotomy tube change prior to establishment of fistula tract

427.5 Cardiac arrest
478.6 Edema of larynx
482.1 Pseudomonal pneumonia
518.5 Post traum pulmonary insufficiency
518.81 Respiratory failure
518.82 Other pulmonary insufficiency
519.8 Respiratory system disease NEC
748.3 Congenital laryngotrach anomaly NEC
770.0 NB Congenital pneumonia
770.1 NB meconium aspiration syndrome
770.2 NB interstitial emphysema
770.6 NB transitory tachypnea
770.8 Post-birth resp problem NEC
770.9 NB respiratory condition NOS
799.1 Respiratory arrest

REIMBURSEMENT INFORMATION

Medicare

- Follow-up Days — 0
- Assistant Surgeon — not paid
- Supply Charges — not allowed
- Outpatient Limit — does not apply
- Minor Surgery Rules Apply

CPT CODE	SERVICE
31505	Laryngoscopy, indirect (separate procedure), diagnostic

CPT NOTES

- For endoscopic procedures, code appropriate endoscopy of each anatomic site examined.

ICD–9–CM

146.9	M-Neoplasm, Oropharynx NOS
148.9	M-Neoplasm, Hypopharynx NOS
161.9	M-Neoplasm, Larynx NOS
210.6	B-Neoplasm, Oropharynx NEC
210.9	B-Neoplasm, Pharynx NOS
212.1	B-Neoplasm, Larynx
235.1	UB-Neoplasm, Oral cavity/pharynx
235.6	UB-Neoplasm, Larynx
461.8	Other acute sinusitis
464.0	Acute laryngitis
464.10	Acute tracheitis, no obstruction
464.11	Acute tracheitis w/obstruction
464.20	Acute laryngotracheitis no obstruct
464.21	Acute laryngotracheitis w/obstruct
464.30	Acute epiglottitis, no obstruction
464.31	Acute epiglottitis w/obstruction
472.1	Chronic pharyngitis
472.2	Chronic nasopharyngitis
473.8	Chronic sinusitis NEC
474.0	Chronic tonsillitis
475	Peritonsillar abscess
476.0	Chronic laryngitis
476.1	Chronic laryngotracheitis
478.1	Nasal and sinus disease NEC
478.30	Vocal cord/larynx paralysis NOS
478.31	Vocal cord paralysis, unilat, part
478.32	Vocal cord paralysis, unilat, total
478.33	Vocal cord paralysis, bilat, part
478.34	Vocal cord paralysis, bilat, total
478.4	Polyp of vocal cord/larynx
478.5	Vocal cord disease NEC
478.6	Edema of larynx
478.70	Disease of larynx NOS
478.71	Laryngeal cellulitis
478.74	Stenosis of larynx
478.75	Laryngeal spasm
478.79	Disease of larynx NEC
519.0	Tracheostomy complication
530.6	Acquired esophageal diverticulum
784.1	Throat pain
784.4x	Voice disturbance
787.2	Dysphagia
933.0	Foreign body in pharynx
935.0	Foreign body in mouth
V10.02	Hx of oral/pharynx malignancy NEC

REIMBURSEMENT INFORMATION

General

- Separate procedure rules apply.

Medicare

- Follow–up Days — 0
- Assistant Surgeon — not paid
- Supply Charges — not allowed
- Outpatient Limit — applies
- Minor Surgery Rules Apply

CPT CODE **SERVICE**

31510 Laryngoscopy, indirect (separate procedure); with biopsy

CPT NOTES

- For endoscopic procedures, code appropriate endoscopy of each anatomic site examined.

ICD–9–CM

146.9	M-Neoplasm, Oropharynx NOS
148.9	M-Neoplasm, Hypopharynx NOS
161.9	M-Neoplasm, Larynx NOS
235.1	UB-Neoplasm, Oral cavity/pharynx
235.6	UB-Neoplasm, Larynx
461.8	Other acute sinusitis
464.0	Acute laryngitis
464.10	Acute tracheitis, no obstruction
464.11	Acute tracheitis w/obstruction
464.20	Acute laryngotracheitis no obstruct
464.21	Acute laryngotracheitis w/obstruct
464.30	Acute epiglottitis, no obstruction
464.31	Acute epiglottitis w/obstruction
472.1	Chronic pharyngitis
472.2	Chronic nasopharyngitis
473.8	Chronic sinusitis NEC
474.0	Chronic tonsillitis
475	Peritonsillar abscess
476.0	Chronic laryngitis
476.1	Chronic laryngotracheitis
478.1	Nasal and sinus disease NEC
478.3	Paralysis of vocal cords or larynx
478.4	Polyp of vocal cord/larynx
478.5	Vocal cord disease NEC
478.6	Edema of larynx
478.7	Disease of larynx NEC
530.6	Acquired esophageal diverticulum
784.1	Throat pain
784.49	Voice disturbance NEC
787.2	Dysphagia
V10.02	Hx of oral/pharynx malignancy NEC

REIMBURSEMENT INFORMATION

General

- Separate procedure rules apply.

Medicare

- Follow–up Days — 0
- Assistant Surgeon — not paid
- Supply Charges — not allowed
- Outpatient Limit — does not apply
- Minor Surgery Rules Apply

CPT CODE	SERVICE	ICD-9-CM

31511 Laryngoscopy, indirect (separate procedure), with removal of foreign body

CPT NOTES

- For endoscopic procedures, code appropriate endoscopy of each anatomic site examined.

519.8	Respiratory system disease NEC
787.2	Dysphagia
933.0	Foreign body in pharynx
933.1	Foreign body in larynx
935.0	Foreign body in mouth

REIMBURSEMENT INFORMATION

General

- Separate procedure rules apply.

Medicare

- Follow–up Days — 0
- Assistant Surgeon — not paid
- Supply Charges — not allowed
- Outpatient Limit — does not apply
- Minor Surgery Rules Apply

31512 Laryngoscopy, indirect (separate procedure); with removal of lesion

CPT NOTES

- For endoscopic procedures, code appropriate endoscopy of each anatomic site examined.

146.9	M-Neoplasm, Oropharynx NOS
148.9	M-Neoplasm, Hypopharynx NOS
161.9	M-Neoplasm, Larynx NOS
212.1	B-Neoplasm, Larynx
235.1	UB-Neoplasm, Oral cavity/pharynx
235.6	UB-Neoplasm, Larynx
748.3	Congenital laryngotrach anomaly NEC

REIMBURSEMENT INFORMATION

General

- Separate procedure rules apply.

Medicare

- Follow–up Days — 0
- Assistant Surgeon — not paid
- Supply Charges — not allowed
- Outpatient Limit — does not apply
- Minor Surgery Rules Apply

CPT CODE **SERVICE**

31513 Laryngoscopy, indirect (separate procedure); with vocal cord injection

CPT NOTES

- For endoscopic procedures, code appropriate endoscopy of each anatomic site examined.

ICD–9–CM

478.30	Vocal cord/larynx paralysis NOS
478.5	Vocal cord disease NEC
507.0	Food/vomit pneumonitis
784.49	Voice disturbance NEC
934.0	Foreign body, trachea

REIMBURSEMENT INFORMATION

General

- Separate procedure rules apply.

Medicare

- Follow–up Days — 0
- Assistant Surgeon — not paid
- Supply Charges — not allowed
- Outpatient Limit — does not apply
- Minor Surgery Rules Apply

31515 Laryngoscopy, direct, with or without tracheoscopy; for aspiration

CPT NOTES

- For endoscopic procedures, code appropriate endoscopy of each anatomic site examined.

466.0	Acute bronchitis
478.30	Vocal cord/larynx paralysis NOS
478.74	Stenosis of larynx
507.0	Food/vomit pneumonitis
518.81	Respiratory failure
787.2	Dysphagia
933.1	Foreign body in larynx
934.0	Foreign body, trachea

REIMBURSEMENT INFORMATION

Medicare

- Follow–up Days — 0
- Assistant Surgeon — not paid
- Supply Charges — not allowed
- Outpatient Limit — does not apply
- Minor Surgery Rules Apply

CPT CODE **SERVICE**

31520 Laryngoscopy, direct, with or without tracheoscopy; diagnostic, newborn

CPT NOTES

- For endoscopic procedures, code appropriate endoscopy of each anatomic site examined.

ICD–9–CM

478.30	Vocal cord/larynx paralysis NOS
478.74	Stenosis of larynx
748.2	Congenital laryngeal web anomaly
748.3	Congenital laryngotrach anomaly NEC
770.1	NB meconium aspiration syndrome
784.41	Aphonia
786.09	Respiratory abnormality NEC
786.1	Stridor
787.2	Dysphagia

REIMBURSEMENT INFORMATION

Medicare

- Follow–up Days — 0
- Assistant Surgeon — not paid
- Supply Charges — not allowed
- Outpatient Limit — does not apply
- Minor Surgery Rules Apply

CPT CODE **SERVICE**

31525 Laryngoscopy, direct, with or without tracheoscopy; diagnostic, except newborn

CPT NOTES

- For endoscopic procedures, code appropriate endoscopy of each anatomic site examined.

ICD–9–CM

141.1	M-Neoplasm, Tongue dorsal surface
146.9	M-Neoplasm, Oropharynx NOS
150.0	M-Neoplasm, Cervical esophagus
161.9	M-Neoplasm, Larynx NOS
195.0	M-Neoplasm, Head/face/neck
196.0	M-Neoplasm, Lymph head/neck/face
210.4	B-Neoplasm, Mouth NEC/NOS
210.6	B-Neoplasm, Oropharynx NEC
210.8	B-Neoplasm, Hypopharynx
212.1	B-Neoplasm, Larynx
229.8	Benign neoplasm NEC
235.1	UB-Neoplasm, Oral cavity/pharynx
464.0	Acute laryngitis
464.30	Acute epiglottitis, no obstruction
472.1	Chronic pharyngitis
478.20	Disease of pharynx NOS
478.21	Cellulitis of pharynx/nasopharynx
478.22	Parapharyngeal abscess
478.24	Retropharyngeal abscess
478.25	Edema of pharynx/nasopharynx
478.26	Cyst of pharynx/nasopharynx
478.29	Disease of pharynx NEC
478.30	Vocal cord/larynx paralysis NOS
478.31	Vocal cord paralysis, unilat, part
478.32	Vocal cord paralysis, unilat, total
478.33	Vocal cord paralysis, bilat, part
478.34	Vocal cord paralysis, bilat, total
478.4	Polyp of vocal cord/larynx
478.5	Vocal cord disease NEC
478.6	Edema of larynx
478.7x	Disease of larynx
519.8	Respiratory system disease NEC
528.7	Oral epithelium disturbance NEC
748.3	Congenital laryngotrach anomaly NEC
780.56	Sleep stage dysfunctions
784.2	Swelling in head/neck
784.4x	Voice disturbance
784.8	Hemorrhage from throat
786.1	Stridor
787.2	Dysphagia
933.0	Foreign body in pharynx
935.1	Foreign body in esophagus
947.2	Burn of Esophagus

REIMBURSEMENT INFORMATION

Medicare

- Follow–up Days — 0
- Assistant Surgeon — not paid
- Supply Charges — not allowed
- Outpatient Limit — does not apply
- Minor Surgery Rules Apply

CPT CODE	SERVICE
31526	Laryngoscopy, direct, with or without tracheoscopy; diagnostic, with operating microscope

CPT NOTES

- For endoscopic procedures, code appropriate endoscopy of each anatomic site examined.

ICD–9–CM

231.0	CA in situ, Larynx
235.1	UB-Neoplasm, Oral cavity/pharynx
464.0	Acute laryngitis
464.30	Acute epiglottitis, no obstruction
465.0	Acute laryngopharyngitis
472.1	Chronic pharyngitis
476.0	Chronic laryngitis
478.29	Disease of pharynx NEC
478.30	Vocal cord/larynx paralysis NOS
478.31	Vocal cord paralysis, unilat, part
478.32	Vocal cord paralysis, unilat, total
478.33	Vocal cord paralysis, bilat, part
478.34	Vocal cord paralysis, bilat, total
478.4	Polyp of vocal cord/larynx
478.5	Vocal cord disease NEC
478.6	Edema of larynx
478.79	Disease of larynx NEC
519.8	Respiratory system disease NEC
528.7	Oral epithelium disturbance NEC
530.6	Acquired esophageal diverticulum
784.40	Voice disturbance NOS
784.41	Aphonia
784.49	Voice disturbance NEC
784.8	Hemorrhage from throat
786.09	Respiratory abnormality NEC
786.1	Stridor
787.2	Dysphagia
933.0	Foreign body in pharynx
935.1	Foreign body in esophagus
947.2	Burn of Esophagus

REIMBURSEMENT INFORMATION

Medicare

- Follow–up Days — 0
- Assistant Surgeon — not paid
- Supply Charges — not allowed
- Outpatient Limit — does not apply
- Minor Surgery Rules Apply

CPT CODE / SERVICE	ICD–9–CM
31527 Laryngoscopy, direct, with or without tracheoscopy; with insertion of obturator **CPT NOTES** ♦ For endoscopic procedures, code appropriate endoscopy of each anatomic site examined.	478.74 Stenosis of larynx 519.0 Tracheostomy complication 784.40 Voice disturbance NOS 784.41 Aphonia 784.49 Voice disturbance NEC 786.09 Respiratory abnormality NEC 786.1 Stridor 959.0 Face and neck injury NOS **REIMBURSEMENT INFORMATION** Medicare ♦ Follow–up Days — 0 ♦ Assistant Surgeon — by report ♦ Supply Charges — not allowed ♦ Outpatient Limit — does not apply ♦ Minor Surgery Rules Apply
31528 Laryngoscopy, direct, with or without tracheoscopy; with dilatation, initial **CPT NOTES** ♦ For endoscopic procedures, code appropriate endoscopy of each anatomic site examined.	478.74 Stenosis of larynx **REIMBURSEMENT INFORMATION** Medicare ♦ Follow–up Days — 0 ♦ Assistant Surgeon — not paid ♦ Supply Charges — not allowed ♦ Outpatient Limit — does not apply ♦ Minor Surgery Rules Apply
31529 Laryngoscopy, direct, with or without tracheoscopy; with dilatation, subsequent **CPT NOTES** ♦ For endoscopic procedures, code appropriate endoscopy of each anatomic site examined.	478.74 Stenosis of larynx **REIMBURSEMENT INFORMATION** Medicare ♦ Follow–up Days — 0 ♦ Assistant Surgeon — by report ♦ Supply Charges — not allowed ♦ Outpatient Limit — does not apply ♦ Minor Surgery Rules Apply

CPT CODE	SERVICE	ICD-9-CM
31530	Laryngoscopy, direct, operative, with foreign body removal	787.2 Dysphagia 933.0 Foreign body in pharynx 933.1 Foreign body in larynx 935.1 Foreign body in esophagus

CPT NOTES

- For endoscopic procedures, code appropriate endoscopy of each anatomic site examined.

REIMBURSEMENT INFORMATION

Medicare

- Follow-up Days — 0
- Assistant Surgeon — not paid
- Supply Charges — not allowed
- Outpatient Limit — does not apply
- Minor Surgery Rules Apply

CPT CODE	SERVICE	ICD-9-CM
31531	Laryngoscopy, direct, operative, with foreign body removal; with operating microscope	787.2 Dysphagia 933.0 Foreign body in pharynx 933.1 Foreign body in larynx 935.1 Foreign body in esophagus

CPT NOTES

- For endoscopic procedures, code appropriate endoscopy of each anatomic site examined.

REIMBURSEMENT INFORMATION

Medicare

- Follow-up Days — 0
- Assistant Surgeon — not paid
- Supply Charges — not allowed
- Outpatient Limit — does not apply
- Minor Surgery Rules Apply

CPT CODE **SERVICE**

31535 Laryngoscopy, direct, operative, with biopsy

CPT NOTES

- For endoscopic procedures, code appropriate endoscopy of each anatomic site examined.

ICD–9–CM

141.0	M-Neoplasm, Tongue base
141.9	M-Neoplasm, Tongue NOS
145.3	M-Neoplasm, Soft palate
146.0	M-Neoplasm, Tonsil
148.9	M-Neoplasm, Hypopharynx NOS
149.0	M-Neoplasm, Pharynx NOS
161.0	M-Neoplasm, Glottis
161.1	M-Neoplasm, Supraglottis
161.8	M-Neoplasm, Larynx NEC
195.0	M-Neoplasm, Head/face/neck
196.0	M-Neoplasm, Lymph head/neck/face
210.4	B-Neoplasm, Mouth NEC/NOS
210.6	B-Neoplasm, Oropharynx NEC
210.8	B-Neoplasm, Hypopharynx
212.1	B-Neoplasm, Larynx
231.0	CA in situ, Larynx
235.1	UB-Neoplasm, Oral cavity/pharynx
235.6	UB-Neoplasm, Larynx
464.0	Acute laryngitis
476.0	Chronic laryngitis
478.29	Disease of pharynx NEC
478.4	Polyp of vocal cord/larynx
478.5	Vocal cord disease NEC
478.74	Stenosis of larynx
478.79	Disease of larynx NEC
784.1	Throat pain
784.2	Swelling in head/neck
784.49	Voice disturbance NEC
787.2	Dysphagia

REIMBURSEMENT INFORMATION

Medicare

- Follow–up Days — 0
- Assistant Surgeon — not paid
- Supply Charges — not allowed
- Outpatient Limit — does not apply
- Minor Surgery Rules Apply

CPT CODE **SERVICE**

31536 Laryngoscopy, direct, operative, with biopsy, with operating microscope

CPT NOTES

- For endoscopic procedures, code appropriate endoscopy of each anatomic site examined.

ICD–9–CM

141.0	M-Neoplasm, Tongue base
141.9	M-Neoplasm, Tongue NOS
146.0	M-Neoplasm, Tonsil
148.9	M-Neoplasm, Hypopharynx NOS
149.0	M-Neoplasm, Pharynx NOS
161.0	M-Neoplasm, Glottis
161.1	M-Neoplasm, Supraglottis
161.8	M-Neoplasm, Larynx NEC
195.0	M-Neoplasm, Head/face/neck
196.0	M-Neoplasm, Lymph head/neck/face
210.4	B-Neoplasm, Mouth NEC/NOS
210.6	B-Neoplasm, Oropharynx NEC
210.8	B-Neoplasm, Hypopharynx
212.1	B-Neoplasm, Larynx
231.0	CA in situ, Larynx
235.1	UB-Neoplasm, Oral cavity/pharynx
235.6	UB-Neoplasm, Larynx
464.0	Acute laryngitis
476.0	Chronic laryngitis
478.29	Disease of pharynx NEC
478.4	Polyp of vocal cord/larynx
478.5	Vocal cord disease NEC
478.74	Stenosis of larynx
478.79	Disease of larynx NEC
784.1	Throat pain
784.2	Swelling in head/neck
784.49	Voice disturbance NEC
787.2	Dysphagia

REIMBURSEMENT INFORMATION

Medicare

- Follow–up Days — 0
- Assistant Surgeon — not paid
- Supply Charges — not allowed
- Outpatient Limit — does not apply
- Minor Surgery Rules Apply
- Fragments — 31535

CPT CODE **SERVICE**

31540 Laryngoscopy, direct, operative, with excision of tumor and/or stripping of vocal cords or epiglottis

CPT NOTES

- For endoscopic procedures, code appropriate endoscopy of each anatomic site examined.

ICD–9–CM

141.0	M-Neoplasm, Tongue base
141.9	M-Neoplasm, Tongue NOS
146.0	M-Neoplasm, Tonsil
148.9	M-Neoplasm, Hypopharynx NOS
149.0	M-Neoplasm, Pharynx NOS
161.0	M-Neoplasm, Glottis
161.1	M-Neoplasm, Supraglottis
161.8	M-Neoplasm, Larynx NEC
195.0	M-Neoplasm, Head/face/neck
196.0	M-Neoplasm, Lymph head/neck/face
210.4	B-Neoplasm, Mouth NEC/NOS
210.6	B-Neoplasm, Oropharynx NEC
210.8	B-Neoplasm, Hypopharynx
210.9	B-Neoplasm, Pharynx NOS
212.1	B-Neoplasm, Larynx
231.0	CA in situ, Larynx
235.1	UB-Neoplasm, Oral cavity/pharynx
235.6	UB-Neoplasm, Larynx
476.0	Chronic laryngitis
478.4	Polyp of vocal cord/larynx
478.5	Vocal cord disease NEC
478.70	Disease of larynx NOS
519.8	Respiratory system disease NEC
528.6	Leukoplakia of oral mucosa/tongue
784.49	Voice disturbance NEC

REIMBURSEMENT INFORMATION

Medicare

- Follow–up Days — 0
- Assistant Surgeon — not paid
- Supply Charges — not allowed
- Outpatient Limit — does not apply
- Minor Surgery Rules Apply

CPT CODE **SERVICE**

31541 Laryngoscopy, direct, operative, with excision of tumor and/or stripping of vocal cords or epiglottis; with operating microscope

CPT NOTES

- For endoscopic procedures, code appropriate endoscopy of each anatomic site examined.

ICD–9–CM

141.0	M-Neoplasm, Tongue base
141.9	M-Neoplasm, Tongue NOS
146.0	M-Neoplasm, Tonsil
148.9	M-Neoplasm, Hypopharynx NOS
149.0	M-Neoplasm, Pharynx NOS
161.0	M-Neoplasm, Glottis
161.1	M-Neoplasm, Supraglottis
161.8	M-Neoplasm, Larynx NEC
195.0	M-Neoplasm, Head/face/neck
196.0	M-Neoplasm, Lymph head/neck/face
210.4	B-Neoplasm, Mouth NEC/NOS
210.6	B-Neoplasm, Oropharynx NEC
210.8	B-Neoplasm, Hypopharynx
210.9	B-Neoplasm, Pharynx NOS
212.1	B-Neoplasm, Larynx
231.0	CA in situ, Larynx
235.1	UB-Neoplasm, Oral cavity/pharynx
235.6	UB-Neoplasm, Larynx
476.0	Chronic laryngitis
478.4	Polyp of vocal cord/larynx
478.5	Vocal cord disease NEC
478.70	Disease of larynx NOS
519.8	Respiratory system disease NEC
528.6	Leukoplakia of oral mucosa/tongue
784.49	Voice disturbance NEC

REIMBURSEMENT INFORMATION

Medicare

- Follow–up Days — 0
- Assistant Surgeon — not paid
- Supply Charges — not allowed
- Outpatient Limit — does not apply
- Minor Surgery Rules Apply
- Fragments — 31525, 31540

CPT CODE **SERVICE**

31560 Laryngoscopy, direct, operative, with arytenoidectomy

CPT NOTES

- For endoscopic procedures, code appropriate endoscopy of each anatomic site examined.

ICD–9–CM

141.0	M-Neoplasm, Tongue base
141.9	M-Neoplasm, Tongue NOS
146.0	M-Neoplasm, Tonsil
148.9	M-Neoplasm, Hypopharynx NOS
149.0	M-Neoplasm, Pharynx NOS
161.0	M-Neoplasm, Glottis
161.1	M-Neoplasm, Supraglottis
161.8	M-Neoplasm, Larynx NEC
195.0	M-Neoplasm, Head/face/neck
196.0	M-Neoplasm, Lymph head/neck/face
210.4	B-Neoplasm, Mouth NEC/NOS
210.6	B-Neoplasm, Oropharynx NEC
210.8	B-Neoplasm, Hypopharynx
210.9	B-Neoplasm, Pharynx NOS
212.1	B-Neoplasm, Larynx
231.0	CA in situ, Larynx
235.1	UB-Neoplasm, Oral cavity/pharynx
235.6	UB-Neoplasm, Larynx
476.0	Chronic laryngitis
478.4	Polyp of vocal cord/larynx
478.5	Vocal cord disease NEC
478.70	Disease of larynx NOS
519.8	Respiratory system disease NEC
528.6	Leukoplakia of oral mucosa/tongue
784.49	Voice disturbance NEC

REIMBURSEMENT INFORMATION

Medicare

- Follow–up Days — 0
- Assistant Surgeon — by report
- Supply Charges — not allowed
- Outpatient Limit — does not apply
- Minor Surgery Rules Apply

CPT CODE	SERVICE
31561	Laryngoscopy, direct, operative, with arytenoidectomy; with operating microscope

CPT NOTES

- For endoscopic procedures, code appropriate endoscopy of each anatomic site examined.

ICD-9-CM

141.0	M-Neoplasm, Tongue base
141.9	M-Neoplasm, Tongue NOS
146.0	M-Neoplasm, Tonsil
148.9	M-Neoplasm, Hypopharynx NOS
149.0	M-Neoplasm, Pharynx NOS
161.0	M-Neoplasm, Glottis
161.1	M-Neoplasm, Supraglottis
161.8	M-Neoplasm, Larynx NEC
195.0	M-Neoplasm, Head/face/neck
196.0	M-Neoplasm, Lymph head/neck/face
210.4	B-Neoplasm, Mouth NEC/NOS
210.6	B-Neoplasm, Oropharynx NEC
210.8	B-Neoplasm, Hypopharynx
210.9	B-Neoplasm, Pharynx NOS
212.1	B-Neoplasm, Larynx
231.0	CA in situ, Larynx
235.1	UB-Neoplasm, Oral cavity/pharynx
235.6	UB-Neoplasm, Larynx
478.4	Polyp of vocal cord/larynx
478.5	Vocal cord disease NEC
478.70	Disease of larynx NOS
519.8	Respiratory system disease NEC
784.49	Voice disturbance NEC

REIMBURSEMENT INFORMATION

Medicare

- Follow–up Days — 0
- Assistant Surgeon — not paid
- Supply Charges — not allowed
- Outpatient Limit — does not apply
- Minor Surgery Rules Apply

CPT CODE	SERVICE
31570	Laryngoscopy, direct, with injection into vocal cord(s), therapeutic

CPT NOTES

- For endoscopic procedures, code appropriate endoscopy of each anatomic site examined.

ICD-9-CM

478.31	Vocal cord paralysis, unilat, part
478.33	Vocal cord paralysis, bilat, part
784.49	Voice disturbance NEC
786.1	Stridor

REIMBURSEMENT INFORMATION

Medicare

- Follow–up Days — 0
- Assistant Surgeon — not paid
- Supply Charges — not allowed
- Outpatient Limit — does not apply
- Minor Surgery Rules Apply

CPT CODE **SERVICE**

31571 Laryngoscopy, direct, with injection into vocal cord(s), therapeutic; with operating microscope

CPT NOTES

- For endoscopic procedures, code appropriate endoscopy of each anatomic site examined.

ICD–9–CM

478.31 Vocal cord paralysis, unilat, part
478.33 Vocal cord paralysis, bilat, part
784.49 Voice disturbance NEC
786.1 Stridor

REIMBURSEMENT INFORMATION

Medicare

- Follow–up Days — 0
- Assistant Surgeon — not paid
- Supply Charges — not allowed
- Outpatient Limit — does not apply
- Minor Surgery Rules Apply

CPT CODE	SERVICE
31575	Laryngoscopy, flexible fiberscopic; diagnostic

CPT NOTES

- For endoscopic procedures, code appropriate endoscopy of each anatomic site examined.

ICD–9–CM

141.1	M-Neoplasm, Tongue dorsal surface
146.9	M-Neoplasm, Oropharynx NOS
150.0	M-Neoplasm, Cervical esophagus
161.9	M-Neoplasm, Larynx NOS
195.0	M-Neoplasm, Head/face/neck
196.0	M-Neoplasm, Lymph head/neck/face
210.4	B-Neoplasm, Mouth NEC/NOS
210.6	B-Neoplasm, Oropharynx NEC
210.8	B-Neoplasm, Hypopharynx
212.1	B-Neoplasm, Larynx
229.8	Benign neoplasm NEC
235.1	UB-Neoplasm, Oral cavity/pharynx
464.0	Acute laryngitis
464.30	Acute epiglottitis, no obstruction
472.1	Chronic pharyngitis
478.20	Disease of pharynx NOS
478.21	Cellulitis of pharynx/nasopharynx
478.22	Parapharyngeal abscess
478.24	Retropharyngeal abscess
478.25	Edema of pharynx/nasopharynx
478.26	Cyst of pharynx/nasopharynx
478.29	Disease of pharynx NEC
478.30	Vocal cord/larynx paralysis NOS
478.31	Vocal cord paralysis, unilat, part
478.32	Vocal cord paralysis, unilat, total
478.33	Vocal cord paralysis, bilat, part
478.34	Vocal cord paralysis, bilat, total
478.4	Polyp of vocal cord/larynx
478.5	Vocal cord disease NEC
478.6	Edema of larynx
478.7x	Disease of larynx
519.8	Respiratory system disease NEC
528.7	Oral epithelium disturbance NEC
748.3	Congenital laryngotrach anomaly NEC
780.56	Sleep stage dysfunctions
784.2	Swelling in head/neck
784.4x	Voice disturbance
784.8	Hemorrhage from throat
786.1	Stridor
787.2	Dysphagia
933.0	Foreign body in pharynx
935.1	Foreign body in esophagus
947.2	Burn of Esophagus

REIMBURSEMENT INFORMATION

Medicare

- Follow–up Days — 0
- Assistant Surgeon — not paid
- Supply Charges — not allowed
- Outpatient Limit — applies
- Minor Surgery Rules Apply

CPT CODE / SERVICE	ICD–9–CM
31576 Laryngoscopy, flexible fiberscopic; with biopsy **CPT NOTES** ♦ For endoscopic procedures, code appropriate endoscopy of each anatomic site examined.	141.0 M-Neoplasm, Tongue base 141.9 M-Neoplasm, Tongue NOS 145.3 M-Neoplasm, Soft palate 146.0 M-Neoplasm, Tonsil 148.9 M-Neoplasm, Hypopharynx NOS 149.0 M-Neoplasm, Pharynx NOS 161.0 M-Neoplasm, Glottis 161.1 M-Neoplasm, Supraglottis 161.3 M-Neoplasm, Laryngeal cartilages 161.8 M-Neoplasm, Larynx NEC 195.0 M-Neoplasm, Head/face/neck 196.0 M-Neoplasm, Lymph head/neck/face 210.4 B-Neoplasm, Mouth NEC/NOS 210.6 B-Neoplasm, Oropharynx NEC 210.8 B-Neoplasm, Hypopharynx 212.1 B-Neoplasm, Larynx 231.0 CA in situ, Larynx 235.1 UB-Neoplasm, Oral cavity/pharynx 235.6 UB-Neoplasm, Larynx 464.0 Acute laryngitis 476.0 Chronic laryngitis 478.4 Polyp of vocal cord/larynx 478.5 Vocal cord disease NEC 478.74 Stenosis of larynx 478.79 Disease of larynx NEC 784.1 Throat pain 784.2 Swelling in head/neck 784.49 Voice disturbance NEC 787.2 Dysphagia **REIMBURSEMENT INFORMATION** Medicare ♦ Follow–up Days — 0 ♦ Assistant Surgeon — not paid ♦ Supply Charges — not allowed ♦ Outpatient Limit — does not apply ♦ Minor Surgery Rules Apply
31577 Laryngoscopy, flexible fiberscopic; with removal of foreign body **CPT NOTES** ♦ For endoscopic procedures, code appropriate endoscopy of each anatomic site examined.	519.8 Respiratory system disease NEC 787.2 Dysphagia 933.0 Foreign body in pharynx 933.1 Foreign body in larynx **REIMBURSEMENT INFORMATION** Medicare ♦ Follow–up Days — 0 ♦ Assistant Surgeon — not paid ♦ Supply Charges — not allowed ♦ Outpatient Limit — does not apply ♦ Minor Surgery Rules Apply

CPT CODE **SERVICE**

31578 Laryngoscopy, flexible fiberscopic; with removal of lesion

CPT NOTES

- For endoscopic procedures, code appropriate endoscopy of each anatomic site examined.

ICD–9–CM

141.0	M-Neoplasm, Tongue base
141.9	M-Neoplasm, Tongue NOS
145.3	M-Neoplasm, Soft palate
146.0	M-Neoplasm, Tonsil
148.9	M-Neoplasm, Hypopharynx NOS
149.0	M-Neoplasm, Pharynx NOS
161.0	M-Neoplasm, Glottis
161.1	M-Neoplasm, Supraglottis
161.8	M-Neoplasm, Larynx NEC
195.0	M-Neoplasm, Head/face/neck
196.0	M-Neoplasm, Lymph head/neck/face
210.6	B-Neoplasm, Oropharynx NEC
210.8	B-Neoplasm, Hypopharynx
212.1	B-Neoplasm, Larynx
231.0	CA in situ, Larynx
235.1	UB-Neoplasm, Oral cavity/pharynx
235.6	UB-Neoplasm, Larynx
464.0	Acute laryngitis
476.0	Chronic laryngitis
478.29	Disease of pharynx NEC
478.4	Polyp of vocal cord/larynx
478.5	Vocal cord disease NEC
478.74	Stenosis of larynx
478.79	Disease of larynx NEC
784.1	Throat pain
784.2	Swelling in head/neck
784.49	Voice disturbance NEC
787.2	Dysphagia

REIMBURSEMENT INFORMATION

Medicare

- Follow–up Days — 0
- Assistant Surgeon — by report
- Supply Charges — not allowed
- Outpatient Limit — does not apply
- Minor Surgery Rules Apply

CPT CODE / SERVICE	ICD-9-CM
31579 Laryngoscopy, flexible fiberoptic; with stroboscopy **CPT NOTES** ♦ For endoscopic procedures, code appropriate endoscopy of each anatomic site examined.	141.0 M-Neoplasm, Tongue base 210.1 B-Neoplasm, Tongue 464.20 Acute laryngotracheitis no obstruct 476.0 Chronic laryngitis 478.20 Disease of pharynx NOS 478.30 Vocal cord/larynx paralysis NOS 478.4 Polyp of vocal cord/larynx 478.5 Vocal cord disease NEC 478.6 Edema of larynx 478.70 Disease of larynx NOS 784.49 Voice disturbance NEC **REIMBURSEMENT INFORMATION** Medicare ♦ Follow-up Days — 0 ♦ Assistant Surgeon — not paid ♦ Supply Charges — not allowed ♦ Outpatient Limit — does not apply ♦ Minor Surgery Rules Apply
31580 Laryngoplasty; for laryngeal web, two stage, with keel insertion and removal	748.2 Congenital laryngeal web anomaly **REIMBURSEMENT INFORMATION** Medicare ♦ Follow-up Days — 90 ♦ Assistant Surgeon — paid ♦ Supply Charges — not allowed ♦ Outpatient Limit — does not apply ♦ Major Surgery Rules Apply
31582 Laryngoplasty; for laryngeal stenosis, with graft or core mold, including tracheotomy	478.74 Stenosis of larynx 519.8 Respiratory system disease NEC 748.3 Congenital laryngotrach anomaly NEC 784.41 Aphonia 784.49 Voice disturbance NEC 959.0 Face and neck injury NOS **REIMBURSEMENT INFORMATION** Medicare ♦ Follow-up Days — 90 ♦ Assistant Surgeon — paid ♦ Supply Charges — not allowed ♦ Outpatient Limit — does not apply ♦ Major Surgery Rules Apply

CPT CODE	SERVICE	ICD–9–CM
31584	Laryngoplasty; with open reduction of fracture	519.8 Respiratory system disease NEC 784.49 Voice disturbance NEC 807.6 Fracture larynx/trachea-open **REIMBURSEMENT INFORMATION** <u>Medicare</u> ♦ Follow–up Days — 90 ♦ Assistant Surgeon — paid ♦ Supply Charges — not allowed ♦ Outpatient Limit — does not apply ♦ Major Surgery Rules Apply
31585	Treatment of closed laryngeal fracture; without manipulation	478.6 Edema of larynx 784.49 Voice disturbance NEC 807.5 Fracture larynx/trachea-closed **REIMBURSEMENT INFORMATION** <u>Medicare</u> ♦ Follow–up Days — 90 ♦ Assistant Surgeon — by report ♦ Supply Charges — not allowed ♦ Outpatient Limit — does not apply ♦ Major Surgery Rules Apply
31586	Treatment of closed laryngeal fracture; with closed manipulative reduction	807.5 Fracture larynx/trachea-closed **REIMBURSEMENT INFORMATION** <u>Medicare</u> ♦ Follow–up Days — 90 ♦ Assistant Surgeon — by report ♦ Supply Charges — not allowed ♦ Outpatient Limit — does not apply ♦ Major Surgery Rules Apply

CPT CODE	SERVICE	ICD–9–CM
31587	Laryngoplasty, cricoid split	478.74 Stenosis of larynx 519.1 Trachea/bronchus disease NEC 519.8 Respiratory system disease NEC 748.3 Congenital laryngotrach anomaly NEC 786.09 Respiratory abnormality NEC 786.1 Stridor **REIMBURSEMENT INFORMATION** Medicare ♦ Follow–up Days — 90 ♦ Assistant Surgeon — paid ♦ Supply Charges — not allowed ♦ Outpatient Limit — does not apply ♦ Major Surgery Rules Apply
31588	Laryngoplasty, not otherwise specified (eg, for burns, reconstruction after partial laryngectomy)	478.32 Vocal cord paralysis, unilat, total 478.33 Vocal cord paralysis, bilat, part 519.8 Respiratory system disease NEC 784.49 Voice disturbance NEC 947.1 Burn of larynx, trachea, and lung **REIMBURSEMENT INFORMATION** Medicare ♦ Follow–up Days — 90 ♦ Assistant Surgeon — paid ♦ Supply Charges — not allowed ♦ Outpatient Limit — does not apply ♦ Major Surgery Rules Apply
31590	Laryngeal reinnervation by neuromuscular pedicle	478.32 Vocal cord paralysis, unilat, total 478.33 Vocal cord paralysis, bilat, part **REIMBURSEMENT INFORMATION** Medicare ♦ Follow–up Days — 90 ♦ Assistant Surgeon — paid ♦ Supply Charges — not allowed ♦ Outpatient Limit — does not apply ♦ Major Surgery Rules Apply

CPT CODE	SERVICE
31599	Unlisted procedure, larynx

ICD–9–CM

193	M-Neoplasm, Thyroid gland
226	B-Neoplasm, Thyroid gland
246.9	Disorder of thyroid NOS
464.0	Acute laryngitis
478.32	Vocal cord paralysis, unilat, total

REIMBURSEMENT INFORMATION

Medicare

- Follow–up Days — determined by local carrier
- Assistant Surgeon — determined by local carrier
- Supply Charges — determined by local carrier
- Outpatient Limit — determined by local carrier

CPT CODE	SERVICE
31600	Tracheostomy, planned (separate procedure)

ICD–9–CM

141.0	M-Neoplasm, Tongue base
145.9	M-Neoplasm, Mouth NOS
146.0	M-Neoplasm, Tonsil
146.9	M-Neoplasm, Oropharynx NOS
148.9	M-Neoplasm, Hypopharynx NOS
161.0	M-Neoplasm, Glottis
161.1	M-Neoplasm, Supraglottis
161.8	M-Neoplasm, Larynx NEC
212.1	B-Neoplasm, Larynx
235.1	UB-Neoplasm, Oral cavity/pharynx
239.1	Respiratory system neoplasm NOS
478.5	Vocal cord disease NEC
478.6	Edema of larynx
478.74	Stenosis of larynx
478.79	Disease of larynx NEC
518.5	Post traum pulmonary insufficiency
518.8	Diseases of lung
518.81	Respiratory failure
518.82	Other pulmonary insufficiency
519.1	Trachea/bronchus disease NEC
519.8	Respiratory system disease NEC
786.09	Respiratory abnormality NEC
799.1	Respiratory arrest
802.20	Mandible Fx NOS, closed
802.30	Mandible Fx NOS, open
802.4	Fx malar/maxillary, closed
802.5	Fx malar/maxillary, open

REIMBURSEMENT INFORMATION

General

- Separate procedure rules apply.

Medicare

- Follow–up Days — 0
- Assistant Surgeon — not paid
- Supply Charges — not allowed
- Outpatient Limit — does not apply
- Minor Surgery Rules Apply

CPT CODE	SERVICE	ICD–9–CM
31601	Tracheostomy, planned (separate procedure); under two years	470.0 Edema of larynx 478.74 Stenosis of larynx 478.79 Disease of larynx NEC 519.0 Tracheostomy complication 519.1 Trachea/bronchus disease NEC 786.09 Respiratory abnormality NEC 786.1 Stridor **REIMBURSEMENT INFORMATION** General ♦ Separate procedure rules apply. Medicare ♦ Follow–up Days — 0 ♦ Assistant Surgeon — paid ♦ Supply Charges — not allowed ♦ Outpatient Limit — does not apply ♦ Minor Surgery Rules Apply
31603	Tracheostomy, emergency procedure; transtracheal	518.81 Respiratory failure 518.82 Other pulmonary insufficiency 519.0 Tracheostomy complication 519.8 Respiratory system disease NEC 784.8 Hemorrhage from throat 786.09 Respiratory abnormality NEC 799.1 Respiratory arrest 933.0 Foreign body in pharynx 933.1 Foreign body in larynx 959.0 Face and neck injury NOS **REIMBURSEMENT INFORMATION** Medicare ♦ Follow–up Days — 0 ♦ Assistant Surgeon — not paid ♦ Supply Charges — not allowed ♦ Outpatient Limit — does not apply ♦ Minor Surgery Rules Apply

CPT CODE	SERVICE	ICD–9–CM
31605	Tracheostomy, emergency procedure; cricothyroid membrane	518.81 Respiratory failure 518.82 Other pulmonary insufficiency 519.0 Tracheostomy complication 519.8 Respiratory system disease NEC 784.8 Hemorrhage from throat 786.09 Respiratory abnormality NEC 799.1 Respiratory arrest 933.0 Foreign body in pharynx 933.1 Foreign body in larynx 959.0 Face and neck injury NOS **REIMBURSEMENT INFORMATION** Medicare ♦ Follow–up Days — 0 ♦ Assistant Surgeon — not paid ♦ Supply Charges — not allowed ♦ Outpatient Limit — does not apply ♦ Minor Surgery Rules Apply
31610	Tracheostomy, fenestration procedure with skin flaps **CPT NOTES** ♦ For endotracheal intubation, see 31500. ♦ For tracheal aspiration under direct vision, see 31515.	141.0 M-Neoplasm, Tongue base 146.0 M-Neoplasm, Tonsil 148.9 M-Neoplasm, Hypopharynx NOS 161.0 M-Neoplasm, Glottis 161.1 M-Neoplasm, Supraglottis 161.8 M-Neoplasm, Larynx NEC 212.1 B-Neoplasm, Larynx 235.1 UB-Neoplasm, Oral cavity/pharynx 239.1 Respiratory system neoplasm NOS 478.5 Vocal cord disease NEC 478.6 Edema of larynx 478.74 Stenosis of larynx 478.79 Disease of larynx NEC 518.5 Post traum pulmonary insufficiency 518.8 Diseases of lung 519.1 Trachea/bronchus disease NEC 519.8 Respiratory system disease NEC 786.09 Respiratory abnormality NEC 799.1 Respiratory arrest 802.20 Mandible Fx NOS, closed 802.30 Mandible Fx NOS, open 802.4 Fx malar/maxillary, closed 802.5 Fx malar/maxillary, open **REIMBURSEMENT INFORMATION** Medicare ♦ Follow–up Days — 90 ♦ Assistant Surgeon — not paid ♦ Supply Charges — not allowed ♦ Outpatient Limit — does not apply ♦ Major Surgery Rules Apply

CPT CODE	SERVICE	ICD–9–CM
31611	Construction of tracheoesophageal fistula and subsequent insertion of an alaryngeal speech prosthesis (eg, voice button, Blom-Singer prosthesis)	161.0 M-Neoplasm, Glottis 161.1 M-Neoplasm, Supraglottis 161.2 M-Neoplasm, Subglottis 161.3 M-Neoplasm, Laryngeal cartilages 161.8 M-Neoplasm, Larynx NEC 161.9 M-Neoplasm, Larynx NOS 784.41 Aphonia

REIMBURSEMENT INFORMATION

Medicare

- Follow–up Days — 90
- Assistant Surgeon — paid
- Supply Charges — not allowed
- Outpatient Limit — does not apply
- Major Surgery Rules Apply

CPT CODE	SERVICE	ICD–9–CM
▲ **31612**	Tracheal puncture, percutaneous with transtracheal aspiration and/or injection	466.0 Acute bronchitis 481 Pneumococcal pneumonia 482.9 Bacterial pneumonia NOS 485 Bronchopneumonia, organism NOS 486 Pneumonia, organism NOS 487.0 Influenza w/pneumonia 490 Bronchitis NOS 491.1 Mucopurulent chronic bronchitis 507.0 Food/vomit pneumonitis 518.89 Other lung disease NEC 519.8 Respiratory system disease NEC

REIMBURSEMENT INFORMATION

General

- Description changed in 1995 CPT.

Medicare

- Follow–up Days — 0
- Assistant Surgeon — not paid
- Supply Charges — not allowed
- Outpatient Limit — does not apply
- Minor Surgery Rules Apply

CPT CODE SERVICE	ICD–9–CM
31613 Tracheostoma revision; simple, without flap rotation	518.89 Other lung disease NEC 519.0 Tracheostomy complication 519.1 Trachea/bronchus disease NEC 519.8 Respiratory system disease NEC **REIMBURSEMENT INFORMATION** Medicare ♦ Follow–up Days — 90 ♦ Assistant Surgeon — not paid ♦ Supply Charges — not allowed ♦ Outpatient Limit — does not apply ♦ Major Surgery Rules Apply
31614 Tracheostoma revision; complex, with flap rotation	518.89 Other lung disease NEC 519.0 Tracheostomy complication 519.1 Trachea/bronchus disease NEC 519.8 Respiratory system disease NEC **REIMBURSEMENT INFORMATION** Medicare ♦ Follow–up Days — 90 ♦ Assistant Surgeon — not paid ♦ Supply Charges — not allowed ♦ Outpatient Limit — does not apply ♦ Major Surgery Rules Apply
31615 Tracheobronchoscopy through established tracheostomy incision **CPT NOTES** ♦ For endoscopic procedures, code appropriate endoscopy of each anatomic site examined. ♦ For tracheoscopy, see laryngoscopy codes 31515–31578.	212.1 B-Neoplasm, Larynx 519.0 Tracheostomy complication 519.1 Trachea/bronchus disease NEC 748.3 Congenital laryngotrach anomaly NEC 786.09 Respiratory abnormality NEC **REIMBURSEMENT INFORMATION** Medicare ♦ Follow–up Days — 0 ♦ Assistant Surgeon — not paid ♦ Supply Charges — not allowed ♦ Outpatient Limit — does not apply ♦ Minor Surgery Rules Apply

CPT CODE **SERVICE**

31622 Bronchoscopy; diagnostic, (flexible or rigid), with or without cell washing or brushing

CPT NOTES

- For endoscopic procedures, code appropriate endoscopy of each anatomic site examined.
- For tracheoscopy, see laryngoscopy codes 31515–31578.

ICD–9–CM

161.9	M-Neoplasm, Larynx NOS
162.9	M-Neoplasm, Bronchus/Lung NOS
212.3	B-Neoplasm, Bronchus/lung
239.1	Respiratory system neoplasm NOS
277.00	Cystic fibrosis w/o meconium ileus
478.30	Vocal cord/larynx paralysis NOS
478.74	Stenosis of larynx
518.81	Respiratory failure
518.82	Other pulmonary insufficiency
519.0	Tracheostomy complication
519.1	Trachea/bronchus disease NEC
519.8	Respiratory system disease NEC
748.3	Congenital laryngotrach anomaly NEC
748.61	Congenital bronchiectasis
759.3	Situs inversus
784.1	Throat pain
784.2	Swelling in head/neck
784.41	Aphonia
784.49	Voice disturbance NEC
786.09	Respiratory abnormality NEC
786.1	Stridor
786.2	Cough
786.3	Hemoptysis
787.2	Dysphagia
799.1	Respiratory arrest

REIMBURSEMENT INFORMATION

Medicare

- Follow–up Days — 0
- Assistant Surgeon — not paid
- Supply Charges — not allowed
- Outpatient Limit — does not apply
- Minor Surgery Rules Apply

CPT CODE **SERVICE**

31625 Bronchoscopy; with biopsy

CPT NOTES

- For endoscopic procedures, code appropriate endoscopy of each anatomic site examined.
- For tracheoscopy, see laryngoscopy codes 31515–31578.

ICD–9–CM

161.9	M-Neoplasm, Larynx NOS
162.9	M-Neoplasm, Bronchus/Lung NOS
212.3	B-Neoplasm, Bronchus/lung
239.1	Respiratory system neoplasm NOS
277.00	Cystic fibrosis w/o meconium ileus
478.30	Vocal cord/larynx paralysis NOS
478.74	Stenosis of larynx
518.81	Respiratory failure
518.82	Other pulmonary insufficiency
519.0	Tracheostomy complication
519.1	Trachea/bronchus disease NEC
519.8	Respiratory system disease NEC
748.3	Congenital laryngotrach anomaly NEC
784.1	Throat pain
784.2	Swelling in head/neck
784.41	Aphonia
784.49	Voice disturbance NEC
786.09	Respiratory abnormality NEC
786.1	Stridor
786.2	Cough
786.3	Hemoptysis
787.2	Dysphagia
799.1	Respiratory arrest

REIMBURSEMENT INFORMATION

Medicare

- Follow–up Days — 0
- Assistant Surgeon — not paid
- Supply Charges — not allowed
- Outpatient Limit — does not apply
- Minor Surgery Rules Apply
- Fragments — 31622

CPT CODE	SERVICE	ICD-9-CM

31630 Bronchoscopy; with tracheal or bronchial dilation or closed reduction of fracture

CPT NOTES

- For endoscopic procedures, code appropriate endoscopy of each anatomic site examined.
- For tracheoscopy, see laryngoscopy codes 31515–31578.

478.74 Stenosis of larynx
519.1 Trachea/bronchus disease NEC
807.5 Fracture larynx/trachea-closed
807.6 Fracture larynx/trachea-open

REIMBURSEMENT INFORMATION

Medicare

- Follow-up Days — 0
- Assistant Surgeon — not paid
- Supply Charges — not allowed
- Outpatient Limit — does not apply
- Minor Surgery Rules Apply

31631 Bronchoscopy; with tracheal dilation and placement of tracheal stent

CPT NOTES

- For endoscopic procedures, code appropriate endoscopy of each anatomic site examined.
- For tracheoscopy, see laryngoscopy codes 31515–31578.

478.74 Stenosis of larynx
519.1 Trachea/bronchus disease NEC
807.5 Fracture larynx/trachea-closed
807.6 Fracture larynx/trachea-open

REIMBURSEMENT INFORMATION

Medicare

- Follow-up Days — 0
- Assistant Surgeon — not paid
- Supply Charges — not allowed
- Outpatient Limit — does not apply
- Minor Surgery Rules Apply

31635 Bronchoscopy; with removal of foreign body

CPT NOTES

- For endoscopic procedures, code appropriate endoscopy of each anatomic site examined.
- For tracheoscopy, see laryngoscopy codes 31515–31578.

934.1 Foreign body, main bronchus
934.8 Foreign body, trachea/bronchus/lung

REIMBURSEMENT INFORMATION

Medicare

- Follow-up Days — 0
- Assistant Surgeon — not paid
- Supply Charges — not allowed
- Outpatient Limit — does not apply
- Minor Surgery Rules Apply

CPT CODE	SERVICE	ICD–9–CM
31641	Bronchoscopy; with destruction of tumor or relief of stenosis by any method other than excision (eg, laser)	162.2 M-Neoplasm, Main bronchus 162.3 M-Neoplasm, Upper lobe, Lung 162.4 M-Neoplasm, Middle lobe, Lung 162.5 M-Neoplasm, Lower lobe, Lung 162.8 M-Neoplasm, Bronchus/Lung NEC 212.3 B-Neoplasm, Bronchus/lung 464.10 Acute tracheitis, no obstruction 478.74 Stenosis of larynx 519.1 Trachea/bronchus disease NEC 701.5 Abnormal granulation tissue NEC

CPT NOTES

- For endoscopic procedures, code appropriate endoscopy of each anatomic site examined.
- For tracheoscopy, see laryngoscopy codes 31515–31578.

REIMBURSEMENT INFORMATION

Medicare

- Follow–up Days — 0
- Assistant Surgeon — not paid
- Supply Charges — not allowed
- Outpatient Limit — does not apply
- Minor Surgery Rules Apply

CPT CODE	SERVICE	ICD–9–CM
31645	Bronchoscopy; with therapeutic aspiration of tracheobronchial tree, initial (eg, drainage of lung abscess)	277.00 Cystic fibrosis w/o meconium ileus 466.0 Acute bronchitis 491.20 Obstr chron bronchitis w/o exacerb 491.21 Obstr chron bronchitis w/exacerb 491.9 Chronic bronchitis NOS 496 Chronic airway obstruction NEC 518.5 Post traum pulmonary insufficiency 518.81 Respiratory failure 518.82 Other pulmonary insufficiency 519.1 Trachea/bronchus disease NEC 519.8 Respiratory system disease NEC 786.09 Respiratory abnormality NEC 786.1 Stridor 786.2 Cough 799.1 Respiratory arrest

CPT NOTES

- For endoscopic procedures, code appropriate endoscopy of each anatomic site examined.
- For tracheoscopy, see laryngoscopy codes 31515–31578.
- For catheter aspiration of tracheobronchial tree at bedside, use 31725.

REIMBURSEMENT INFORMATION

Medicare

- Follow–up Days — 0
- Assistant Surgeon — not paid
- Supply Charges — not allowed
- Outpatient Limit — does not apply
- Minor Surgery Rules Apply
- Fragments — 31622

CPT CODE **SERVICE**

31646 Bronchoscopy; with therapeutic aspiration of tracheobronchial tree, subsequent

CPT NOTES

- For endoscopic procedures, code appropriate endoscopy of each anatomic site examined.
- For tracheoscopy, see laryngoscopy codes 31515–31578.
- For catheter aspiration of tracheobronchial tree at bedside, use 31725.

ICD–9–CM

466.0	Acute bronchitis
491.20	Obstr chron bronchitis w/o exacerb
491.21	Obstr chron bronchitis w/exacerb
491.9	Chronic bronchitis NOS
496	Chronic airway obstruction NEC
518.5	Post traum pulmonary insufficiency
518.81	Respiratory failure
518.82	Other pulmonary insufficiency
519.1	Trachea/bronchus disease NEC
519.8	Respiratory system disease NEC
786.09	Respiratory abnormality NEC
786.1	Stridor
786.2	Cough
799.1	Respiratory arrest

REIMBURSEMENT INFORMATION

Medicare

- Follow–up Days — 0
- Assistant Surgeon — not paid
- Supply Charges — not allowed
- Outpatient Limit — does not apply
- Minor Surgery Rules Apply

31656 Bronchoscopy; with injection of contrast material for segmental bronchography (fiberscope only)

CPT NOTES

- For endoscopic procedures, code appropriate endoscopy of each anatomic site examined.
- For tracheoscopy, see laryngoscopy codes 31515–31578.
- For radiological supervision and interpretation, see 71040, 71060.

466.0	Acute bronchitis
491.20	Obstr chron bronchitis w/o exacerb
491.21	Obstr chron bronchitis w/exacerb
491.9	Chronic bronchitis NOS
496	Chronic airway obstruction NEC
518.5	Post traum pulmonary insufficiency
518.81	Respiratory failure
518.82	Other pulmonary insufficiency
519.1	Trachea/bronchus disease NEC
519.8	Respiratory system disease NEC
786.09	Respiratory abnormality NEC
786.1	Stridor
786.2	Cough
799.1	Respiratory arrest

REIMBURSEMENT INFORMATION

Medicare

- Follow–up Days — 0
- Assistant Surgeon — not paid
- Supply Charges — not allowed
- Outpatient Limit — does not apply
- Minor Surgery Rules Apply

CPT CODE **SERVICE**

31700 Catheterization, transglottic (separate procedure)

CPT NOTES

- For endotracheal intubation, see 31500.
- For tracheal aspiration under direct vision, see 31515.

ICD–9–CM

427.5	Cardiac arrest
466.0	Acute bronchitis
478.30	Vocal cord/larynx paralysis NOS
478.6	Edema of larynx
478.74	Stenosis of larynx
482.1	Pseudomonal pneumonia
518.5	Post traum pulmonary insufficiency
518.81	Respiratory failure
518.82	Other pulmonary insufficiency
748.3	Congenital laryngotrach anomaly NEC
770.0	NB Congenital pneumonia
770.1	NB meconium aspiration syndrome
770.2	NB interstitial emphysema
770.6	NB transitory tachypnea
770.8	Post-birth resp problem NEC
770.9	NB respiratory condition NOS
776.1	Neonatal thrombocytopenia
799.1	Respiratory arrest

REIMBURSEMENT INFORMATION

General

- Separate procedure rules apply.

Medicare

- Follow–up Days — 0
- Assistant Surgeon — not paid
- Supply Charges — not allowed
- Outpatient Limit — does not apply
- Minor Surgery Rules Apply

CPT CODE	SERVICE
31708	Instillation of contrast material for laryngography or bronchography, without catheterization

CPT NOTES

- For endotracheal intubation, see 31500.
- For tracheal aspiration under direct vision, see 31515.
- For radiological supervision and interpretation, see 70373, 71040, 71060.

ICD–9–CM

466.0	Acute bronchitis
491.20	Obstr chron bronchitis w/o exacerb
491.21	Obstr chron bronchitis w/exacerb
491.9	Chronic bronchitis NOS
496	Chronic airway obstruction NEC
518.1	Interstitial emphysema
518.5	Post traum pulmonary insufficiency
518.81	Respiratory failure
518.82	Other pulmonary insufficiency
519.1	Trachea/bronchus disease NEC
519.8	Respiratory system disease NEC
786.09	Respiratory abnormality NEC
786.1	Stridor
786.2	Cough
799.1	Respiratory arrest

REIMBURSEMENT INFORMATION

Medicare

- Follow–up Days — 0
- Assistant Surgeon — by report
- Supply Charges — not allowed
- Outpatient Limit — does not apply
- Minor Surgery Rules Apply

CPT CODE **SERVICE**

31710 Catheterization for bronchography, with or without instillation of contrast material

CPT NOTES

- For endotracheal intubation, see 31500.
- For tracheal aspiration under direct vision, see 31515.
- For bronchoscopic catheterization for bronchography, fiberscope only, see 31656.
- For radiological supervision and interpretation, see 71040, 71060.

ICD–9–CM

466.0	Acute bronchitis
481	Pneumococcal pneumonia
482.9	Bacterial pneumonia NOS
485	Bronchopneumonia, organism NOS
486	Pneumonia, organism NOS
487.0	Influenza w/pneumonia
491.20	Obstr chron bronchitis w/o exacerb
491.21	Obstr chron bronchitis w/exacerb
491.9	Chronic bronchitis NOS
496	Chronic airway obstruction NEC
507.0	Food/vomit pneumonitis
507.1	Oil/essence pneumonitis
507.8	Solid/liquid pneumonitis NEC
513.0	Abscess of lung
518.5	Post traum pulmonary insufficiency
518.81	Respiratory failure
518.82	Other pulmonary insufficiency
519.1	Trachea/bronchus disease NEC
519.8	Respiratory system disease NEC
748.61	Congenital bronchiectasis
786.09	Respiratory abnormality NEC
786.1	Stridor
786.2	Cough
799.1	Respiratory arrest

REIMBURSEMENT INFORMATION

Medicare

- Follow–up Days — 0
- Assistant Surgeon — not paid
- Supply Charges — not allowed
- Outpatient Limit — does not apply
- Minor Surgery Rules Apply

CPT CODE **SERVICE**

31715 Transtracheal injection for bronchography

CPT NOTES

- For endotracheal intubation, see 31500.
- For tracheal aspiration under direct vision, see 31515.
- For radiological supervision and interpretation, see 71040, 71060.
- For prolonged services, see 99354–99360.

ICD–9–CM

466.0	Acute bronchitis
481	Pneumococcal pneumonia
482.9	Bacterial pneumonia NOS
485	Bronchopneumonia, organism NOS
486	Pneumonia, organism NOS
487.0	Influenza w/pneumonia
491.20	Obstr chron bronchitis w/o exacerb
491.21	Obstr chron bronchitis w/exacerb
491.9	Chronic bronchitis NOS
496	Chronic airway obstruction NEC
507.0	Food/vomit pneumonitis
507.1	Oil/essence pneumonitis
507.8	Solid/liquid pneumonitis NEC
513.0	Abscess of lung
518.5	Post traum pulmonary insufficiency
518.81	Respiratory failure
518.82	Other pulmonary insufficiency
519.1	Trachea/bronchus disease NEC
519.8	Respiratory system disease NEC
748.61	Congenital bronchiectasis
786.09	Respiratory abnormality NEC
786.1	Stridor
786.2	Cough
799.1	Respiratory arrest

REIMBURSEMENT INFORMATION

Medicare

- Follow–up Days — 0
- Assistant Surgeon — not paid
- Supply Charges — not allowed
- Outpatient Limit — does not apply
- Minor Surgery Rules Apply

CPT CODE **SERVICE**

▲ **31720** Catheter aspiration (separate procedure); nasotracheal

CPT NOTES

- For endotracheal intubation, see 31500.
- For tracheal aspiration under direct vision, see 31515.

ICD-9-CM

466.0	Acute bronchitis
481	Pneumococcal pneumonia
482.9	Bacterial pneumonia NOS
485	Bronchopneumonia, organism NOS
486	Pneumonia, organism NOS
491.20	Obstr chron bronchitis w/o exacerb
491.21	Obstr chron bronchitis w/exacerb
491.9	Chronic bronchitis NOS
496	Chronic airway obstruction NEC
507.0	Food/vomit pneumonitis
507.1	Oil/essence pneumonitis
507.8	Solid/liquid pneumonitis NEC

REIMBURSEMENT INFORMATION

General

- Separate procedure rules apply.
- Description changed in 1995 CPT.

Medicare

- Follow–up Days — 0
- Assistant Surgeon — not paid
- Supply Charges — not allowed
- Outpatient Limit — does not apply
- Minor Surgery Rules Apply

31725 Catheter aspiration (separate procedure); tracheobronchial with fiberscope, bedside

CPT NOTES

- For endotracheal intubation, see 31500.
- For tracheal aspiration under direct vision, see 31515.

466.0	Acute bronchitis
481	Pneumococcal pneumonia
482.9	Bacterial pneumonia NOS
485	Bronchopneumonia, organism NOS
486	Pneumonia, organism NOS
487.0	Influenza w/pneumonia
491.20	Obstr chron bronchitis w/o exacerb
491.21	Obstr chron bronchitis w/exacerb
491.9	Chronic bronchitis NOS
496	Chronic airway obstruction NEC
507.0	Food/vomit pneumonitis
507.1	Oil/essence pneumonitis
507.8	Solid/liquid pneumonitis NEC

REIMBURSEMENT INFORMATION

General

- Separate procedure rules apply.

Medicare

- Follow–up Days — 0
- Assistant Surgeon — not paid
- Supply Charges — not allowed
- Outpatient Limit — does not apply
- Minor Surgery Rules Apply

CPT CODE **SERVICE** | **ICD–9–CM**

31730 Transtracheal (percutaneous) introduction of needle wire dilator/stent or indwelling tube for oxygen therapy

CPT NOTES

- For endotracheal intubation, see 31500.
- For tracheal aspiration under direct vision, see 31515.

478.74 Stenosis of larynx
478.79 Disease of larynx NEC
519.8 Respiratory system disease NEC

REIMBURSEMENT INFORMATION

Medicare

- Follow–up Days — 0
- Assistant Surgeon — paid
- Supply Charges — not allowed
- Outpatient Limit — does not apply
- Minor Surgery Rules Apply

31750 Tracheoplasty; cervical

161.0 M-Neoplasm, Glottis
161.1 M-Neoplasm, Supraglottis
161.2 M-Neoplasm, Subglottis
161.3 M-Neoplasm, Laryngeal cartilages
161.8 M-Neoplasm, Larynx NEC
519.1 Trachea/bronchus disease NEC

REIMBURSEMENT INFORMATION

Medicare

- Follow–up Days — 90
- Assistant Surgeon — paid
- Supply Charges — not allowed
- Outpatient Limit — does not apply
- Major Surgery Rules Apply

31755 Tracheoplasty; tracheopharyngeal fistulization, each stage

161.0 M-Neoplasm, Glottis
161.1 M-Neoplasm, Supraglottis
161.2 M-Neoplasm, Subglottis
161.3 M-Neoplasm, Laryngeal cartilages
161.8 M-Neoplasm, Larynx NEC
784.41 Aphonia

REIMBURSEMENT INFORMATION

Medicare

- Follow–up Days — 90
- Assistant Surgeon — paid
- Supply Charges — not allowed
- Outpatient Limit — does not apply
- Major Surgery Rules Apply

CPT CODE	SERVICE	ICD–9–CM
31775	Bronchoplasty; excision stenosis and anastomosis	518.81 Respiratory failure 518.82 Other pulmonary insufficiency 519.1 Trachea/bronchus disease NEC 748.3 Congenital laryngotrach anomaly NEC

CPT NOTES

- For lobectomy and bronchoplasty, see 32485.

REIMBURSEMENT INFORMATION

Medicare

- Follow–up Days — 90
- Assistant Surgeon — paid
- Supply Charges — not allowed
- Outpatient Limit — does not apply
- Major Surgery Rules Apply

31780	Excision tracheal stenosis and anastomosis; cervical	519.0 Tracheostomy complication 519.1 Trachea/bronchus disease NEC 748.3 Congenital laryngotrach anomaly NEC

REIMBURSEMENT INFORMATION

Medicare

- Follow–up Days — 90
- Assistant Surgeon — paid
- Supply Charges — not allowed
- Outpatient Limit — does not apply
- Major Surgery Rules Apply

31781	Excision tracheal stenosis and anastomosis; cervicothoracic	519.0 Tracheostomy complication 519.1 Trachea/bronchus disease NEC 748.3 Congenital laryngotrach anomaly NEC

REIMBURSEMENT INFORMATION

Medicare

- Follow–up Days — 90
- Assistant Surgeon — paid
- Supply Charges — not allowed
- Outpatient Limit — does not apply
- Major Surgery Rules Apply

CPT CODE **SERVICE**

ICD–9–CM

31820 Surgical closure tracheostomy or fistula; without plastic repair

CPT NOTES

- For repair tracheoesophageal fistula, see 43305, 43312.

519.0 Tracheostomy complication
519.1 Trachea/bronchus disease NEC
748.3 Congenital laryngotrach anomaly NEC
786.09 Respiratory abnormality NEC

REIMBURSEMENT INFORMATION

Medicare

- Follow–up Days — 90
- Assistant Surgeon — not paid
- Supply Charges — not allowed
- Outpatient Limit — does not apply
- Major Surgery Rules Apply

31825 Surgical closure tracheostomy or fistula; with plastic repair

CPT NOTES

- For repair tracheoesophageal fistula, see 43305, 43312.

519.0 Tracheostomy complication
519.1 Trachea/bronchus disease NEC
748.3 Congenital laryngotrach anomaly NEC
786.09 Respiratory abnormality NEC

REIMBURSEMENT INFORMATION

Medicare

- Follow–up Days — 90
- Assistant Surgeon — not paid
- Supply Charges — not allowed
- Outpatient Limit — does not apply
- Major Surgery Rules Apply

31830 Revision of tracheostomy scar

519.0 Tracheostomy complication
701.4 Keloid scar

REIMBURSEMENT INFORMATION

Medicare

- Follow–up Days — 90
- Assistant Surgeon — not paid
- Supply Charges — not allowed
- Outpatient Limit — does not apply
- Major Surgery Rules Apply

CPT CODE	SERVICE	ICD–9–CM
31899	Unlisted procedure, trachea, bronchi	464.10 Acute tracheitis, no obstruction 476.0 Chronic laryngitis 478.34 Vocal cord paralysis, bilat, total 478.74 Stenosis of larynx 478.79 Disease of larynx NEC 519.0 Tracheostomy complication 786.09 Respiratory abnormality NEC 787.2 Dysphagia **REIMBURSEMENT INFORMATION** Medicare ♦ Follow–up Days — determined by local carrier ♦ Assistant Surgeon — determined by local carrier ♦ Supply Charges — determined by local carrier ♦ Outpatient Limit — determined by local carrier
38500	Biopsy or excision of lymph node(s); superficial (separate procedure) **CPT NOTES** ♦ For fine needle aspiration, use 88170.	196.0 M-Neoplasm, Lymph head/neck/face 200.81 Mixed lymphosarcoma, head/neck/face 202.81 Lymphoma NEC, head/neck 229.0 B-Neoplasm, Lymph nodes 229.9 Benign neoplasm NOS 239.7 Endocrine/CNS neoplasm NOS **REIMBURSEMENT INFORMATION** General ♦ Separate procedure rules apply. Medicare ♦ Follow–up Days — 10 ♦ Assistant Surgeon — not paid ♦ Supply Charges — allowed ♦ Outpatient Limit — does not apply ♦ Minor Surgery Rules Apply
38505	Biopsy or excision of lymph node(s); by needle, superficial (eg, cervical, inguinal, axillary) **CPT NOTES** ♦ For fine needle aspiration, use 88170.	196.0 M-Neoplasm, Lymph head/neck/face 200.81 Mixed lymphosarcoma, head/neck/face 202.81 Lymphoma NEC, head/neck 229.0 B-Neoplasm, Lymph nodes 229.9 Benign neoplasm NOS 239.7 Endocrine/CNS neoplasm NOS **REIMBURSEMENT INFORMATION** Medicare ♦ Follow–up Days — 0 ♦ Assistant Surgeon — not paid ♦ Supply Charges — not allowed ♦ Outpatient Limit — does not apply ♦ Minor Surgery Rules Apply

CPT CODE	SERVICE	ICD-9-CM

40490 Biopsy of lip

CPT NOTES

- For procedures on skin of lips, see 10040 et seq.

079.9	Viral/chlamydial infection NOS
140.0	M-Neoplasm, Upper lip, vermilion
140.1	M-Neoplasm, Lower lip, vermilion
140.3	M-Neoplasm, Upper lip, inner aspect
140.4	M-Neoplasm, Lower lip, inner aspect
140.5	M-Neoplasm, Lip NOS, inner NOS
140.6	M-Neoplasm, lip, commissure
140.8	M-Neoplasm, Lip NEC
140.9	M-Neoplasm, Lip/vermilion NOS
173.0	M-Neoplasm, Skin of lip
210.0	B-Neoplasm, Lip
210.4	B-Neoplasm, Mouth NEC/NOS
230.0	CA in situ, Oral cavity/pharynx
232.0	CA in situ, Skin of lip
235.1	UB-Neoplasm, Oral cavity/pharynx
238.2	UB-Neoplasm, Skin
527.2	Sialoadenitis
527.6	Salivary gland mucocele
527.7	Salivary secretion disturbance
528.0	Stomatitis
528.5	Diseases of lips
528.6	Leukoplakia of oral mucosa/tongue
528.7	Oral epithelium disturbance NEC
528.9	Oral soft tissue disease NEC
706.2	Sebaceous cyst
710.2	Sicca syndrome

REIMBURSEMENT INFORMATION

Medicare

- Follow-up Days — 0
- Assistant Surgeon — not paid
- Supply Charges — not allowed
- Outpatient Limit — applies
- Minor Surgery Rules Apply

40500 Vermilionectomy (lip shave), with mucosal advancement

CPT NOTES

- For procedures on skin of lips, see 10040 et seq.

140.0	M-Neoplasm, Upper lip, vermilion
210.0	B-Neoplasm, Lip
230.0	CA in situ, Oral cavity/pharynx
232.0	CA in situ, Skin of lip
528.6	Leukoplakia of oral mucosa/tongue

REIMBURSEMENT INFORMATION

Medicare

- Follow-up Days — 90
- Assistant Surgeon — not paid
- Supply Charges — not allowed
- Outpatient Limit — does not apply
- Major Surgery Rules Apply

CPT CODE	SERVICE	ICD–9–CM
40510	Excision of lip; transverse wedge excision with primary closure	140.0 M-Neoplasm, Upper lip, vermilion 140.1 M-Neoplasm, Lower lip, vermilion 140.3 M-Neoplasm, Upper lip, inner aspect 140.4 M-Neoplasm, Lower lip, inner aspect 140.5 M-Neoplasm, Lip NOS, inner NOS 140.6 M-Neoplasm, lip, commissure 140.8 M-Neoplasm, Lip NEC 140.9 M-Neoplasm, Lip/vermilion NOS 173.0 M-Neoplasm, Skin of lip 195.0 M-Neoplasm, Head/face/neck 210.0 B-Neoplasm, Lip 230.0 CA in situ, Oral cavity/pharynx 235.1 UB-Neoplasm, Oral cavity/pharynx 528.5 Diseases of lips 873.43 Open wound of lip 873.53 Open wound of lip, complicated 941.33 3rd deg burn, lip 959.0 Face and neck injury NOS

CPT NOTES

- For procedures on skin of lips, see 10040 et seq.
- For excision of mucous lesions, see 40810–40816.

REIMBURSEMENT INFORMATION

Medicare

- Follow–up Days — 90
- Assistant Surgeon — not paid
- Supply Charges — not allowed
- Outpatient Limit — does not apply
- Major Surgery Rules Apply

CPT CODE	SERVICE	ICD–9–CM
40520	Excision of lip; V-excision with primary direct linear closure	140.0 M-Neoplasm, Upper lip, vermilion 140.1 M-Neoplasm, Lower lip, vermilion 140.3 M-Neoplasm, Upper lip, inner aspect 140.4 M-Neoplasm, Lower lip, inner aspect 140.5 M-Neoplasm, Lip NOS, inner NOS 140.6 M-Neoplasm, lip, commissure 140.8 M-Neoplasm, Lip NEC 140.9 M-Neoplasm, Lip/vermilion NOS 173.0 M-Neoplasm, Skin of lip 195.0 M-Neoplasm, Head/face/neck 235.1 UB-Neoplasm, Oral cavity/pharynx 873.43 Open wound of lip 873.53 Open wound of lip, complicated 941.33 3rd deg burn, lip 959.0 Face and neck injury NOS

CPT NOTES

- For procedures on skin of lips, see 10040 et seq.
- For excision of mucous lesions, see 40810–40816.

REIMBURSEMENT INFORMATION

Medicare

- Follow–up Days — 90
- Assistant Surgeon — not paid
- Supply Charges — not allowed
- Outpatient Limit — does not apply
- Major Surgery Rules Apply

CPT CODE	SERVICE	ICD-9-CM

40525 Excision of lip; full thickness, reconstruction with local flap (eg, Estlander or fan)

CPT NOTES

- For procedures on skin of lips, see 10040 et seq.

140.0	M-Neoplasm, Upper lip, vermilion
140.1	M-Neoplasm, Lower lip, vermilion
140.3	M-Neoplasm, Upper lip, inner aspect
140.4	M-Neoplasm, Lower lip, inner aspect
140.5	M-Neoplasm, Lip NOS, inner NOS
140.6	M-Neoplasm, lip, commissure
140.8	M-Neoplasm, Lip NEC
140.9	M-Neoplasm, Lip/vermilion NOS
173.0	M-Neoplasm, Skin of lip
195.0	M-Neoplasm, Head/face/neck
235.1	UB-Neoplasm, Oral cavity/pharynx
873.43	Open wound of lip
873.53	Open wound of lip, complicated
941.33	3rd deg burn, lip
959.0	Face and neck injury NOS

REIMBURSEMENT INFORMATION

Medicare

- Follow–up Days — 90
- Assistant Surgeon — not paid
- Supply Charges — not allowed
- Outpatient Limit — does not apply
- Major Surgery Rules Apply

40527 Excision of lip; full thickness, reconstruction with cross lip flap (Abbe-Estlander)

CPT NOTES

- For procedures on skin of lips, see 10040 et seq.

140.0	M-Neoplasm, Upper lip, vermilion
140.1	M-Neoplasm, Lower lip, vermilion
140.3	M-Neoplasm, Upper lip, inner aspect
140.4	M-Neoplasm, Lower lip, inner aspect
140.5	M-Neoplasm, Lip NOS, inner NOS
140.6	M-Neoplasm, lip, commissure
140.8	M-Neoplasm, Lip NEC
140.9	M-Neoplasm, Lip/vermilion NOS
173.0	M-Neoplasm, Skin of lip
195.0	M-Neoplasm, Head/face/neck
235.1	UB-Neoplasm, Oral cavity/pharynx
873.43	Open wound of lip
873.53	Open wound of lip, complicated
941.33	3rd deg burn, lip
959.0	Face and neck injury NOS

REIMBURSEMENT INFORMATION

Medicare

- Follow–up Days — 90
- Assistant Surgeon — not paid
- Supply Charges — not allowed
- Outpatient Limit — does not apply
- Major Surgery Rules Apply

CPT CODE	SERVICE	ICD–9–CM
40530	Resection of lip, more than one-fourth, without reconstruction	140.0 M-Neoplasm, Upper lip, vermilion 140.1 M-Neoplasm, Lower lip, vermilion 140.3 M-Neoplasm, Upper lip, inner aspect 140.4 M-Neoplasm, Lower lip, inner aspect 140.5 M-Neoplasm, Lip NOS, inner NOS 140.6 M-Neoplasm, lip, commissure 140.8 M-Neoplasm, Lip NEC 140.9 M-Neoplasm, Lip/vermilion NOS 173.0 M-Neoplasm, Skin of lip 195.0 M-Neoplasm, Head/face/neck 210.0 B-Neoplasm, Lip 235.1 UB-Neoplasm, Oral cavity/pharynx 873.43 Open wound of lip 873.53 Open wound of lip, complicated 941.33 3rd deg burn, lip 959.0 Face and neck injury NOS

CPT NOTES

- For procedures on skin of lips, see 10040 et seq.
- For reconstruction, see 13131 et seq.

REIMBURSEMENT INFORMATION

Medicare

- Follow–up Days — 90
- Assistant Surgeon — not paid
- Supply Charges — not allowed
- Outpatient Limit — does not apply
- Major Surgery Rules Apply

CPT CODE	SERVICE	ICD–9–CM
40650	Repair lip, full thickness; vermilion only	140.0 M-Neoplasm, Upper lip, vermilion 140.1 M-Neoplasm, Lower lip, vermilion 140.9 M-Neoplasm, Lip/vermilion NOS 173.0 M-Neoplasm, Skin of lip 210.0 B-Neoplasm, Lip 873.43 Open wound of lip 873.53 Open wound of lip, complicated

CPT NOTES

- For procedures on skin of lips, see 10040 et seq.

REIMBURSEMENT INFORMATION

Medicare

- Follow–up Days — 90
- Assistant Surgeon — not paid
- Supply Charges — not allowed
- Outpatient Limit — does not apply
- Major Surgery Rules Apply

CPT CODE	SERVICE	ICD-9-CM

40652 Repair lip, full thickness; up to half vertical height

CPT NOTES

- For procedures on skin of lips, see 10040 et seq.

140.0 M-Neoplasm, Upper lip, vermilion
140.1 M-Neoplasm, Lower lip, vermilion
140.3 M-Neoplasm, Upper lip, inner aspect
140.4 M-Neoplasm, Lower lip, inner aspect
140.5 M-Neoplasm, Lip NOS, inner NOS
140.6 M-Neoplasm, lip, commissure
140.8 M-Neoplasm, Lip NEC
173.0 M-Neoplasm, Skin of lip
873.43 Open wound of lip
873.53 Open wound of lip, complicated

REIMBURSEMENT INFORMATION

Medicare

- Follow-up Days — 90
- Assistant Surgeon — not paid
- Supply Charges — not allowed
- Outpatient Limit — does not apply
- Major Surgery Rules Apply

40654 Repair lip, full thickness; over one half vertical height, or complex

CPT NOTES

- For procedures on skin of lips, see 10040 et seq.

140.0 M-Neoplasm, Upper lip, vermilion
140.1 M-Neoplasm, Lower lip, vermilion
140.3 M-Neoplasm, Upper lip, inner aspect
140.4 M-Neoplasm, Lower lip, inner aspect
140.5 M-Neoplasm, Lip NOS, inner NOS
140.6 M-Neoplasm, lip, commissure
140.8 M-Neoplasm, Lip NEC
173.0 M-Neoplasm, Skin of lip
873.43 Open wound of lip
873.53 Open wound of lip, complicated

REIMBURSEMENT INFORMATION

Medicare

- Follow-up Days — 90
- Assistant Surgeon — not paid
- Supply Charges — not allowed
- Outpatient Limit — does not apply
- Major Surgery Rules Apply

CPT CODE	SERVICE	ICD-9-CM

40700 Plastic repair of cleft lip/nasal deformity; primary, partial or complete, unilateral

CPT NOTES

- For procedures on skin of lips, see 10040 et seq.
- To report rhinoplasty only for nasal deformity secondary to congenital cleft lip, see 30460, 30462.
- For repair cleft palate, see 42200 et seq.
- For other reconstructive procedures, see 14060, 14061, 15120–15261, 15574, 15576, 15630.

749.10 Cleft lip NOS
749.11 Unilateral cleft lip, complete
749.12 Unilateral cleft lip, incomplete
749.20 Cleft palate w/cleft lip NOS
749.21 Unilat cleft palate/lip, complete
749.22 Unilat cleft palate/lip, incomplete
749.25 Cleft palate w/cleft lip NEC

REIMBURSEMENT INFORMATION

Medicare

- Follow–up Days — 90
- Assistant Surgeon — not paid
- Supply Charges — not allowed
- Outpatient Limit — does not apply
- Major Surgery Rules Apply

40701 Plastic repair of cleft lip/nasal deformity; primary bilateral, one stage procedure

CPT NOTES

- For procedures on skin of lips, see 10040 et seq.
- To report rhinoplasty only for nasal deformity secondary to congenital cleft lip, see 30460, 30462.
- For repair cleft palate, see 42200 et seq.
- For other reconstructive procedures, see 14060, 14061, 15120–15261, 15574, 15576, 15630.

749.10 Cleft lip NOS
749.13 Bilateral cleft lip, complete
749.14 Bilateral cleft lip, incomplete
749.20 Cleft palate w/cleft lip NOS
749.23 Bilat cleft palate/lip, complete
749.24 Bilat cleft palate/lip, incomplete
749.25 Cleft palate w/cleft lip NEC

REIMBURSEMENT INFORMATION

Medicare

- Follow–up Days — 90
- Assistant Surgeon — paid
- Supply Charges — not allowed
- Outpatient Limit — does not apply
- Major Surgery Rules Apply

40702 Plastic repair of cleft lip/nasal deformity; primary bilateral, one of two stages

CPT NOTES

- For procedures on skin of lips, see 10040 et seq.
- To report rhinoplasty only for nasal deformity secondary to congenital cleft lip, see 30460, 30462.
- For repair cleft palate, see 42200 et seq.
- For other reconstructive procedures, see 14060, 14061, 15120–15261, 15574, 15576, 15630.

749.10 Cleft lip NOS
749.13 Bilateral cleft lip, complete
749.14 Bilateral cleft lip, incomplete
749.20 Cleft palate w/cleft lip NOS
749.21 Unilat cleft palate/lip, complete
749.22 Unilat cleft palate/lip, incomplete
749.23 Bilat cleft palate/lip, complete
749.24 Bilat cleft palate/lip, incomplete
749.25 Cleft palate w/cleft lip NEC

REIMBURSEMENT INFORMATION

Medicare

- Follow–up Days — 90
- Assistant Surgeon — paid
- Supply Charges — not allowed
- Outpatient Limit — does not apply
- Major Surgery Rules Apply

CPT CODE **SERVICE**

40720 Plastic repair of cleft lip/nasal deformity; secondary, by recreation of defect and reclosure

CPT NOTES

- For procedures on skin of lips, see 10040 et seq.
- To report rhinoplasty only for nasal deformity secondary to congenital cleft lip, see 30460, 30462.
- For repair cleft palate, see 42200 et seq.
- For other reconstructive procedures, see 14060, 14061, 15120–15261, 15574, 15576, 15630.

ICD–9–CM

749.10 Cleft lip NOS
749.11 Unilateral cleft lip, complete
749.12 Unilateral cleft lip, incomplete
749.20 Cleft palate w/cleft lip NOS
749.21 Unilat cleft palate/lip, complete
749.22 Unilat cleft palate/lip, incomplete
749.23 Bilat cleft palate/lip, complete
749.24 Bilat cleft palate/lip, incomplete
749.25 Cleft palate w/cleft lip NEC

REIMBURSEMENT INFORMATION

Medicare

- Follow–up Days — 90
- Assistant Surgeon — by report
- Supply Charges — not allowed
- Outpatient Limit — does not apply
- Major Surgery Rules Apply

40761 Plastic repair of cleft lip; with cross lip pedicle flap (Abbe- Estlander type), including sectioning and inserting of pedicle

CPT NOTES

- For procedures on skin of lips, see 10040 et seq.
- For repair cleft palate, see 42200 et seq.
- For other reconstructive procedures, see 14060, 14061, 15120–15261, 15574, 15576, 15630.

749.10 Cleft lip NOS
749.11 Unilateral cleft lip, complete
749.13 Bilateral cleft lip, complete
749.14 Bilateral cleft lip, incomplete
749.20 Cleft palate w/cleft lip NOS
749.21 Unilat cleft palate/lip, complete
749.23 Bilat cleft palate/lip, complete
749.24 Bilat cleft palate/lip, incomplete
749.25 Cleft palate w/cleft lip NEC

REIMBURSEMENT INFORMATION

Medicare

- Follow–up Days — 90
- Assistant Surgeon — paid
- Supply Charges — not allowed
- Outpatient Limit — does not apply
- Major Surgery Rules Apply

40799 Unlisted procedure, lips

CPT NOTES

- For procedures on skin of lips, see 10040 et seq.

144.0 M-Neoplasm, Anterior floor of mouth
160.2 M-Neoplasm, Maxillary sinus
229.8 Benign neoplasm NEC

REIMBURSEMENT INFORMATION

Medicare

- Follow–up Days — determined by local carrier
- Assistant Surgeon — determined by local carrier
- Supply Charges — determined by local carrier
- Outpatient Limit — determined by local carrier

CPT CODE **SERVICE**

40800* Drainage of abscess, cyst, hematoma, vestibule of mouth; simple

CPT NOTES

- The vestibule is the part of the oral cavity outside the dentoalveolar structures; it includes the mucosal and submucosal tissue of lips and cheeks.

ICD–9–CM

522.0	Pulpitis
522.5	Periapical abscess w/o sinus
522.7	Periapical abscess w/sinus
522.8	Radicular cyst
523.3	Acute periodontitis
525.2	Atrophy, edentulous alveolar ridge
526.0	Developmental odontogenic cysts
526.4	Inflammation of jaw
527.2	Sialoadenitis
527.3	Salivary gland abscess
527.6	Salivary gland mucocele
528.3	Cellulitis/abscess of mouth
528.4	Oral soft tissue cyst
528.5	Diseases of lips
528.7	Oral epithelium disturbance NEC
528.9	Oral soft tissue disease NEC
920	Contusion face/scalp/neck

REIMBURSEMENT INFORMATION

General

- Starred procedure.

Medicare

- Follow–up Days — 10
- Assistant Surgeon — not paid
- Supply Charges — not allowed
- Outpatient Limit — does not apply
- Minor Surgery Rules Apply

CPT CODE **SERVICE**

40801 Drainage of abscess, cyst, hematoma, vestibule of mouth; complicated

CPT NOTES

- The vestibule is the part of the oral cavity outside the dentoalveolar structures; it includes the mucosal and submucosal tissue of lips and cheeks.

ICD-9-CM

522.0	Pulpitis
522.5	Periapical abscess w/o sinus
522.7	Periapical abscess w/sinus
522.8	Radicular cyst
523.3	Acute periodontitis
525.2	Atrophy, edentulous alveolar ridge
526.0	Developmental odontogenic cysts
526.4	Inflammation of jaw
527.3	Salivary gland abscess
527.6	Salivary gland mucocele
528.3	Cellulitis/abscess of mouth
528.4	Oral soft tissue cyst
528.5	Diseases of lips
528.9	Oral soft tissue disease NEC
920	Contusion face/scalp/neck

REIMBURSEMENT INFORMATION

Medicare

- Follow-up Days — 10
- Assistant Surgeon — not paid
- Supply Charges — not allowed
- Outpatient Limit — does not apply
- Minor Surgery Rules Apply

40804* Removal of embedded foreign body, vestibule of mouth; simple

CPT NOTES

- The vestibule is the part of the oral cavity outside the dentoalveolar structures; it includes the mucosal and submucosal tissue of lips and cheeks.

873.79	Open wound of mouth NEC, complic
935.0	Foreign body in mouth

REIMBURSEMENT INFORMATION

General

- Starred procedure.

Medicare

- Follow-up Days — 10
- Assistant Surgeon — not paid
- Supply Charges — not allowed
- Outpatient Limit — does not apply
- Minor Surgery Rules Apply

CPT CODE	SERVICE	ICD–9–CM

40805 Removal of embedded foreign body, vestibule of mouth; complicated

873.79 Open wound of mouth NEC, complic
935.0 Foreign body in mouth

CPT NOTES

- The vestibule is the part of the oral cavity outside the dentoalveolar structures; it includes the mucosal and submucosal tissue of lips and cheeks.

REIMBURSEMENT INFORMATION

Medicare

- Follow–up Days — 10
- Assistant Surgeon — by report
- Supply Charges — not allowed
- Outpatient Limit — does not apply
- Minor Surgery Rules Apply

40806 Incision of labial frenum (frenotomy)

528.9 Oral soft tissue disease NEC
750.26 Mouth anomaly NEC

CPT NOTES

- The vestibule is the part of the oral cavity outside the dentoalveolar structures; it includes the mucosal and submucosal tissue of lips and cheeks.

REIMBURSEMENT INFORMATION

Medicare

- Follow–up Days — 10
- Assistant Surgeon — by report
- Supply Charges — not allowed
- Outpatient Limit — does not apply
- Minor Surgery Rules Apply

CPT CODE	SERVICE
40808	Biopsy, vestibule of mouth

CPT NOTES

- The vestibule is the part of the oral cavity outside the dentoalveolar structures; it includes the mucosal and submucosal tissue of lips and cheeks.

ICD–9–CM

145.0	M-Neoplasm, Cheek mucosa
145.1	M-Neoplasm, Mouth vestibule
145.9	M-Neoplasm, Mouth NOS
210.0	B-Neoplasm, Lip
210.4	B-Neoplasm, Mouth NEC/NOS
230.0	CA in situ, Oral cavity/pharynx
235.1	UB-Neoplasm, Oral cavity/pharynx
523.1	Chronic gingivitis
523.9	Gingival/periodontal disease NOS
526.0	Developmental odontogenic cysts
527.2	Sialoadenitis
527.5	Sialolithiasis
527.9	Salivary gland disease NOS
528.0	Stomatitis
528.4	Oral soft tissue cyst
528.5	Diseases of lips
528.6	Leukoplakia of oral mucosa/tongue
528.7	Oral epithelium disturbance NEC
528.9	Oral soft tissue disease NEC
701.5	Abnormal granulation tissue NEC
706.2	Sebaceous cyst

REIMBURSEMENT INFORMATION

<u>Medicare</u>

- Follow–up Days — 10
- Assistant Surgeon — not paid
- Supply Charges — not allowed
- Outpatient Limit — applies
- Minor Surgery Rules Apply

CPT CODE **SERVICE**

40810 Excision of lesion of mucosa and submucosa, vestibule of mouth; without repair

CPT NOTES

- The vestibule is the part of the oral cavity outside the dentoalveolar structures; it includes the mucosal and submucosal tissue of lips and cheeks.

ICD–9–CM

145.0	M-Neoplasm, Cheek mucosa
145.1	M-Neoplasm, Mouth vestibule
145.9	M-Neoplasm, Mouth NOS
171.0	M-Neoplasm, Soft tissue, head
171.8	M-Neoplasm, Soft tissue NEC
195.0	M-Neoplasm, Head/face/neck
210.0	B-Neoplasm, Lip
210.4	B-Neoplasm, Mouth NEC/NOS
215.0	B-Neoplasm, Soft tissue, head
230.0	CA in situ, Oral cavity/pharynx
235.1	UB-Neoplasm, Oral cavity/pharynx
238.1	UB-Neoplasm, Soft tissue
526.4	Inflammation of jaw
527.6	Salivary gland mucocele
527.8	Salivary gland disease NEC
528.5	Diseases of lips
528.6	Leukoplakia of oral mucosa/tongue
528.7	Oral epithelium disturbance NEC
528.9	Oral soft tissue disease NEC
706.2	Sebaceous cyst

REIMBURSEMENT INFORMATION

Medicare

- Follow–up Days — 10
- Assistant Surgeon — not paid
- Supply Charges — not allowed
- Outpatient Limit — applies
- Minor Surgery Rules Apply

CPT CODE	SERVICE
40012	Excision of lesion of mucosa and submucosa, vestibule of mouth; with simple repair

CPT NOTES

- The vestibule is the part of the oral cavity outside the dentoalveolar structures; it includes the mucosal and submucosal tissue of lips and cheeks.

ICD–9–CM

145.0	M-Neoplasm, Cheek mucosa
145.1	M-Neoplasm, Mouth vestibule
145.9	M-Neoplasm, Mouth NOS
171.0	M-Neoplasm, Soft tissue, head
171.8	M-Neoplasm, Soft tissue NEC
195.0	M-Neoplasm, Head/face/neck
202.81	Lymphoma NEC, head/neck
210.0	B-Neoplasm, Lip
210.2	B-Neoplasm, Major salivary glands
210.4	B-Neoplasm, Mouth NEC/NOS
215.0	B-Neoplasm, Soft tissue, head
230.0	CA in situ, Oral cavity/pharynx
235.1	UB-Neoplasm, Oral cavity/pharynx
238.1	UB-Neoplasm, Soft tissue
239.2	Bone/Skin neoplasm NOS
526.4	Inflammation of jaw
527.2	Sialoadenitis
527.5	Sialolithiasis
527.6	Salivary gland mucocele
527.8	Salivary gland disease NEC
528.0	Stomatitis
528.6	Leukoplakia of oral mucosa/tongue
528.7	Oral epithelium disturbance NEC
528.9	Oral soft tissue disease NEC
706.2	Sebaceous cyst

REIMBURSEMENT INFORMATION

Medicare

- Follow–up Days — 10
- Assistant Surgeon — not paid
- Supply Charges — not allowed
- Outpatient Limit — does not apply
- Minor Surgery Rules Apply

CPT CODE **SERVICE**

40814 Excision of lesion of mucosa and submucosa, vestibule of mouth; with complex repair

CPT NOTES

- The vestibule is the part of the oral cavity outside the dentoalveolar structures; it includes the mucosal and submucosal tissue of lips and cheeks.

ICD–9–CM

140.4	M-Neoplasm, Lower lip, inner aspect
145.0	M-Neoplasm, Cheek mucosa
145.1	M-Neoplasm, Mouth vestibule
145.9	M-Neoplasm, Mouth NOS
171.0	M-Neoplasm, Soft tissue, head
171.8	M-Neoplasm, Soft tissue NEC
195.0	M-Neoplasm, Head/face/neck
210.0	B-Neoplasm, Lip
210.4	B-Neoplasm, Mouth NEC/NOS
213.0	B-Neoplasm, Skull/Face bone
215.0	B-Neoplasm, Soft tissue, head
230.0	CA in situ, Oral cavity/pharynx
235.1	UB-Neoplasm, Oral cavity/pharynx
238.1	UB-Neoplasm, Soft tissue
239.2	Bone/Skin neoplasm NOS
525.2	Atrophy, edentulous alveolar ridge
526.4	Inflammation of jaw
527.2	Sialoadenitis
527.6	Salivary gland mucocele
527.8	Salivary gland disease NEC
528.4	Oral soft tissue cyst
528.5	Diseases of lips
528.6	Leukoplakia of oral mucosa/tongue
528.7	Oral epithelium disturbance NEC
528.9	Oral soft tissue disease NEC
706.2	Sebaceous cyst

REIMBURSEMENT INFORMATION

Medicare

- Follow–up Days — 90
- Assistant Surgeon — not paid
- Supply Charges — not allowed
- Outpatient Limit — does not apply
- Major Surgery Rules Apply

CPT CODE **SERVICE**

40816 Excision of lesion of mucosa and submucosa, vestibule of mouth; complex, with excision of underlying muscle

CPT NOTES

- The vestibule is the part of the oral cavity outside the dentoalveolar structures; it includes the mucosal and submucosal tissue of lips and cheeks.

ICD–9–CM

145.0	M-Neoplasm, Cheek mucosa
145.1	M-Neoplasm, Mouth vestibule
145.9	M-Neoplasm, Mouth NOS
171.0	M-Neoplasm, Soft tissue, head
171.8	M-Neoplasm, Soft tissue NEC
195.0	M-Neoplasm, Head/face/neck
210.0	B-Neoplasm, Lip
210.3	B-Neoplasm, Floor of mouth
210.4	B-Neoplasm, Mouth NEC/NOS
215.0	B-Neoplasm, Soft tissue, head
230.0	CA in situ, Oral cavity/pharynx
235.1	UB-Neoplasm, Oral cavity/pharynx
238.1	UB-Neoplasm, Soft tissue
523.1	Chronic gingivitis
526.4	Inflammation of jaw
527.6	Salivary gland mucocele
527.8	Salivary gland disease NEC
528.6	Leukoplakia of oral mucosa/tongue
528.7	Oral epithelium disturbance NEC
528.9	Oral soft tissue disease NEC
706.2	Sebaceous cyst

REIMBURSEMENT INFORMATION

Medicare

- Follow–up Days — 90
- Assistant Surgeon — not paid
- Supply Charges — not allowed
- Outpatient Limit — does not apply
- Major Surgery Rules Apply

40818 Excision of mucosa of vestibule of mouth as donor graft

CPT NOTES

- The vestibule is the part of the oral cavity outside the dentoalveolar structures; it includes the mucosal and submucosal tissue of lips and cheeks.

752.49	Female genital anomaly NEC
752.8	Genital organ anomaly NEC

REIMBURSEMENT INFORMATION

Medicare

- Follow–up Days — 90
- Assistant Surgeon — not paid
- Supply Charges — not allowed
- Outpatient Limit — does not apply
- Major Surgery Rules Apply

CPT CODE	SERVICE	ICD-9-CM
40819	Excision of frenum, labial or buccal (frenumectomy, frenulectomy, frenectomy)	140.3 M-Neoplasm, Upper lip, inner aspect 140.4 M-Neoplasm, Lower lip, inner aspect 140.5 M-Neoplasm, Lip NOS, inner NOS 140.8 M-Neoplasm, Lip NEC 210.0 B-Neoplasm, Lip 210.4 B-Neoplasm, Mouth NEC/NOS 235.1 UB-Neoplasm, Oral cavity/pharynx 523.9 Gingival/periodontal disease NOS 528.9 Oral soft tissue disease NEC V51 Aftercare w/plastic surgery

CPT NOTES

- The vestibule is the part of the oral cavity outside the dentoalveolar structures; it includes the mucosal and submucosal tissue of lips and cheeks.

REIMBURSEMENT INFORMATION

Medicare

- Follow-up Days — 90
- Assistant Surgeon — not paid
- Supply Charges — not allowed
- Outpatient Limit — does not apply
- Major Surgery Rules Apply

CPT CODE	SERVICE	ICD-9-CM
40820	Destruction of lesion or scar of vestibule of mouth by physical methods (eg, laser, thermal, cryo, chemical)	210.4 B-Neoplasm, Mouth NEC/NOS 230.0 CA in situ, Oral cavity/pharynx 232.0 CA in situ, Skin of lip 235.1 UB-Neoplasm, Oral cavity/pharynx 239.2 Bone/Skin neoplasm NOS V51 Aftercare w/plastic surgery

CPT NOTES

- The vestibule is the part of the oral cavity outside the dentoalveolar structures; it includes the mucosal and submucosal tissue of lips and cheeks.

REIMBURSEMENT INFORMATION

Medicare

- Follow-up Days — 10
- Assistant Surgeon — not paid
- Supply Charges — not allowed
- Outpatient Limit — does not apply
- Minor Surgery Rules Apply

CPT CODE **SERVICE**

40830 Closure of laceration, vestibule of mouth; 2.5 cm or less

CPT NOTES

- The vestibule is the part of the oral cavity outside the dentoalveolar structures; it includes the mucosal and submucosal tissue of lips and cheeks.

ICD–9–CM

145.1	M-Neoplasm, Mouth vestibule
198.89	M2-Neoplasm NEC
873.61	Open wound of buccal mucosa
873.62	Open wound of gum
873.64	Open wound of tongue/mouth floor
873.69	Open wound of mouth NEC
873.71	Open wound of buccal mucosa, compl
873.72	Open wound of gum, complicated
873.74	Open wound of tongue, complicated
873.79	Open wound of mouth NEC, complic

REIMBURSEMENT INFORMATION

Medicare

- Follow–up Days — 10
- Assistant Surgeon — not paid
- Supply Charges — not allowed
- Outpatient Limit — does not apply
- Minor Surgery Rules Apply

40831 Closure of laceration, vestibule of mouth; over 2.5 cm or complex

CPT NOTES

- The vestibule is the part of the oral cavity outside the dentoalveolar structures; it includes the mucosal and submucosal tissue of lips and cheeks.

145.1	M-Neoplasm, Mouth vestibule
198.89	M2-Neoplasm NEC
873.61	Open wound of buccal mucosa
873.62	Open wound of gum
873.64	Open wound of tongue/mouth floor
873.69	Open wound of mouth NEC
873.71	Open wound of buccal mucosa, compl
873.72	Open wound of gum, complicated
873.74	Open wound of tongue, complicated
873.79	Open wound of mouth NEC, complic

REIMBURSEMENT INFORMATION

Medicare

- Follow–up Days — 10
- Assistant Surgeon — not paid
- Supply Charges — not allowed
- Outpatient Limit — does not apply
- Minor Surgery Rules Apply

CPT CODE	SERVICE	ICD–9–CM

40840 Vestibuloplasty; anterior

CPT NOTES

- The vestibule is the part of the oral cavity outside the dentoalveolar structures; it includes the mucosal and submucosal tissue of lips and cheeks.
- For skin grafts, see 15000 et seq.

145.1	M-Neoplasm, Mouth vestibule
198.89	M2-Neoplasm NEC
525.2	Atrophy, edentulous alveolar ridge
749.20	Cleft palate w/cleft lip NOS
749.21	Unilat cleft palate/lip, complete
749.22	Unilat cleft palate/lip, incomplete
749.23	Bilat cleft palate/lip, complete
749.24	Bilat cleft palate/lip, incomplete
749.25	Cleft palate w/cleft lip NEC
905.0	Late effect, skull/face fracture

REIMBURSEMENT INFORMATION

Medicare

- Follow–up Days — global concept does not apply
- Assistant Surgeon — paid
- Supply Charges — not allowed
- Outpatient Limit — does not apply

40842 Vestibuloplasty; posterior, unilateral

CPT NOTES

- The vestibule is the part of the oral cavity outside the dentoalveolar structures; it includes the mucosal and submucosal tissue of lips and cheeks.
- For skin grafts, see 15000 et seq.

145.1	M-Neoplasm, Mouth vestibule
198.89	M2-Neoplasm NEC
525.2	Atrophy, edentulous alveolar ridge
749.21	Unilat cleft palate/lip, complete
749.22	Unilat cleft palate/lip, incomplete
905.0	Late effect, skull/face fracture
909.3	Late effect of surg/med complic

REIMBURSEMENT INFORMATION

Medicare

- Follow–up Days — global concept does not apply
- Assistant Surgeon — by report
- Supply Charges — not allowed
- Outpatient Limit — does not apply

CPT CODE **SERVICE**

40843 Vestibuloplasty; posterior, bilateral

CPT NOTES

- The vestibule is the part of the oral cavity outside the dentoalveolar structures; it includes the mucosal and submucosal tissue of lips and cheeks.
- For skin grafts, see 15000 et seq.

ICD–9–CM

145.1 M-Neoplasm, Mouth vestibule
198.89 M2-Neoplasm NEC
525.2 Atrophy, edentulous alveolar ridge
749.23 Bilat cleft palate/lip, complete
749.24 Bilat cleft palate/lip, incomplete
905.0 Late effect, skull/face fracture
909.3 Late effect of surg/med complic

REIMBURSEMENT INFORMATION

Medicare

- Follow–up Days — global concept does not apply
- Assistant Surgeon — paid
- Supply Charges — not allowed
- Outpatient Limit — does not apply

40844 Vestibuloplasty; entire arch

CPT NOTES

- The vestibule is the part of the oral cavity outside the dentoalveolar structures; it includes the mucosal and submucosal tissue of lips and cheeks.
- For skin grafts, see 15000 et seq.

145.1 M-Neoplasm, Mouth vestibule
198.89 M2-Neoplasm NEC
525.2 Atrophy, edentulous alveolar ridge
528.9 Oral soft tissue disease NEC
905.0 Late effect, skull/face fracture
909.3 Late effect of surg/med complic

REIMBURSEMENT INFORMATION

Medicare

- Follow–up Days — global concept does not apply
- Assistant Surgeon — paid
- Supply Charges — not allowed
- Outpatient Limit — does not apply

CPT CODE	SERVICE	ICD–9–CM

40845 Vestibuloplasty; complex (including ridge extension, muscle repositioning)

CPT NOTES

- The vestibule is the part of the oral cavity outside the dentoalveolar structures; it includes the mucosal and submucosal tissue of lips and cheeks.
- For skin grafts, see 15000 et seq.

ICD–9–CM

145.1	M-Neoplasm, Mouth vestibule
198.89	M2-Neoplasm NEC
524.00	Anomaly of jaw size NOS
524.01	Maxillary hyperplasia
524.02	Mandibular hyperplasia
524.03	Maxillary hypoplasia
524.04	Mandibular hypoplasia
524.05	Macrogenia
524.06	Microgenia
524.09	Anomaly of jaw size NEC
525.2	Atrophy, edentulous alveolar ridge
749.20	Cleft palate w/cleft lip NOS
749.21	Unilat cleft palate/lip, complete
749.22	Unilat cleft palate/lip, incomplete
749.23	Bilat cleft palate/lip, complete
749.24	Bilat cleft palate/lip, incomplete
749.25	Cleft palate w/cleft lip NEC
905.0	Late effect, skull/face fracture
909.3	Late effect of surg/med complic

REIMBURSEMENT INFORMATION

Medicare

- Follow–up Days — global concept does not apply
- Assistant Surgeon — by report
- Supply Charges — not allowed
- Outpatient Limit — does not apply

40899 Unlisted procedure, vestibule of mouth

CPT NOTES

- The vestibule is the part of the oral cavity outside the dentoalveolar structures; it includes the mucosal and submucosal tissue of lips and cheeks.

210.4	B-Neoplasm, Mouth NEC/NOS
520.6	Tooth eruption disturbances
526.81	Exostosis of jaw

REIMBURSEMENT INFORMATION

Medicare

- Follow–up Days — global concept does not apply
- Assistant Surgeon — not paid
- Supply Charges — not allowed
- Outpatient Limit — does not apply

CPT CODE	SERVICE
41000*	Intraoral incision and drainage of abscess, cyst, or hematoma of tongue or floor of mouth; lingual

ICD-9-CM

101	Vincent's angina
522.0	Pulpitis
522.5	Periapical abscess w/o sinus
522.7	Periapical abscess w/sinus
522.8	Radicular cyst
523.3	Acute periodontitis
526.0	Developmental odontogenic cysts
526.4	Inflammation of jaw
527.3	Salivary gland abscess
527.6	Salivary gland mucocele
528.3	Cellulitis/abscess of mouth
528.4	Oral soft tissue cyst
528.5	Diseases of lips
529.0	Glossitis
529.8	Tongue disorder NEC
910.8	Superficial injury, head NEC
910.9	Superficial inj, head NEC, infected

REIMBURSEMENT INFORMATION

General

- Starred procedure.

Medicare

- Follow-up Days — 10
- Assistant Surgeon — not paid
- Supply Charges — not allowed
- Outpatient Limit — does not apply
- Minor Surgery Rules Apply

CPT CODE	SERVICE
41005*	Intraoral incision and drainage of abscess, cyst, or hematoma of tongue or floor of mouth; sublingual, superficial

ICD–9–CM

101	Vincent's angina
210.3	B-Neoplasm, Floor of mouth
522.0	Pulpitis
522.5	Periapical abscess w/o sinus
522.7	Periapical abscess w/sinus
522.8	Radicular cyst
523.3	Acute periodontitis
526.0	Developmental odontogenic cysts
526.4	Inflammation of jaw
527.3	Salivary gland abscess
527.6	Salivary gland mucocele
528.3	Cellulitis/abscess of mouth
528.4	Oral soft tissue cyst
528.5	Diseases of lips
528.9	Oral soft tissue disease NEC
529.0	Glossitis
529.8	Tongue disorder NEC
683	Acute lymphadenitis
910.8	Superficial injury, head NEC
910.9	Superficial inj, head NEC, infected

REIMBURSEMENT INFORMATION

General

- Starred procedure.

Medicare

- Follow–up Days — 10
- Assistant Surgeon — by report
- Supply Charges — not allowed
- Outpatient Limit — does not apply
- MInor Surgery Rules Apply

CPT CODE	SERVICE
41006	Intraoral incision and drainage of abscess, cyst, or hematoma of tongue or floor of mouth; sublingual, deep, supramylohyoid

ICD–9–CM

145.0	M Neoplasm, Mouth NOC
522.0	Pulpitis
522.5	Periapical abscess w/o sinus
522.7	Periapical abscess w/sinus
522.8	Radicular cyst
523.3	Acute periodontitis
526.0	Developmental odontogenic cysts
526.4	Inflammation of jaw
527.3	Salivary gland abscess
527.6	Salivary gland mucocele
528.3	Cellulitis/abscess of mouth
528.4	Oral soft tissue cyst
528.5	Diseases of lips
529.0	Glossitis
529.8	Tongue disorder NEC
683	Acute lymphadenitis
910.8	Superficial injury, head NEC
910.9	Superficial inj, head NEC, infected

REIMBURSEMENT INFORMATION

Medicare

- Follow–up Days — 90
- Assistant Surgeon — by report
- Supply Charges — not allowed
- Outpatient Limit — does not apply
- Major Surgery Rules Apply

CPT CODE	SERVICE
41007	Intraoral incision and drainage of abscess, cyst, or hematoma of tongue or floor of mouth; submental space

ICD–9–CM

522.0	Pulpitis
522.5	Periapical abscess w/o sinus
522.7	Periapical abscess w/sinus
522.8	Radicular cyst
523.3	Acute periodontitis
526.0	Developmental odontogenic cysts
526.4	Inflammation of jaw
527.3	Salivary gland abscess
527.6	Salivary gland mucocele
528.3	Cellulitis/abscess of mouth
528.4	Oral soft tissue cyst
528.5	Diseases of lips
529.0	Glossitis
529.8	Tongue disorder NEC
683	Acute lymphadenitis
910.8	Superficial injury, head NEC
910.9	Superficial inj, head NEC, infected

REIMBURSEMENT INFORMATION

Medicare

- ♦ Follow–up Days — 90
- ♦ Assistant Surgeon — by report
- ♦ Supply Charges — not allowed
- ♦ Outpatient Limit — does not apply
- ♦ Major Surgery Rules Apply

CPT CODE	SERVICE
41008	Intraoral incision and drainage of abscess, cyst, or hematoma of tongue or floor of mouth; submandibular space

ICD–9–CM

145.9	M-Neoplasm, Mouth NOS
522.0	Pulpitis
522.5	Periapical abscess w/o sinus
522.7	Periapical abscess w/sinus
522.8	Radicular cyst
523.3	Acute periodontitis
526.0	Developmental odontogenic cysts
526.4	Inflammation of jaw
527.3	Salivary gland abscess
527.6	Salivary gland mucocele
528.3	Cellulitis/abscess of mouth
528.4	Oral soft tissue cyst
528.5	Diseases of lips
529.0	Glossitis
529.8	Tongue disorder NEC
683	Acute lymphadenitis
910.8	Superficial injury, head NEC
910.9	Superficial inj, head NEC, infected

REIMBURSEMENT INFORMATION

Medicare

- Follow–up Days — 90
- Assistant Surgeon — not paid
- Supply Charges — not allowed
- Outpatient Limit — does not apply
- Major Surgery Rules Apply

CPT CODE	SERVICE	ICD–9–CM
41009	Intraoral incision and drainage of abscess, cyst, or hematoma of tongue or floor of mouth; masticator space	522.0 Pulpitis 522.5 Periapical abscess w/o sinus 522.7 Periapical abscess w/sinus 522.8 Radicular cyst 523.3 Acute periodontitis 526.0 Developmental odontogenic cysts 526.4 Inflammation of jaw 527.3 Salivary gland abscess 527.6 Salivary gland mucocele 528.3 Cellulitis/abscess of mouth 528.4 Oral soft tissue cyst 528.5 Diseases of lips 529.0 Glossitis 529.8 Tongue disorder NEC 683 Acute lymphadenitis 910.8 Superficial injury, head NEC 910.9 Superficial inj, head NEC, infected **REIMBURSEMENT INFORMATION** <u>Medicare</u> ♦ Follow–up Days — 90 ♦ Assistant Surgeon — by report ♦ Supply Charges — not allowed ♦ Outpatient Limit — does not apply ♦ Major Surgery Rules Apply
41010	Incision of lingual frenum (frenotomy)	529.8 Tongue disorder NEC 750.0 Tongue tie 784.5 Speech disturbance NEC **REIMBURSEMENT INFORMATION** <u>Medicare</u> ♦ Follow–up Days — 10 ♦ Assistant Surgeon — by report ♦ Supply Charges — not allowed ♦ Outpatient Limit — does not apply ♦ Minor Surgery Rules Apply

CPT CODE	SERVICE
41015	Extraoral incision and drainage of abscess, cyst, or hematoma of floor of mouth; sublingual

CPT NOTES

- For frenosplasty, see 41520.

ICD–9–CM

145.9	M-Neoplasm, Mouth NOS
522.0	Pulpitis
522.5	Periapical abscess w/o sinus
522.7	Periapical abscess w/sinus
522.8	Radicular cyst
523.3	Acute periodontitis
526.0	Developmental odontogenic cysts
526.4	Inflammation of jaw
527.3	Salivary gland abscess
527.6	Salivary gland mucocele
528.3	Cellulitis/abscess of mouth
528.4	Oral soft tissue cyst
528.5	Diseases of lips
529.0	Glossitis
529.8	Tongue disorder NEC
683	Acute lymphadenitis
910.8	Superficial injury, head NEC
910.9	Superficial inj, head NEC, infected

REIMBURSEMENT INFORMATION

Medicare

- Follow–up Days — 90
- Assistant Surgeon — by report
- Supply Charges — not allowed
- Outpatient Limit — does not apply
- Major Surgery Rules Apply

CPT CODE	SERVICE
41016	Extraoral incision and drainage of abscess, cyst, or hematoma of floor of mouth; submental

CPT NOTES

- For frenoplasty, see 41520.

ICD–9–CM

522.0	Pulpitis
522.5	Periapical abscess w/o sinus
522.7	Periapical abscess w/sinus
522.8	Radicular cyst
523.3	Acute periodontitis
526.0	Developmental odontogenic cysts
526.4	Inflammation of jaw
527.3	Salivary gland abscess
527.6	Salivary gland mucocele
528.3	Cellulitis/abscess of mouth
528.4	Oral soft tissue cyst
528.5	Diseases of lips
529.0	Glossitis
529.8	Tongue disorder NEC
683	Acute lymphadenitis
910.8	Superficial injury, head NEC
910.9	Superficial inj, head NEC, infected

REIMBURSEMENT INFORMATION

Medicare

- Follow–up Days — 90
- Assistant Surgeon — by report
- Supply Charges — not allowed
- Outpatient Limit — does not apply
- Major Surgery Rules Apply

CPT CODE **SERVICE**

41017 Extraoral incision and drainage of abscess, cyst, or hematoma of floor of mouth; submandibular

CPT NOTES

- For frenoplasty, see 41520.

ICD–9–CM

145.9	M-Neoplasm, Mouth NOS
210.4	B-Neoplasm, Mouth NEC/NOS
522.0	Pulpitis
522.5	Periapical abscess w/o sinus
522.7	Periapical abscess w/sinus
522.8	Radicular cyst
523.3	Acute periodontitis
526.0	Developmental odontogenic cysts
526.4	Inflammation of jaw
527.3	Salivary gland abscess
527.6	Salivary gland mucocele
528.3	Cellulitis/abscess of mouth
528.4	Oral soft tissue cyst
528.5	Diseases of lips
529.0	Glossitis
529.8	Tongue disorder NEC
683	Acute lymphadenitis
910.8	Superficial injury, head NEC
910.9	Superficial inj, head NEC, infected

REIMBURSEMENT INFORMATION

Medicare

- Follow–up Days — 90
- Assistant Surgeon — not paid
- Supply Charges — not allowed
- Outpatient Limit — does not apply
- Major Surgery Rules Apply

CPT CODE **SERVICE**

41018 Extraoral incision and drainage of abscess, cyst, or hematoma of floor of mouth; masticator space

CPT NOTES

- For frenoplasty, see 41520.

ICD–9–CM

522.0	Pulpitis
522.5	Periapical abscess w/o sinus
522.7	Periapical abscess w/sinus
522.8	Radicular cyst
523.3	Acute periodontitis
526.0	Developmental odontogenic cysts
526.4	Inflammation of jaw
527.3	Salivary gland abscess
527.6	Salivary gland mucocele
528.3	Cellulitis/abscess of mouth
528.4	Oral soft tissue cyst
528.5	Diseases of lips
529.0	Glossitis
529.8	Tongue disorder NEC
683	Acute lymphadenitis
910.8	Superficial injury, head NEC
910.9	Superficial inj, head NEC, infected

REIMBURSEMENT INFORMATION

<u>Medicare</u>

- Follow–up Days — 90
- Assistant Surgeon — by report
- Supply Charges — not allowed
- Outpatient Limit — does not apply
- Major Surgery Rules Apply

CPT CODE	SERVICE
41100	Biopsy of tongue; anterior two thirds

ICD–9–CM

141.1	M-Neoplasm, Tongue dorsal surface
141.2	M-Neoplasm, Tongue tip/lat border
141.3	M-Neoplasm, Tongue ventral surface
141.4	M-Neoplasm, Tongue anterior 2/3 NOS
141.5	M-Neoplasm, Tongue junctional zone
141.8	M-Neoplasm, Tongue NEC
141.9	M-Neoplasm, Tongue NOS
144.0	M-Neoplasm, Anterior floor of mouth
144.9	M-Neoplasm, Floor of mouth NOS
198.89	M2-Neoplasm NEC
210.0	B-Neoplasm, Lip
210.1	B-Neoplasm, Tongue
210.4	B-Neoplasm, Mouth NEC/NOS
230.0	CA in situ, Oral cavity/pharynx
235.1	UB-Neoplasm, Oral cavity/pharynx
528.6	Leukoplakia of oral mucosa/tongue
528.7	Oral epithelium disturbance NEC
528.9	Oral soft tissue disease NEC
529.0	Glossitis
529.8	Tongue disorder NEC

REIMBURSEMENT INFORMATION

Medicare

- Follow–up Days — 10
- Assistant Surgeon — not paid
- Supply Charges — not allowed
- Outpatient Limit — applies
- Minor Surgery Rules Apply

CPT CODE	SERVICE
41105	Biopsy of tongue; posterior one-third

ICD–9–CM

141.0	M-Neoplasm, Tongue base
141.5	M-Neoplasm, Tongue junctional zone
141.6	M-Neoplasm, Lingual tonsil
141.8	M-Neoplasm, Tongue NEC
141.9	M-Neoplasm, Tongue NOS
144.1	M-Neoplasm, Lateral floor of mouth
144.9	M-Neoplasm, Floor of mouth NOS
146.1	M-Neoplasm, Tonsillar fossa
146.2	M-Neoplasm, Tonsillar pillars
198.89	M2-Neoplasm NEC
210.1	B-Neoplasm, Tongue
230.0	CA in situ, Oral cavity/pharynx
235.1	UB-Neoplasm, Oral cavity/pharynx
528.6	Leukoplakia of oral mucosa/tongue
528.7	Oral epithelium disturbance NEC
528.9	Oral soft tissue disease NEC
529.0	Glossitis
529.1	Geographic tongue

REIMBURSEMENT INFORMATION

Medicare

- Follow–up Days — 10
- Assistant Surgeon — not paid
- Supply Charges — not allowed
- Outpatient Limit — does not apply
- Minor Surgery Rules Apply

CPT CODE **SERVICE**

41108 Biopsy of floor of mouth

ICD–9–CM

141.0 M-Neoplasm, Tongue base
141.6 M-Neoplasm, Lingual tonsil
141.9 M-Neoplasm, Tongue NOS
144.0 M-Neoplasm, Anterior floor of mouth
144.1 M-Neoplasm, Lateral floor of mouth
144.8 M-Neoplasm, Floor of mouth NEC
144.9 M-Neoplasm, Floor of mouth NOS
145.9 M-Neoplasm, Mouth NOS
146.0 M-Neoplasm, Tonsil
210.1 B-Neoplasm, Tongue
210.3 B-Neoplasm, Floor of mouth
210.5 B-Neoplasm, Tonsil
230.0 CA in situ, Oral cavity/pharynx
235.1 UB-Neoplasm, Oral cavity/pharynx
527.6 Salivary gland mucocele
528.4 Oral soft tissue cyst
528.6 Leukoplakia of oral mucosa/tongue
528.7 Oral epithelium disturbance NEC
528.9 Oral soft tissue disease NEC

REIMBURSEMENT INFORMATION

Medicare

- Follow–up Days — 10
- Assistant Surgeon — not paid
- Supply Charges — not allowed
- Outpatient Limit — applies
- Minor Surgery Rules Apply

CPT CODE	SERVICE	ICD–9–CM
41110	Excision of lesion of tongue without closure	

141.0	M-Neoplasm, Tongue base
141.1	M-Neoplasm, Tongue dorsal surface
141.2	M-Neoplasm, Tongue tip/lat border
141.3	M-Neoplasm, Tongue ventral surface
141.4	M-Neoplasm, Tongue anterior 2/3 NOS
141.5	M-Neoplasm, Tongue junctional zone
141.6	M-Neoplasm, Lingual tonsil
141.8	M-Neoplasm, Tongue NEC
141.9	M-Neoplasm, Tongue NOS
210.1	B-Neoplasm, Tongue
210.4	B-Neoplasm, Mouth NEC/NOS
230.0	CA in situ, Oral cavity/pharynx
235.1	UB-Neoplasm, Oral cavity/pharynx
528.6	Leukoplakia of oral mucosa/tongue
528.7	Oral epithelium disturbance NEC
528.9	Oral soft tissue disease NEC
529.0	Glossitis
529.8	Tongue disorder NEC

REIMBURSEMENT INFORMATION

Medicare

- Follow–up Days — 10
- Assistant Surgeon — not paid
- Supply Charges — not allowed
- Outpatient Limit — does not apply
- Minor Surgery Rules Apply

41112 Excision of lesion of tongue with closure; anterior two-thirds

CPT NOTES

- List 41114 in addition to this code.

141.1	M-Neoplasm, Tongue dorsal surface
141.2	M-Neoplasm, Tongue tip/lat border
141.3	M-Neoplasm, Tongue ventral surface
141.4	M-Neoplasm, Tongue anterior 2/3 NOS
141.8	M-Neoplasm, Tongue NEC
141.9	M-Neoplasm, Tongue NOS
210.1	B-Neoplasm, Tongue
210.4	B-Neoplasm, Mouth NEC/NOS
230.0	CA in situ, Oral cavity/pharynx
235.1	UB-Neoplasm, Oral cavity/pharynx
528.6	Leukoplakia of oral mucosa/tongue
528.7	Oral epithelium disturbance NEC
528.9	Oral soft tissue disease NEC
529.0	Glossitis

REIMBURSEMENT INFORMATION

Medicare

- Follow–up Days — 90
- Assistant Surgeon — not paid
- Supply Charges — not allowed
- Outpatient Limit — does not apply
- Major Surgery Rules Apply

CPT CODE	SERVICE	ICD-9-CM

41113 Excision of lesion of tongue with closure; posterior one-third

CPT NOTES

- List 41114 in addition to this code.

141.0 M-Neoplasm, Tongue base
141.1 M-Neoplasm, Tongue dorsal surface
141.3 M-Neoplasm, Tongue ventral surface
141.5 M-Neoplasm, Tongue junctional zone
141.6 M-Neoplasm, Lingual tonsil
141.8 M-Neoplasm, Tongue NEC
141.9 M-Neoplasm, Tongue NOS
210.0 B-Neoplasm, Lip
210.1 B-Neoplasm, Tongue
210.4 B-Neoplasm, Mouth NEC/NOS
230.0 CA in situ, Oral cavity/pharynx
235.1 UB-Neoplasm, Oral cavity/pharynx
528.6 Leukoplakia of oral mucosa/tongue
528.7 Oral epithelium disturbance NEC
528.9 Oral soft tissue disease NEC
529.0 Glossitis

REIMBURSEMENT INFORMATION

Medicare

- Follow–up Days — 90
- Assistant Surgeon — not paid
- Supply Charges — not allowed
- Outpatient Limit — does not apply
- Major Surgery Rules Apply

41114 Excision of lesion of tongue with closure; with local tongue flap

CPT NOTES

- List in addition to code 41112 or 41113.

141.0 M-Neoplasm, Tongue base
141.1 M-Neoplasm, Tongue dorsal surface
141.2 M-Neoplasm, Tongue tip/lat border
141.3 M-Neoplasm, Tongue ventral surface
141.4 M-Neoplasm, Tongue anterior 2/3 NOS
141.5 M-Neoplasm, Tongue junctional zone
141.6 M-Neoplasm, Lingual tonsil
141.8 M-Neoplasm, Tongue NEC
141.9 M-Neoplasm, Tongue NOS
210.1 B-Neoplasm, Tongue
230.0 CA in situ, Oral cavity/pharynx
528.6 Leukoplakia of oral mucosa/tongue
528.7 Oral epithelium disturbance NEC
528.9 Oral soft tissue disease NEC
529.0 Glossitis

REIMBURSEMENT INFORMATION

Medicare

- Follow–up Days — 90
- Assistant Surgeon — not paid
- Supply Charges — not allowed
- Outpatient Limit — does not apply
- Major Surgery Rules Apply

CPT CODE	SERVICE	ICD–9–CM
41115	Excision of lingual frenum (frenectomy)	141.3 M-Neoplasm, Tongue ventral surface 141.8 M-Neoplasm, Tongue NEC 528.6 Leukoplakia of oral mucosa/tongue 528.7 Oral epithelium disturbance NEC 529.8 Tongue disorder NEC 750.0 Tongue tie 784.5 Speech disturbance NEC

REIMBURSEMENT INFORMATION

Medicare

- Follow–up Days — 10
- Assistant Surgeon — by report
- Supply Charges — not allowed
- Outpatient Limit — does not apply
- Minor Surgery Rules Apply

CPT CODE	SERVICE	ICD–9–CM
41116	Excision, lesion of floor of mouth	141.0 M-Neoplasm, Tongue base 144.0 M-Neoplasm, Anterior floor of mouth 144.1 M-Neoplasm, Lateral floor of mouth 144.8 M-Neoplasm, Floor of mouth NEC 144.9 M-Neoplasm, Floor of mouth NOS 210.2 B-Neoplasm, Major salivary glands 210.3 B-Neoplasm, Floor of mouth 210.4 B-Neoplasm, Mouth NEC/NOS 230.0 CA in situ, Oral cavity/pharynx 235.1 UB-Neoplasm, Oral cavity/pharynx 520.6 Tooth eruption disturbances 522.5 Periapical abscess w/o sinus 527.6 Salivary gland mucocele 528.6 Leukoplakia of oral mucosa/tongue 528.7 Oral epithelium disturbance NEC 528.9 Oral soft tissue disease NEC

REIMBURSEMENT INFORMATION

Medicare

- Follow–up Days — 90
- Assistant Surgeon — not paid
- Supply Charges — not allowed
- Outpatient Limit — does not apply
- Major Surgery Rules Apply

CPT CODE	SERVICE	ICD-9-CM

41120 Glossectomy; less than one-half tongue

141.0 M-Neoplasm, Tongue base
141.1 M-Neoplasm, Tongue dorsal surface
141.2 M-Neoplasm, Tongue tip/lat border
141.3 M-Neoplasm, Tongue ventral surface
141.4 M-Neoplasm, Tongue anterior 2/3 NOS
141.5 M-Neoplasm, Tongue junctional zone
141.8 M-Neoplasm, Tongue NEC
141.9 M-Neoplasm, Tongue NOS
144.0 M-Neoplasm, Anterior floor of mouth
144.1 M-Neoplasm, Lateral floor of mouth
144.8 M-Neoplasm, Floor of mouth NEC
144.9 M-Neoplasm, Floor of mouth NOS
146.0 M-Neoplasm, Tonsil
161.8 M-Neoplasm, Larynx NEC
210.1 B-Neoplasm, Tongue
750.19 Tongue anomaly NEC

REIMBURSEMENT INFORMATION

Medicare

- Follow–up Days — 90
- Assistant Surgeon — paid
- Supply Charges — not allowed
- Outpatient Limit — does not apply
- Major Surgery Rules Apply

41130 Glossectomy; hemiglossectomy

141.0 M-Neoplasm, Tongue base
141.1 M-Neoplasm, Tongue dorsal surface
141.2 M-Neoplasm, Tongue tip/lat border
141.3 M-Neoplasm, Tongue ventral surface
141.4 M-Neoplasm, Tongue anterior 2/3 NOS
141.5 M-Neoplasm, Tongue junctional zone
141.6 M-Neoplasm, Lingual tonsil
141.8 M-Neoplasm, Tongue NEC
141.9 M-Neoplasm, Tongue NOS
144.0 M-Neoplasm, Anterior floor of mouth
144.1 M-Neoplasm, Lateral floor of mouth
144.8 M-Neoplasm, Floor of mouth NEC
144.9 M-Neoplasm, Floor of mouth NOS
161.8 M-Neoplasm, Larynx NEC
210.1 B-Neoplasm, Tongue

REIMBURSEMENT INFORMATION

Medicare

- Follow–up Days — 90
- Assistant Surgeon — paid
- Supply Charges — not allowed
- Outpatient Limit — does not apply
- Major Surgery Rules Apply

CPT CODE	SERVICE	ICD–9–CM
41135	Glossectomy; partial, with unilateral radical neck dissection	141.0 M-Neoplasm, Tongue base 141.1 M-Neoplasm, Tongue dorsal surface 141.3 M-Neoplasm, Tongue ventral surface 141.4 M-Neoplasm, Tongue anterior 2/3 NOS 141.5 M-Neoplasm, Tongue junctional zone 141.8 M-Neoplasm, Tongue NEC 141.9 M-Neoplasm, Tongue NOS 161.8 M-Neoplasm, Larynx NEC **REIMBURSEMENT INFORMATION** Medicare ♦ Follow–up Days — 90 ♦ Assistant Surgeon — paid ♦ Supply Charges — not allowed ♦ Outpatient Limit — does not apply ♦ Major Surgery Rules Apply
41140	Glossectomy; complete or total, with or without tracheostomy, without radical neck dissection	141.0 M-Neoplasm, Tongue base 141.1 M-Neoplasm, Tongue dorsal surface 141.2 M-Neoplasm, Tongue tip/lat border 141.3 M-Neoplasm, Tongue ventral surface 141.4 M-Neoplasm, Tongue anterior 2/3 NOS 141.5 M-Neoplasm, Tongue junctional zone 141.6 M-Neoplasm, Lingual tonsil 141.8 M-Neoplasm, Tongue NEC 141.9 M-Neoplasm, Tongue NOS 144.0 M-Neoplasm, Anterior floor of mouth 144.1 M-Neoplasm, Lateral floor of mouth 144.8 M-Neoplasm, Floor of mouth NEC 144.9 M-Neoplasm, Floor of mouth NOS 161.8 M-Neoplasm, Larynx NEC **REIMBURSEMENT INFORMATION** Medicare ♦ Follow–up Days — 90 ♦ Assistant Surgeon — paid ♦ Supply Charges — not allowed ♦ Outpatient Limit — does not apply ♦ Major Surgery Rules Apply

CPT CODE	SERVICE	ICD–9–CM
41145	Glossectomy; complete or total, with or without tracheostomy, with unilateral radical neck dissection	

141.0	M-Neoplasm, Tongue base
141.1	M-Neoplasm, Tongue dorsal surface
141.3	M-Neoplasm, Tongue ventral surface
141.4	M-Neoplasm, Tongue anterior 2/3 NOS
141.5	M-Neoplasm, Tongue junctional zone
141.8	M-Neoplasm, Tongue NEC
141.9	M-Neoplasm, Tongue NOS
161.8	M-Neoplasm, Larynx NEC

REIMBURSEMENT INFORMATION

Medicare

- Follow–up Days — 90
- Assistant Surgeon — paid
- Supply Charges — not allowed
- Outpatient Limit — does not apply
- Major Surgery Rules Apply

41150 Glossectomy; composite procedure with resection floor of mouth and mandibular resection, without radical neck dissection

144.0	M-Neoplasm, Anterior floor of mouth
144.1	M-Neoplasm, Lateral floor of mouth
144.8	M-Neoplasm, Floor of mouth NEC
144.9	M-Neoplasm, Floor of mouth NOS
161.8	M-Neoplasm, Larynx NEC

REIMBURSEMENT INFORMATION

Medicare

- Follow–up Days — 90
- Assistant Surgeon — paid
- Supply Charges — not allowed
- Outpatient Limit — does not apply
- Major Surgery Rules Apply

41153 Glossectomy; composite procedure with resection floor of mouth, with suprahyoid neck dissection

144.0	M-Neoplasm, Anterior floor of mouth
144.1	M-Neoplasm, Lateral floor of mouth
144.8	M-Neoplasm, Floor of mouth NEC
144.9	M-Neoplasm, Floor of mouth NOS
161.8	M-Neoplasm, Larynx NEC
230.0	CA in situ, Oral cavity/pharynx

REIMBURSEMENT INFORMATION

Medicare

- Follow–up Days — 90
- Assistant Surgeon — paid
- Supply Charges — not allowed
- Outpatient Limit — does not apply
- Major Surgery Rules Apply

CPT CODE	SERVICE	ICD–9–CM
41155	Glossectomy; composite procedure with resection floor of mouth, mandibular resection, and radical neck dissection (Commando type)	141.0 M-Neoplasm, Tongue base 144.0 M-Neoplasm, Anterior floor of mouth 144.1 M-Neoplasm, Lateral floor of mouth 144.8 M-Neoplasm, Floor of mouth NEC 144.9 M-Neoplasm, Floor of mouth NOS **REIMBURSEMENT INFORMATION** Medicare ♦ Follow–up Days — 90 ♦ Assistant Surgeon — paid ♦ Supply Charges — not allowed ♦ Outpatient Limit — does not apply ♦ Major Surgery Rules Apply
41250*	Repair of laceration 2.5 cm or less; floor of mouth and/or anterior two-thirds of tongue	141.1 M-Neoplasm, Tongue dorsal surface 141.3 M-Neoplasm, Tongue ventral surface 141.4 M-Neoplasm, Tongue anterior 2/3 NOS 141.5 M-Neoplasm, Tongue junctional zone 141.6 M-Neoplasm, Lingual tonsil 141.8 M-Neoplasm, Tongue NEC 141.9 M-Neoplasm, Tongue NOS 146.0 M-Neoplasm, Tonsil 146.8 M-Neoplasm, Oropharynx NEC 146.9 M-Neoplasm, Oropharynx NOS 210.1 B-Neoplasm, Tongue 210.5 B-Neoplasm, Tonsil 873.64 Open wound of tongue/mouth floor 873.69 Open wound of mouth NEC 873.74 Open wound of tongue, complicated 873.79 Open wound of mouth NEC, complic **REIMBURSEMENT INFORMATION** General ♦ Starred procedure. Medicare ♦ Follow–up Days — 10 ♦ Assistant Surgeon — not paid ♦ Supply Charges — not allowed ♦ Outpatient Limit — does not apply ♦ Minor Surgery Rules Apply

CPT CODE	SERVICE	ICD–9–CM
41251*	Repair of laceration 2.5 cm or less; floor of mouth and/or posterior one-third of tongue	141.5 M-Neoplasm, Tongue junctional zone 141.6 M-Neoplasm, Lingual tonsil 141.8 M-Neoplasm, Tongue NEC 141.9 M-Neoplasm, Tongue NOS 146.0 M-Neoplasm, Tonsil 146.8 M-Neoplasm, Oropharynx NEC 146.9 M-Neoplasm, Oropharynx NOS 210.1 B-Neoplasm, Tongue 210.5 B-Neoplasm, Tonsil 873.64 Open wound of tongue/mouth floor 873.69 Open wound of mouth NEC 873.74 Open wound of tongue, complicated 873.79 Open wound of mouth NEC, complic

REIMBURSEMENT INFORMATION

General

- Starred procedure.

Medicare

- Follow–up Days — 10
- Assistant Surgeon — by report
- Supply Charges — not allowed
- Outpatient Limit — does not apply
- Minor Surgery Rules Apply

CPT CODE	SERVICE	ICD–9–CM
41252*	Repair of laceration of tongue, floor of mouth, over 2.6 cm or complex	873.64 Open wound of tongue/mouth floor 873.69 Open wound of mouth NEC 873.71 Open wound of buccal mucosa, compl 873.72 Open wound of gum, complicated 873.74 Open wound of tongue, complicated 873.79 Open wound of mouth NEC, complic

REIMBURSEMENT INFORMATION

General

- Starred procedure.

Medicare

- Follow–up Days — 10
- Assistant Surgeon — not paid
- Supply Charges — not allowed
- Outpatient Limit — does not apply
- Minor Surgery Rules Apply

CPT CODE	SERVICE	ICD–9–CM
41500	Fixation of tongue, mechanical, other than suture (eg, K-wire)	802.20 Mandible Fx NOS, closed 802.30 Mandible Fx NOS, open 873.64 Open wound of tongue/mouth floor **REIMBURSEMENT INFORMATION** Medicare ♦ Follow–up Days — 90 ♦ Assistant Surgeon — by report ♦ Supply Charges — not allowed ♦ Outpatient Limit — does not apply ♦ Major Surgery Rules Apply
41510	Suture of tongue to lip for micrognathia (Douglas type procedure)	519.8 Respiratory system disease NEC 524.00 Anomaly of jaw size NOS 524.01 Maxillary hyperplasia 524.02 Mandibular hyperplasia 524.03 Maxillary hypoplasia 524.04 Mandibular hypoplasia 524.05 Macrogenia 524.06 Microgenia 524.09 Anomaly of jaw size NEC 756.0 Anomaly of skull/face bones 786.09 Respiratory abnormality NEC 786.1 Stridor **REIMBURSEMENT INFORMATION** Medicare ♦ Follow–up Days — 90 ♦ Assistant Surgeon — by report ♦ Supply Charges — not allowed ♦ Outpatient Limit — does not apply ♦ Major Surgery Rules Apply
41520	Frenoplasty (surgical revision of frenum, eg, with Z-plasty) **CPT NOTES** ♦ For frenotomy, see 40806, 41010.	750.0 Tongue tie 784.5 Speech disturbance NEC 873.64 Open wound of tongue/mouth floor 873.74 Open wound of tongue, complicated V51 Aftercare w/plastic surgery **REIMBURSEMENT INFORMATION** Medicare ♦ Follow–up Days — 90 ♦ Assistant Surgeon — by report ♦ Supply Charges — not allowed ♦ Outpatient Limit — does not apply ♦ Major Surgery Rules Apply

CPT CODE	SERVICE	ICD-9-CM
41599	Unlisted procedure, tongue, floor of mouth	141.0 M-Neoplasm, Tongue base 141.9 M-Neoplasm, Tongue NOS 750.0 Tongue tie

REIMBURSEMENT INFORMATION

Medicare

- ♦ Follow–up Days — determined by local carrier
- ♦ Assistant Surgeon — not paid
- ♦ Supply Charges — not allowed
- ♦ Outpatient Limit — does not apply

CPT CODE	SERVICE	ICD-9-CM
41800*	Drainage of abscess, cyst, hematoma from dentoalveolar structures	522.0 Pulpitis 522.5 Periapical abscess w/o sinus 522.7 Periapical abscess w/sinus 522.8 Radicular cyst 523.3 Acute periodontitis 526.0 Developmental odontogenic cysts 526.4 Inflammation of jaw 527.3 Salivary gland abscess 527.6 Salivary gland mucocele 528.3 Cellulitis/abscess of mouth 528.4 Oral soft tissue cyst 528.5 Diseases of lips 873.62 Open wound of gum 873.72 Open wound of gum, complicated

REIMBURSEMENT INFORMATION

General

- ♦ Starred procedure.

Medicare

- ♦ Follow–up Days — 10
- ♦ Assistant Surgeon — not paid
- ♦ Supply Charges — not allowed
- ♦ Outpatient Limit — does not apply
- ♦ Minor Surgery Rules Apply

CPT CODE	SERVICE	ICD-9-CM
41805	Removal of embedded foreign body from dentoalveolar structures; soft tissues	873.79 Open wound of mouth NEC, complic 935.0 Foreign body in mouth

REIMBURSEMENT INFORMATION

Medicare

- ♦ Follow–up Days — 10
- ♦ Assistant Surgeon — not paid
- ♦ Supply Charges — not allowed
- ♦ Outpatient Limit — does not apply
- ♦ Minor Surgery Rules Apply

CPT CODE	SERVICE	ICD–9–CM
41806	Removal of embedded foreign body from dentoalveolar structures; bone	873.79 Open wound of mouth NEC, complic 935.0 Foreign body in mouth **REIMBURSEMENT INFORMATION** Medicare ♦ Follow–up Days — 10 ♦ Assistant Surgeon — not paid ♦ Supply Charges — not allowed ♦ Outpatient Limit — does not apply ♦ Minor Surgery Rules Apply
41820	Gingivectomy, excision gingiva, each quadrant	523.1 Chronic gingivitis 523.9 Gingival/periodontal disease NOS **REIMBURSEMENT INFORMATION** Medicare ♦ Follow–up Days — global concept does not apply ♦ Assistant Surgeon — by report ♦ Supply Charges — not allowed ♦ Outpatient Limit — does not apply
41821	Operculectomy, excision pericoronal tissues	523.1 Chronic gingivitis 523.3 Acute periodontitis 523.4 Chronic periodontitis 523.5 Periodontosis 528.6 Leukoplakia of oral mucosa/tongue 528.9 Oral soft tissue disease NEC **REIMBURSEMENT INFORMATION** Medicare ♦ Follow–up Days — global concept does not apply ♦ Assistant Surgeon — by report ♦ Supply Charges — not allowed ♦ Outpatient Limit — does not apply

CPT CODE	SERVICE	ICD–9–CM	
41822	Excision of fibrous tuberosities, dentoalveolar structures	170.0	M-Neoplasm, Skull/Face bone
		170.1	M-Neoplasm, Mandible
		210.4	B-Neoplasm, Mouth NEC/NOS
		213.0	B-Neoplasm, Skull/Face bone
		213.1	B-Neoplasm, Lower jaw bone
		523.9	Gingival/periodontal disease NOS
		525.2	Atrophy, edentulous alveolar ridge
		526.0	Developmental odontogenic cysts
		528.7	Oral epithelium disturbance NEC
		528.9	Oral soft tissue disease NEC

REIMBURSEMENT INFORMATION

Medicare

- Follow–up Days — global concept does not apply
- Assistant Surgeon — by report
- Supply Charges — not allowed
- Outpatient Limit — does not apply

CPT CODE	SERVICE	ICD–9–CM	
41823	Excision of osseous tuberosities, dentoalveolar structures	170.0	M-Neoplasm, Skull/Face bone
		170.1	M-Neoplasm, Mandible
		213.0	B-Neoplasm, Skull/Face bone
		213.1	B-Neoplasm, Lower jaw bone
		523.3	Acute periodontitis
		523.4	Chronic periodontitis
		523.5	Periodontosis
		523.9	Gingival/periodontal disease NOS
		526.81	Exostosis of jaw

REIMBURSEMENT INFORMATION

Medicare

- Follow–up Days — global concept does not apply
- Assistant Surgeon — by report
- Supply Charges — not allowed
- Outpatient Limit — does not apply

CPT CODE	SERVICE	ICD–9–CM
41825	Excision of lesion or tumor (except listed above), dentoalveolar structures; without repair **CPT RULES** ♦ For nonexcisional destruction, see 41850.	145.9 M-Neoplasm, Mouth NOS 210.4 B-Neoplasm, Mouth NEC/NOS 230.0 CA in situ, Oral cavity/pharynx 235.1 UB-Neoplasm, Oral cavity/pharynx 522.5 Periapical abscess w/o sinus 522.7 Periapical abscess w/sinus 522.8 Radicular cyst 523.1 Chronic gingivitis 523.5 Periodontosis 526.0 Developmental odontogenic cysts 527.6 Salivary gland mucocele 528.0 Stomatitis 528.4 Oral soft tissue cyst 528.6 Leukoplakia of oral mucosa/tongue 528.7 Oral epithelium disturbance NEC 528.9 Oral soft tissue disease NEC **REIMBURSEMENT INFORMATION** <u>Medicare</u> ♦ Follow–up Days — 10 ♦ Assistant Surgeon — not paid ♦ Supply Charges — not allowed ♦ Outpatient Limit — does not apply ♦ Minor Surgery Rules Apply
41826	Excision of lesion or tumor (except listed above), dentoalveolar structures; with simple repair **CPT RULES** ♦ For nonexcisional destruction, see 41850.	145.9 M-Neoplasm, Mouth NOS 210.4 B-Neoplasm, Mouth NEC/NOS 230.0 CA in situ, Oral cavity/pharynx 235.1 UB-Neoplasm, Oral cavity/pharynx 522.5 Periapical abscess w/o sinus 522.7 Periapical abscess w/sinus 522.8 Radicular cyst 523.5 Periodontosis 523.9 Gingival/periodontal disease NOS 524.3 Tooth position anomaly 526.0 Developmental odontogenic cysts 527.6 Salivary gland mucocele 528.4 Oral soft tissue cyst 528.6 Leukoplakia of oral mucosa/tongue 528.7 Oral epithelium disturbance NEC 528.9 Oral soft tissue disease NEC **REIMBURSEMENT INFORMATION** <u>Medicare</u> ♦ Follow–up Days — 10 ♦ Assistant Surgeon — not paid ♦ Supply Charges — not allowed ♦ Outpatient Limit — does not apply ♦ Minor Surgery Rules Apply

CPT CODE **SERVICE**

41827 Excision of lesion or tumor (except listed above), dentoalveolar structures; with complex repair

CPT RULES

- For nonexcisional destruction, see 41850.

ICD–9–CM

145.9	M-Neoplasm, Mouth NOS
210.4	B-Neoplasm, Mouth NEC/NOS
230.0	CA in situ, Oral cavity/pharynx
235.1	UB-Neoplasm, Oral cavity/pharynx
522.5	Periapical abscess w/o sinus
522.7	Periapical abscess w/sinus
522.8	Radicular cyst
526.0	Developmental odontogenic cysts
527.6	Salivary gland mucocele
528.4	Oral soft tissue cyst
528.6	Leukoplakia of oral mucosa/tongue
528.7	Oral epithelium disturbance NEC
528.9	Oral soft tissue disease NEC

REIMBURSEMENT INFORMATION

Medicare

- Follow–up Days — 90
- Assistant Surgeon — not paid
- Supply Charges — not allowed
- Outpatient Limit — does not apply
- Major Surgery Rules Apply

CPT CODE	SERVICE
▲ 41828	Excision of hyperplastic alveolar mucosa, each quadrant (specify)

ICD–9–CM

141.0	M-Neoplasm, Tongue base
141.3	M-Neoplasm, Tongue ventral surface
144.8	M-Neoplasm, Floor of mouth NEC
145.8	M-Neoplasm, Mouth NEC
145.9	M-Neoplasm, Mouth NOS
210.4	B-Neoplasm, Mouth NEC/NOS
213.0	B-Neoplasm, Skull/Face bone
213.1	B-Neoplasm, Lower jaw bone
523.3	Acute periodontitis
523.4	Chronic periodontitis
523.5	Periodontosis
523.9	Gingival/periodontal disease NOS
524.0	Major anomaly of jaw size
524.00	Anomaly of jaw size NOS
524.01	Maxillary hyperplasia
524.02	Mandibular hyperplasia
524.03	Maxillary hypoplasia
524.04	Mandibular hypoplasia
524.05	Macrogenia
524.06	Microgenia
524.09	Anomaly of jaw size NEC
524.3	Tooth position anomaly
525.2	Atrophy, edentulous alveolar ridge
526.81	Exostosis of jaw
528.6	Leukoplakia of oral mucosa/tongue
528.9	Oral soft tissue disease NEC

REIMBURSEMENT INFORMATION

General

- Description changed in 1995 CPT.

Medicare

- Follow–up Days — global concept does not apply
- Assistant Surgeon — not paid
- Supply Charges — not allowed
- Outpatient Limit — does not apply

CPT CODE	SERVICE	ICD–9–CM

41830 Alveolectomy, including curettage of osteitis or sequestrectomy

526.4	Inflammation of jaw
526.81	Exostosis of jaw
990	Effects of radiation NOS
V10.02	Hx of oral/pharynx malignancy NEC

REIMBURSEMENT INFORMATION

Medicare

- ♦ Follow–up Days — global concept does not apply
- ♦ Assistant Surgeon — by report
- ♦ Supply Charges — not allowed
- ♦ Outpatient Limit — does not apply

41850 Destruction of lesion (except excision), dentoalveolar structures

210.3	B-Neoplasm, Floor of mouth
210.4	B-Neoplasm, Mouth NEC/NOS
230.0	CA in situ, Oral cavity/pharynx
235.1	UB-Neoplasm, Oral cavity/pharynx

REIMBURSEMENT INFORMATION

Medicare

- ♦ Follow–up Days — global concept does not apply
- ♦ Assistant Surgeon — by report
- ♦ Supply Charges — not allowed
- ♦ Outpatient Limit — does not apply

41870 Periodontal mucosal grafting

523.1	Chronic gingivitis
523.3	Acute periodontitis
523.4	Chronic periodontitis
523.5	Periodontosis
528.6	Leukoplakia of oral mucosa/tongue
528.9	Oral soft tissue disease NEC

REIMBURSEMENT INFORMATION

Medicare

- ♦ Follow–up Days — global concept does not apply
- ♦ Assistant Surgeon — by report
- ♦ Supply Charges — not allowed
- ♦ Outpatient Limit — does not apply

CPT CODE	SERVICE
▲ **41872**	Gingivoplasty, each quadrant (specify)

ICD–9–CM

523.1	Chronic gingivitis
523.3	Acute periodontitis
523.4	Chronic periodontitis
523.5	Periodontosis
523.9	Gingival/periodontal disease NOS

REIMBURSEMENT INFORMATION

General

- ♦ Description changed in 1995 CPT.

Medicare

- ♦ Follow–up Days — global concept does not apply
- ♦ Assistant Surgeon — by report
- ♦ Supply Charges — not allowed
- ♦ Outpatient Limit — does not apply

CPT CODE **SERVICE**

▲ **41874** Alveoplasty, each quadrant (specify)

CPT NOTES

- For closure of lacerations, see 40830, 40831.
- For segmental osteotomy, see 21206.
- For reduction of fractures, see 21421–21490.

ICD–9–CM

141.0	M-Neoplasm, Tongue base
141.3	M-Neoplasm, Tongue ventral surface
144.8	M-Neoplasm, Floor of mouth NEC
145.9	M-Neoplasm, Mouth NOS
213.0	B-Neoplasm, Skull/Face bone
213.1	B-Neoplasm, Lower jaw bone
523.3	Acute periodontitis
523.4	Chronic periodontitis
523.5	Periodontosis
523.9	Gingival/periodontal disease NOS
524.0	Major anomaly of jaw size
524.00	Anomaly of jaw size NOS
524.01	Maxillary hyperplasia
524.02	Mandibular hyperplasia
524.03	Maxillary hypoplasia
524.04	Mandibular hypoplasia
524.05	Macrogenia
524.06	Microgenia
524.09	Anomaly of jaw size NEC
524.3	Tooth position anomaly
525.2	Atrophy, edentulous alveolar ridge
526.4	Inflammation of jaw
526.81	Exostosis of jaw

REIMBURSEMENT INFORMATION

General

- Description changed in 1995 CPT.

Medicare

- Follow–up Days — global concept does not apply
- Assistant Surgeon — by report
- Supply Charges — not allowed
- Outpatient Limit — does not apply

CPT CODE	SERVICE
41899	Unlisted procedure, dentoalveolar structures

ICD–9–CM

141.0	M-Neoplasm, Tongue base
144.8	M-Neoplasm, Floor of mouth NEC
145.2	M-Neoplasm, Hard palate
145.9	M-Neoplasm, Mouth NOS
195.0	M-Neoplasm, Head/face/neck
213.1	B-Neoplasm, Lower jaw bone
473.0	Chronic maxillary sinusitis
520.6	Tooth eruption disturbances
520.7	Teething syndrome
524.3	Tooth position anomaly
525.2	Atrophy, edentulous alveolar ridge
526.4	Inflammation of jaw
526.8	Jaw disease
526.81	Exostosis of jaw
528.6	Leukoplakia of oral mucosa/tongue
528.9	Oral soft tissue disease NEC
749.2	Cleft palate w/cleft lip
873.61	Open wound of buccal mucosa
873.62	Open wound of gum

REIMBURSEMENT INFORMATION

Medicare

- ♦ Follow–up Days — determined by local carrier
- ♦ Assistant Surgeon — determined by local carrier
- ♦ Supply Charges — determined by local carrier
- ♦ Outpatient Limit — determined by local carrier

CPT CODE	SERVICE	ICD–9–CM
42000*	Drainage of abscess of palate, uvula	034.0 Streptococcal sore throat 475 Peritonsillar abscess 526.4 Inflammation of jaw 528.3 Cellulitis/abscess of mouth

REIMBURSEMENT INFORMATION

General

- ♦ Starred procedure.

Medicare

- ♦ Follow–up Days — 10
- ♦ Assistant Surgeon — not paid
- ♦ Supply Charges — not allowed
- ♦ Outpatient Limit — does not apply
- ♦ Minor Surgery Rules Apply

CPT CODE	SERVICE	ICD–9–CM
42100	Biopsy of palate, uvula	145.2 M-Neoplasm, Hard palate 145.3 M-Neoplasm, Soft palate 145.4 M-Neoplasm, Uvula 145.5 M-Neoplasm, Palate NOS 210.4 B-Neoplasm, Mouth NEC/NOS 230.0 CA in situ, Oral cavity/pharynx 235.1 UB-Neoplasm, Oral cavity/pharynx 522.7 Periapical abscess w/sinus 523.9 Gingival/periodontal disease NOS 527.2 Sialoadenitis 528.0 Stomatitis 528.4 Oral soft tissue cyst 528.6 Leukoplakia of oral mucosa/tongue 528.7 Oral epithelium disturbance NEC 528.9 Oral soft tissue disease NEC

REIMBURSEMENT INFORMATION

Medicare

- ♦ Follow–up Days — 10
- ♦ Assistant Surgeon — not paid
- ♦ Supply Charges — not allowed
- ♦ Outpatient Limit — applies
- ♦ Minor Surgery Rules Apply

CPT CODE	SERVICE	ICD–9–CM

42104 Excision, lesion of palate, uvula; without closure

CPT NOTES

- ♦ For skin graft, see 14040–14300.
- ♦ For mucosal graft, see 40818.

145.2	M-Neoplasm, Hard palate
145.3	M-Neoplasm, Soft palate
145.4	M-Neoplasm, Uvula
145.5	M-Neoplasm, Palate NOS
210.4	B-Neoplasm, Mouth NEC/NOS
230.0	CA in situ, Oral cavity/pharynx
235.1	UB-Neoplasm, Oral cavity/pharynx
528.6	Leukoplakia of oral mucosa/tongue
528.7	Oral epithelium disturbance NEC
528.9	Oral soft tissue disease NEC

REIMBURSEMENT INFORMATION

Medicare

- ♦ Follow–up Days — 10
- ♦ Assistant Surgeon — not paid
- ♦ Supply Charges — not allowed
- ♦ Outpatient Limit — does not apply
- ♦ Minor Surgery Rules Apply

42106 Excision, lesion of palate, uvula; with simple primary closure

CPT NOTES

- ♦ For skin graft, see 14040–14300.
- ♦ For mucosal graft, see 40818.

145.2	M-Neoplasm, Hard palate
145.3	M-Neoplasm, Soft palate
145.4	M-Neoplasm, Uvula
145.5	M-Neoplasm, Palate NOS
210.4	B-Neoplasm, Mouth NEC/NOS
230.0	CA in situ, Oral cavity/pharynx
235.1	UB-Neoplasm, Oral cavity/pharynx
527.2	Sialoadenitis
527.7	Salivary secretion disturbance
528.6	Leukoplakia of oral mucosa/tongue
528.7	Oral epithelium disturbance NEC
528.9	Oral soft tissue disease NEC

REIMBURSEMENT INFORMATION

Medicare

- ♦ Follow–up Days — 10
- ♦ Assistant Surgeon — not paid
- ♦ Supply Charges — not allowed
- ♦ Outpatient Limit — does not apply
- ♦ Minor Surgery Rules Apply

CPT CODE	SERVICE	ICD–9–CM

42107 Excision, lesion of palate, uvula; with local flap closure

CPT NOTES

- For skin graft, see 14040–14300.
- For mucosal graft, see 40818.

145.2	M-Neoplasm, Hard palate
145.3	M-Neoplasm, Soft palate
145.4	M-Neoplasm, Uvula
145.5	M-Neoplasm, Palate NOS
210.4	B-Neoplasm, Mouth NEC/NOS
230.0	CA in situ, Oral cavity/pharynx
235.1	UB-Neoplasm, Oral cavity/pharynx
528.7	Oral epithelium disturbance NEC
528.9	Oral soft tissue disease NEC

REIMBURSEMENT INFORMATION

Medicare

- Follow–up Days — 90
- Assistant Surgeon — not paid
- Supply Charges — not allowed
- Outpatient Limit — does not apply
- Major Surgery Rules Apply

42120 Resection of palate or extensive resection of lesion

CPT NOTES

- For reconstruction of palate with extraoral tissue, see 14040–14300, 15050, 15120, 15240, 15576.

145.2	M-Neoplasm, Hard palate
145.3	M-Neoplasm, Soft palate
145.4	M-Neoplasm, Uvula
145.5	M-Neoplasm, Palate NOS
210.4	B-Neoplasm, Mouth NEC/NOS
230.0	CA in situ, Oral cavity/pharynx
235.1	UB-Neoplasm, Oral cavity/pharynx
528.7	Oral epithelium disturbance NEC
528.9	Oral soft tissue disease NEC

REIMBURSEMENT INFORMATION

Medicare

- Follow–up Days — 90
- Assistant Surgeon — paid
- Supply Charges — not allowed
- Outpatient Limit — does not apply
- Major Surgery Rules Apply

CPT CODE	SERVICE	ICD–9–CM
42140	Uvulectomy, excision of uvula	145.4 M-Neoplasm, Uvula 210.4 B-Neoplasm, Mouth NEC/NOS 230.0 CA in situ, Oral cavity/pharynx 528.7 Oral epithelium disturbance NEC 528.9 Oral soft tissue disease NEC 780.57 Sleep apnea NOS 786.09 Respiratory abnormality NEC **REIMBURSEMENT INFORMATION** Medicare ♦ Follow–up Days — 90 ♦ Assistant Surgeon — not paid ♦ Supply Charges — not allowed ♦ Outpatient Limit — does not apply ♦ Major Surgery Rules Apply
42145	Palatopharyngoplasty (eg, uvulopalatopharyngoplasty, uvulopharyngoplasty)	145.2 M-Neoplasm, Hard palate 145.3 M-Neoplasm, Soft palate 145.4 M-Neoplasm, Uvula 145.5 M-Neoplasm, Palate NOS 780.57 Sleep apnea NOS 786.09 Respiratory abnormality NEC **REIMBURSEMENT INFORMATION** Medicare ♦ Follow–up Days — 90 ♦ Assistant Surgeon — not paid ♦ Supply Charges — not allowed ♦ Outpatient Limit — does not apply ♦ Major Surgery Rules Apply
42180	Repair, laceration of palate; up to 2 cm	873.65 Open wound of palate 873.75 Open wound of palate, complicated **REIMBURSEMENT INFORMATION** Medicare ♦ Follow–up Days — 10 ♦ Assistant Surgeon — by report ♦ Supply Charges — not allowed ♦ Outpatient Limit — does not apply ♦ Minor Surgery Rules Apply

CPT CODE	SERVICE	ICD–9–CM
42182	Repair, laceration of palate, over 2 cm or complex	873.65 Open wound of palate 873.75 Open wound of palate, complicated **REIMBURSEMENT INFORMATION** Medicare ♦ Follow–up Days — 10 ♦ Assistant Surgeon — by report ♦ Supply Charges — not allowed ♦ Outpatient Limit — does not apply ♦ Minor Surgery Rules Apply
42200	Palatoplasty for cleft palate, soft and/or hard palate only	749.00 Cleft palate NOS 749.01 Unilateral cleft palate, complete 749.02 Unilateral cleft palate, incomplete 749.03 Bilateral cleft palate, complete 749.04 Bilateral cleft palate, incomplete 749.20 Cleft palate w/cleft lip NOS 749.21 Unilat cleft palate/lip, complete 749.22 Unilat cleft palate/lip, incomplete 749.23 Bilat cleft palate/lip, complete 749.24 Bilat cleft palate/lip, incomplete **REIMBURSEMENT INFORMATION** Medicare ♦ Follow–up Days — 90 ♦ Assistant Surgeon — paid ♦ Supply Charges — not allowed ♦ Outpatient Limit — does not apply ♦ Major Surgery Rules Apply
42205	Palatoplasty for cleft palate, with closure of alveolar ridge; soft tissue only	749.00 Cleft palate NOS 749.01 Unilateral cleft palate, complete 749.02 Unilateral cleft palate, incomplete 749.03 Bilateral cleft palate, complete 749.04 Bilateral cleft palate, incomplete 749.20 Cleft palate w/cleft lip NOS 749.21 Unilat cleft palate/lip, complete 749.22 Unilat cleft palate/lip, incomplete 749.23 Bilat cleft palate/lip, complete 749.24 Bilat cleft palate/lip, incomplete **REIMBURSEMENT INFORMATION** Medicare ♦ Follow–up Days — 90 ♦ Assistant Surgeon — paid ♦ Supply Charges — not allowed ♦ Outpatient Limit — does not apply ♦ Major Surgery Rules Apply

CPT CODE	SERVICE	ICD–9–CM
42210	Palatoplasty for cleft palate, with closure of alveolar ridge; with bone graft to alveolar ridge (includes obtaining graft)	749.00 Cleft palate NOS 749.01 Unilateral cleft palate, complete 749.02 Unilateral cleft palate, incomplete 749.03 Bilateral cleft palate, complete 749.04 Bilateral cleft palate, incomplete 749.20 Cleft palate w/cleft lip NOS 749.21 Unilat cleft palate/lip, complete 749.22 Unilat cleft palate/lip, incomplete 749.23 Bilat cleft palate/lip, complete 749.24 Bilat cleft palate/lip, incomplete **REIMBURSEMENT INFORMATION** Medicare ♦ Follow–up Days — 90 ♦ Assistant Surgeon — paid ♦ Supply Charges — not allowed ♦ Outpatient Limit — does not apply ♦ Major Surgery Rules Apply
42215	Palatoplasty for cleft palate; major revision	749.00 Cleft palate NOS 749.01 Unilateral cleft palate, complete 749.02 Unilateral cleft palate, incomplete 749.03 Bilateral cleft palate, complete 749.04 Bilateral cleft palate, incomplete 749.20 Cleft palate w/cleft lip NOS 749.21 Unilat cleft palate/lip, complete 749.22 Unilat cleft palate/lip, incomplete 749.23 Bilat cleft palate/lip, complete 749.24 Bilat cleft palate/lip, incomplete **REIMBURSEMENT INFORMATION** Medicare ♦ Follow–up Days — 90 ♦ Assistant Surgeon — paid ♦ Supply Charges — not allowed ♦ Outpatient Limit — does not apply ♦ Major Surgery Rules Apply

CPT CODE	SERVICE	ICD-9-CM
42220	Palatoplasty for cleft palate; secondary lengthening procedure	749.00 Cleft palate NOS 749.01 Unilateral cleft palate, complete 749.02 Unilateral cleft palate, incomplete 749.03 Bilateral cleft palate, complete 749.04 Bilateral cleft palate, incomplete 749.20 Cleft palate w/cleft lip NOS 749.21 Unilat cleft palate/lip, complete 749.22 Unilat cleft palate/lip, incomplete 749.23 Bilat cleft palate/lip, complete 749.24 Bilat cleft palate/lip, incomplete **REIMBURSEMENT INFORMATION** Medicare ♦ Follow–up Days — 90 ♦ Assistant Surgeon — paid ♦ Supply Charges — not allowed ♦ Outpatient Limit — does not apply ♦ Major Surgery Rules Apply
42225	Palatoplasty for cleft palate; attachment pharyngeal flap	749.00 Cleft palate NOS 749.01 Unilateral cleft palate, complete 749.02 Unilateral cleft palate, incomplete 749.03 Bilateral cleft palate, complete 749.04 Bilateral cleft palate, incomplete 749.20 Cleft palate w/cleft lip NOS 749.21 Unilat cleft palate/lip, complete 749.22 Unilat cleft palate/lip, incomplete 749.23 Bilat cleft palate/lip, complete 749.24 Bilat cleft palate/lip, incomplete **REIMBURSEMENT INFORMATION** Medicare ♦ Follow–up Days — 90 ♦ Assistant Surgeon — paid ♦ Supply Charges — not allowed ♦ Outpatient Limit — does not apply ♦ Major Surgery Rules Apply
42226	Lengthening of palate, and pharyngeal flap	749.00 Cleft palate NOS **REIMBURSEMENT INFORMATION** Medicare ♦ Follow–up Days — 90 ♦ Assistant Surgeon — paid ♦ Supply Charges — not allowed ♦ Outpatient Limit — does not apply ♦ Major Surgery Rules Apply

CPT CODE	SERVICE	ICD–9–CM

42227 Lengthening of palate, with island flap

749.00 Cleft palate NOS
749.01 Unilateral cleft palate, complete
749.02 Unilateral cleft palate, incomplete
749.03 Bilateral cleft palate, complete
749.04 Bilateral cleft palate, incomplete
749.20 Cleft palate w/cleft lip NOS
749.21 Unilat cleft palate/lip, complete
749.22 Unilat cleft palate/lip, incomplete
749.23 Bilat cleft palate/lip, complete
749.24 Bilat cleft palate/lip, incomplete

REIMBURSEMENT INFORMATION

Medicare

- Follow–up Days — 90
- Assistant Surgeon — paid
- Supply Charges — not allowed
- Outpatient Limit — does not apply
- Major Surgery Rules Apply

42235 Repair of anterior palate, including vomer flap

749.00 Cleft palate NOS
749.01 Unilateral cleft palate, complete
749.02 Unilateral cleft palate, incomplete
749.03 Bilateral cleft palate, complete
749.04 Bilateral cleft palate, incomplete
749.20 Cleft palate w/cleft lip NOS
749.21 Unilat cleft palate/lip, complete
749.22 Unilat cleft palate/lip, incomplete
749.23 Bilat cleft palate/lip, complete
749.24 Bilat cleft palate/lip, incomplete
873.65 Open wound of palate
873.75 Open wound of palate, complicated

REIMBURSEMENT INFORMATION

Medicare

- Follow–up Days — 90
- Assistant Surgeon — paid
- Supply Charges — not allowed
- Outpatient Limit — does not apply
- Major Surgery Rules Apply

CPT CODE	SERVICE	ICD-9-CM
42260	Repair of nasolabial fistula	528.5 Diseases of lips 749.00 Cleft palate NOS 750.25 Congenital fistula, lip

CPT NOTES

- For repair of cleft lip, see 40700 et seq.

REIMBURSEMENT INFORMATION

Medicare

- Follow-up Days — 90
- Assistant Surgeon — paid
- Supply Charges — not allowed
- Outpatient Limit — does not apply
- Major Surgery Rules Apply

42280 Maxillary impression for palatal prosthesis

145.5	M-Neoplasm, Palate NOS
160.2	M-Neoplasm, Maxillary sinus
524.00	Anomaly of jaw size NOS
524.01	Maxillary hyperplasia
524.02	Mandibular hyperplasia
524.03	Maxillary hypoplasia
524.04	Mandibular hypoplasia
524.05	Macrogenia
524.06	Microgenia
524.09	Anomaly of jaw size NEC
524.3	Tooth position anomaly
749.00	Cleft palate NOS
749.01	Unilateral cleft palate, complete
749.02	Unilateral cleft palate, incomplete
749.03	Bilateral cleft palate, complete
749.04	Bilateral cleft palate, incomplete
749.20	Cleft palate w/cleft lip NOS
749.21	Unilat cleft palate/lip, complete
749.22	Unilat cleft palate/lip, incomplete
749.23	Bilat cleft palate/lip, complete
749.24	Bilat cleft palate/lip, incomplete
749.25	Cleft palate w/cleft lip NEC

REIMBURSEMENT INFORMATION

Medicare

- Follow-up Days — 10
- Assistant Surgeon — by report
- Supply Charges — not allowed
- Outpatient Limit — does not apply
- Minor Surgery Rules Apply

CPT CODE	SERVICE	ICD-9-CM
42281	Insertion of pin-retained palatal prosthesis	145.5 M-Neoplasm, Palate NOS 160.2 M-Neoplasm, Maxillary sinus 524.0 Major anomaly of jaw size 524.00 Anomaly of jaw size NOS 524.01 Maxillary hyperplasia 524.02 Mandibular hyperplasia 524.03 Maxillary hypoplasia 524.04 Mandibular hypoplasia 524.05 Macrogenia 524.06 Microgenia 524.09 Anomaly of jaw size NEC 524.3 Tooth position anomaly 749.00 Cleft palate NOS 749.01 Unilateral cleft palate, complete 749.02 Unilateral cleft palate, incomplete 749.03 Bilateral cleft palate, complete 749.04 Bilateral cleft palate, incomplete 749.20 Cleft palate w/cleft lip NOS 749.21 Unilat cleft palate/lip, complete 749.22 Unilat cleft palate/lip, incomplete 749.23 Bilat cleft palate/lip, complete 749.24 Bilat cleft palate/lip, incomplete 749.25 Cleft palate w/cleft lip NEC **REIMBURSEMENT INFORMATION** <u>Medicare</u> ♦ Follow-up Days — 10 ♦ Assistant Surgeon — by report ♦ Supply Charges — not allowed ♦ Outpatient Limit — does not apply ♦ Minor Surgery Rules Apply
42300*	Drainage of abscess; parotid, simple	527.3 Salivary gland abscess 528.3 Cellulitis/abscess of mouth **REIMBURSEMENT INFORMATION** <u>General</u> ♦ Starred procedure. <u>Medicare</u> ♦ Follow-up Days — 10 ♦ Assistant Surgeon — not paid ♦ Supply Charges — not allowed ♦ Outpatient Limit — does not apply ♦ Minor Surgery Rules Apply

CPT CODE	SERVICE	ICD-9-CM
42005	Drainage of abscess; parotid, complicated	527.3 Salivary gland abscess 528.3 Cellulitis/abscess of mouth **REIMBURSEMENT INFORMATION** Medicare ♦ Follow-up Days — 90 ♦ Assistant Surgeon — not paid ♦ Supply Charges — not allowed ♦ Outpatient Limit — does not apply ♦ Major Surgery Rules Apply
42310*	Drainage of abscess; submaxillary or sublingual, intraoral	527.3 Salivary gland abscess 528.3 Cellulitis/abscess of mouth 528.9 Oral soft tissue disease NEC **REIMBURSEMENT INFORMATION** General ♦ Starred procedure. Medicare ♦ Follow-up Days — 10 ♦ Assistant Surgeon — not paid ♦ Supply Charges — not allowed ♦ Outpatient Limit — does not apply ♦ Minor Surgery Rules Apply
42320*	Drainage of abscess; submaxillary, external	527.3 Salivary gland abscess **REIMBURSEMENT INFORMATION** General ♦ Starred procedure. Medicare ♦ Follow-up Days — 10 ♦ Assistant Surgeon — by report ♦ Supply Charges — not allowed ♦ Outpatient Limit — does not apply ♦ Minor Surgery Rules Apply

CPT CODE	SERVICE	ICD–9–CM
42325	Fistulization of sublingual salivary cyst (ranula)	527.6 Salivary gland mucocele **REIMBURSEMENT INFORMATION** Medicare ♦ Follow–up Days — 90 ♦ Assistant Surgeon — paid ♦ Supply Charges — not allowed ♦ Outpatient Limit — does not apply ♦ Major Surgery Rules Apply
42326	Fistulization of sublingual salivary cyst (ranula); with prothesis	527.6 Salivary gland mucocele **REIMBURSEMENT INFORMATION** Medicare ♦ Follow–up Days — 90 ♦ Assistant Surgeon — paid ♦ Supply Charges — not allowed ♦ Outpatient Limit — does not apply ♦ Major Surgery Rules Apply
42330	Sialolithotomy; submandibular (submaxillary), sublingual or parotid, uncomplicated, intraoral	527.2 Sialoadenitis 527.4 Salivary gland fistula 527.5 Sialolithiasis 527.6 Salivary gland mucocele 527.8 Salivary gland disease NEC 527.9 Salivary gland disease NOS **REIMBURSEMENT INFORMATION** Medicare ♦ Follow–up Days — 10 ♦ Assistant Surgeon — not paid ♦ Supply Charges — not allowed ♦ Outpatient Limit — does not apply ♦ Minor Surgery Rules Apply

CPT CODE	SERVICE	ICD–9–CM	
42335	Sialolithotomy; submandibular (submaxillary), complicated, intraoral	527.2	Sialoadenitis
		527.4	Salivary gland fistula
		527.5	Sialolithiasis
		527.6	Salivary gland mucocele
		527.8	Salivary gland disease NEC

REIMBURSEMENT INFORMATION

Medicare

- ♦ Follow–up Days — 90
- ♦ Assistant Surgeon — not paid
- ♦ Supply Charges — not allowed
- ♦ Outpatient Limit — does not apply
- ♦ Major Surgery Rules Apply

CPT CODE	SERVICE	ICD–9–CM	
42340	Sialolithotomy; parotid, extraoral or complicated intraoral	527.2	Sialoadenitis
		527.4	Salivary gland fistula
		527.5	Sialolithiasis
		527.6	Salivary gland mucocele
		527.8	Salivary gland disease NEC

REIMBURSEMENT INFORMATION

Medicare

- ♦ Follow–up Days — 90
- ♦ Assistant Surgeon — not paid
- ♦ Supply Charges — not allowed
- ♦ Outpatient Limit — does not apply
- ♦ Major Surgery Rules Apply

CPT CODE **SERVICE**

42400* Biopsy of salivary gland; needle

ICD–9–CM

135	Sarcoidosis
142.0	M-Neoplasm, Parotid gland
142.1	M-Neoplasm, Submandibular gland
142.2	M-Neoplasm, Sublingual gland
142.8	M-Neoplasm, Major salivary glnd NEC
142.9	M-Neoplasm, Salivary gland NOS
145.1	M-Neoplasm, Mouth vestibule
198.89	M2-Neoplasm NEC
210.2	B-Neoplasm, Major salivary glands
230.0	CA in situ, Oral cavity/pharynx
235.0	UB-Neoplasm, Major salivary glands
527.1	Salivary gland hypertrophy
527.6	Salivary gland mucocele
527.8	Salivary gland disease NEC
527.9	Salivary gland disease NOS

REIMBURSEMENT INFORMATION

General

- ♦ Starred procedure.

Medicare

- ♦ Follow–up Days — 0
- ♦ Assistant Surgeon — not paid
- ♦ Supply Charges — not allowed
- ♦ Outpatient Limit — does not apply
- ♦ Minor Surgery Rules Apply

CPT CODE	SERVICE	ICD–9–CM
42405	Biopsy of salivary gland; incisional	135 Sarcoidosis 142.0 M-Neoplasm, Parotid gland 142.1 M-Neoplasm, Submandibular gland 142.2 M-Neoplasm, Sublingual gland 142.8 M-Neoplasm, Major salivary glnd NEC 142.9 M-Neoplasm, Salivary gland NOS 198.89 M2-Neoplasm NEC 210.2 B-Neoplasm, Major salivary glands 230.0 CA in situ, Oral cavity/pharynx 235.0 UB-Neoplasm, Major salivary glands 527.1 Salivary gland hypertrophy 527.5 Sialolithiasis 527.6 Salivary gland mucocele 527.8 Salivary gland disease NEC 527.9 Salivary gland disease NOS **REIMBURSEMENT INFORMATION** <u>Medicare</u> ♦ Follow–up Days — 10 ♦ Assistant Surgeon — not paid ♦ Supply Charges — not allowed ♦ Outpatient Limit — does not apply ♦ Minor Surgery Rules Apply
42408	Excision of sublingual salivary cyst (ranula)	527.6 Salivary gland mucocele **REIMBURSEMENT INFORMATION** <u>Medicare</u> ♦ Follow–up Days — 90 ♦ Assistant Surgeon — not paid ♦ Supply Charges — not allowed ♦ Outpatient Limit — does not apply ♦ Major Surgery Rules Apply
42409	Marsupialization of sublingual salivary cyst (ranula) **CPT NOTES** ♦ For fistulization of sublingual salivary cyst, see 42325.	527.4 Salivary gland fistula 527.6 Salivary gland mucocele **REIMBURSEMENT INFORMATION** <u>Medicare</u> ♦ Follow–up Days — 90 ♦ Assistant Surgeon — paid ♦ Supply Charges — not allowed ♦ Outpatient Limit — does not apply ♦ Major Surgery Rules Apply

CPT CODE	SERVICE	ICD–9–CM

42410 Excision of parotid tumor or parotid gland; lateral lobe, without nerve dissection

CPT NOTES

- For suture or grafting of facial nerve, see 64864, 64865, 69740, 69745.

142.0	M-Neoplasm, Parotid gland
198.89	M2-Neoplasm NEC
210.2	B-Neoplasm, Major salivary glands
230.0	CA in situ, Oral cavity/pharynx
235.0	UB-Neoplasm, Major salivary glands
527.1	Salivary gland hypertrophy
527.2	Sialoadenitis
527.6	Salivary gland mucocele
527.8	Salivary gland disease NEC
527.9	Salivary gland disease NOS
785.6	Enlargement of lymph nodes

REIMBURSEMENT INFORMATION

Medicare

- Follow–up Days — 90
- Assistant Surgeon — paid
- Supply Charges — not allowed
- Outpatient Limit — does not apply
- Major Surgery Rules Apply

42415 Excision of parotid tumor or parotid gland; lateral lobe, with dissection and preservation of facial nerve

CPT NOTES

- For suture or grafting of facial nerve, see 64864, 64865, 69740, 69745.

142.0	M-Neoplasm, Parotid gland
198.89	M2-Neoplasm NEC
210.2	B-Neoplasm, Major salivary glands
230.0	CA in situ, Oral cavity/pharynx
235.0	UB-Neoplasm, Major salivary glands
527.1	Salivary gland hypertrophy
527.2	Sialoadenitis
527.6	Salivary gland mucocele
527.8	Salivary gland disease NEC
527.9	Salivary gland disease NOS
785.6	Enlargement of lymph nodes

REIMBURSEMENT INFORMATION

Medicare

- Follow–up Days — 90
- Assistant Surgeon — paid
- Supply Charges — not allowed
- Outpatient Limit — does not apply
- Major Surgery Rules Apply

CPT CODE **SERVICE**

42420 Excision of parotid tumor or parotid gland; total, with dissection and preservation of facial nerve

CPT NOTES

- For suture or grafting of facial nerve, see 64864, 64865, 69740, 69745.

ICD–9–CM

142.0	M-Neoplasm, Parotid gland
198.89	M2-Neoplasm NEC
210.2	B-Neoplasm, Major salivary glands
230.0	CA in situ, Oral cavity/pharynx
234.8	CA in situ NEC
235.0	UB-Neoplasm, Major salivary glands
527.1	Salivary gland hypertrophy
527.2	Sialoadenitis
527.8	Salivary gland disease NEC
527.9	Salivary gland disease NOS
785.6	Enlargement of lymph nodes

REIMBURSEMENT INFORMATION

Medicare

- Follow–up Days — 90
- Assistant Surgeon — paid
- Supply Charges — not allowed
- Outpatient Limit — does not apply
- Major Surgery Rules Apply

42425 Excision of parotid tumor or parotid gland; total, en bloc removal with sacrifice of facial nerve

CPT NOTES

- For suture or grafting of facial nerve, see 64864, 64865, 69740, 69745.

142.0	M-Neoplasm, Parotid gland
198.89	M2-Neoplasm NEC
235.0	UB-Neoplasm, Major salivary glands
527.1	Salivary gland hypertrophy
527.2	Sialoadenitis
527.8	Salivary gland disease NEC
527.9	Salivary gland disease NOS
785.6	Enlargement of lymph nodes

REIMBURSEMENT INFORMATION

Medicare

- Follow–up Days — 90
- Assistant Surgeon — paid
- Supply Charges — not allowed
- Outpatient Limit — does not apply
- Major Surgery Rules Apply

CPT CODE	SERVICE	ICD–9–CM
42426	Excision of parotid tumor or parotid gland; total, with unilateral radical neck dissection **CPT NOTES** ♦ For suture or grafting of facial nerve, see 64864, 64865, 69740, 69745.	142.0 M-Neoplasm, Parotid gland 198.89 M2-Neoplasm NEC 234.8 CA in situ NEC 527.9 Salivary gland disease NOS **REIMBURSEMENT INFORMATION** Medicare ♦ Follow–up Days — 90 ♦ Assistant Surgeon — paid ♦ Supply Charges — not allowed ♦ Outpatient Limit — does not apply ♦ Major Surgery Rules Apply
42440	Excision of submandibular (submaxillary) gland	142.1 M-Neoplasm, Submandibular gland 210.2 B-Neoplasm, Major salivary glands 230.0 CA in situ, Oral cavity/pharynx 235.0 UB-Neoplasm, Major salivary glands 527.2 Sialoadenitis 527.5 Sialolithiasis 527.9 Salivary gland disease NOS **REIMBURSEMENT INFORMATION** Medicare ♦ Follow–up Days — 90 ♦ Assistant Surgeon — paid ♦ Supply Charges — not allowed ♦ Outpatient Limit — does not apply ♦ Major Surgery Rules Apply
42450	Excision of sublingual gland	142.1 M-Neoplasm, Submandibular gland 142.2 M-Neoplasm, Sublingual gland 210.2 B-Neoplasm, Major salivary glands 210.3 B-Neoplasm, Floor of mouth 230.0 CA in situ, Oral cavity/pharynx 235.0 UB-Neoplasm, Major salivary glands 527.6 Salivary gland mucocele 527.9 Salivary gland disease NOS **REIMBURSEMENT INFORMATION** Medicare ♦ Follow–up Days — 90 ♦ Assistant Surgeon — not paid ♦ Supply Charges — not allowed ♦ Outpatient Limit — does not apply ♦ Major Surgery Rules Apply

CPT CODE **SERVICE**

42500 Plastic repair of salivary duct, sialodochoplasty; primary or simple

ICD–9–CM

135	Sarcoidosis
142.0	M-Neoplasm, Parotid gland
142.1	M-Neoplasm, Submandibular gland
142.2	M-Neoplasm, Sublingual gland
142.8	M-Neoplasm, Major salivary glnd NEC
142.9	M-Neoplasm, Salivary gland NOS
198.89	M2-Neoplasm NEC
210.2	B-Neoplasm, Major salivary glands
235.0	UB-Neoplasm, Major salivary glands
527.1	Salivary gland hypertrophy
527.5	Sialolithiasis
527.8	Salivary gland disease NEC
527.9	Salivary gland disease NOS

REIMBURSEMENT INFORMATION

Medicare

- ♦ Follow–up Days — 90
- ♦ Assistant Surgeon — not paid
- ♦ Supply Charges — not allowed
- ♦ Outpatient Limit — does not apply
- ♦ Major Surgery Rules Apply

42505 Plastic repair of salivary duct, sialodochoplasty; secondary or complicated

135	Sarcoidosis
142.0	M-Neoplasm, Parotid gland
142.1	M-Neoplasm, Submandibular gland
142.2	M-Neoplasm, Sublingual gland
142.8	M-Neoplasm, Major salivary glnd NEC
142.9	M-Neoplasm, Salivary gland NOS
198.89	M2-Neoplasm NEC
210.2	B-Neoplasm, Major salivary glands
235.0	UB-Neoplasm, Major salivary glands
527.1	Salivary gland hypertrophy
527.5	Sialolithiasis
527.8	Salivary gland disease NEC
527.9	Salivary gland disease NOS

REIMBURSEMENT INFORMATION

Medicare

- ♦ Follow–up Days — 90
- ♦ Assistant Surgeon — paid
- ♦ Supply Charges — not allowed
- ♦ Outpatient Limit — does not apply
- ♦ Major Surgery Rules Apply

CPT CODE	SERVICE	ICD–9–CM
42507	Parotid duct diversion, bilateral (Wilke type procedure)	527.7 Salivary secretion disturbance **REIMBURSEMENT INFORMATION** Medicare ♦ Follow–up Days — 90 ♦ Assistant Surgeon — paid ♦ Supply Charges — not allowed ♦ Outpatient Limit — does not apply ♦ Major Surgery Rules Apply
42508	Parotid duct diversion, bilateral (Wilke type procedure); with excision of one submandibular gland	527.7 Salivary secretion disturbance **REIMBURSEMENT INFORMATION** Medicare ♦ Follow–up Days — 90 ♦ Assistant Surgeon — paid ♦ Supply Charges — not allowed ♦ Outpatient Limit — does not apply ♦ Major Surgery Rules Apply
42509	Parotid duct diversion, bilateral (Wilke type procedure); with excision of both submandibular glands	527.7 Salivary secretion disturbance **REIMBURSEMENT INFORMATION** Medicare ♦ Follow–up Days — 90 ♦ Assistant Surgeon — by report ♦ Supply Charges — not allowed ♦ Outpatient Limit — does not apply ♦ Major Surgery Rules Apply
42510	Parotid duct diversion, bilateral (Wilke type procedure); with ligation of both submandibular (Wharton's) ducts	527.7 Salivary secretion disturbance **REIMBURSEMENT INFORMATION** Medicare ♦ Follow–up Days — 90 ♦ Assistant Surgeon — paid ♦ Supply Charges — not allowed ♦ Outpatient Limit — does not apply ♦ Major Surgery Rules Apply

CPT CODE	SERVICE	ICD–9–CM	
42550	Injection procedure for sialography	142.1	M-Neoplasm, Submandibular gland
		142.2	M-Neoplasm, Sublingual gland
		142.8	M-Neoplasm, Major salivary glnd NEC
		142.9	M-Neoplasm, Salivary gland NOS
		210.2	B-Neoplasm, Major salivary glands
		230.0	CA in situ, Oral cavity/pharynx
		235.0	UB-Neoplasm, Major salivary glands
		527.0	Salivary gland atrophy
		527.1	Salivary gland hypertrophy
		527.2	Sialoadenitis
		527.3	Salivary gland abscess
		527.4	Salivary gland fistula
		527.5	Sialolithiasis
		527.6	Salivary gland mucocele
		527.7	Salivary secretion disturbance
		527.8	Salivary gland disease NEC
		527.9	Salivary gland disease NOS
		710.2	Sicca syndrome

CPT NOTES

- For radiological supervision and interpretation, see 70390.

REIMBURSEMENT INFORMATION

Medicare

- Follow–up Days — 0
- Assistant Surgeon — not paid
- Supply Charges — not allowed
- Outpatient Limit — does not apply
- Minor Surgery Rules Apply

CPT CODE	SERVICE	ICD–9–CM	
42600	Closure salivary fistula	527.4	Salivary gland fistula
		527.6	Salivary gland mucocele
		527.9	Salivary gland disease NOS
		873.69	Open wound of mouth NEC
		873.79	Open wound of mouth NEC, complic
		959.0	Face and neck injury NOS

REIMBURSEMENT INFORMATION

Medicare

- Follow–up Days — 90
- Assistant Surgeon — by report
- Supply Charges — not allowed
- Outpatient Limit — does not apply
- Major Surgery Rules Apply

CPT CODE	SERVICE	ICD–9–CM
42650*	Dilation salivary duct	527.2 Sialoadenitis 527.3 Salivary gland abscess 527.4 Salivary gland fistula 527.5 Sialolithiasis 527.6 Salivary gland mucocele 527.8 Salivary gland disease NEC 527.9 Salivary gland disease NOS **REIMBURSEMENT INFORMATION** General ♦ Starred procedure. Medicare ♦ Follow–up Days — 0 ♦ Assistant Surgeon — not paid ♦ Supply Charges — not allowed ♦ Outpatient Limit — applies ♦ Minor Surgery Rules Apply
42660*	Dilation and catheterization of salivary duct, with or without injection	210.2 B-Neoplasm, Major salivary glands 527.5 Sialolithiasis 527.8 Salivary gland disease NEC 527.9 Salivary gland disease NOS **REIMBURSEMENT INFORMATION** General ♦ Starred procedure. Medicare ♦ Follow–up Days — 0 ♦ Assistant Surgeon — by report ♦ Supply Charges — not allowed ♦ Outpatient Limit — does not apply ♦ Minor Surgery Rules Apply
42665	Ligation salivary duct, intraoral	527.7 Salivary secretion disturbance **REIMBURSEMENT INFORMATION** Medicare ♦ Follow–up Days — 90 ♦ Assistant Surgeon — by report ♦ Supply Charges — not allowed ♦ Outpatient Limit — does not apply ♦ Major Surgery Rules Apply

CPT CODE **SERVICE** | **ICD–9–CM**

42699 Unlisted procedure, salivary glands or ducts

210.2 B-Neoplasm, Major salivary glands
527.5 Sialolithiasis
527.6 Salivary gland mucocele

REIMBURSEMENT INFORMATION

Medicare

- Follow–up Days — determined by local carrier
- Assistant Surgeon — determined by local carrier
- Supply Charges — determined by local carrier
- Outpatient Limit — determined by local carrier

42700* Incision and drainage abscess; peritonsillar

475 Peritonsillar abscess

REIMBURSEMENT INFORMATION

General

- Starred procedure.

Medicare

- Follow–up Days — 10
- Assistant Surgeon — not paid
- Supply Charges — not allowed
- Outpatient Limit — does not apply
- Minor Surgery Rules Apply

42720 Incision and drainage abscess; retropharyngeal or parapharyngeal, intraoral approach

478.22 Parapharyngeal abscess
478.24 Retropharyngeal abscess

REIMBURSEMENT INFORMATION

Medicare

- Follow–up Days — 10
- Assistant Surgeon — not paid
- Supply Charges — not allowed
- Outpatient Limit — does not apply
- Minor Surgery Rules Apply

CPT CODE	SERVICE	ICD–9–CM
42725	Incision and drainage abscess; retropharyngeal or parapharyngeal, external approach	478.22 Parapharyngeal abscess 478.24 Retropharyngeal abscess

REIMBURSEMENT INFORMATION

Medicare

- Follow–up Days — 90
- Assistant Surgeon — paid
- Supply Charges — not allowed
- Outpatient Limit — does not apply
- Major Surgery Rules Apply

42800 Biopsy; oropharynx

CPT NOTES

- For laryngoscopic biopsy, see 31510, 31535, 31536.

141.6	M-Neoplasm, Lingual tonsil
141.9	M-Neoplasm, Tongue NOS
146.0	M-Neoplasm, Tonsil
146.1	M-Neoplasm, Tonsillar fossa
146.2	M-Neoplasm, Tonsillar pillars
146.3	M-Neoplasm, Vallecula
146.4	M-Neoplasm, Epiglottis, anterior
146.5	M-Neoplasm, Epiglottis, junctional
146.6	M-Neoplasm, Oropharynx lateral
146.7	M-Neoplasm, Oropharynx posterior
146.8	M-Neoplasm, Oropharynx NEC
149.0	M-Neoplasm, Pharynx NOS
210.1	B-Neoplasm, Tongue
210.4	B-Neoplasm, Mouth NEC/NOS
210.5	B-Neoplasm, Tonsil
210.6	B-Neoplasm, Oropharynx NEC
210.9	B-Neoplasm, Pharynx NOS
230.0	CA in situ, Oral cavity/pharynx
235.1	UB-Neoplasm, Oral cavity/pharynx
474.8	Chronic tonsil/adenoid disease NEC
478.29	Disease of pharynx NEC

REIMBURSEMENT INFORMATION

Medicare

- Follow–up Days — 10
- Assistant Surgeon — not paid
- Supply Charges — not allowed
- Outpatient Limit — applies
- Minor Surgery Rules Apply

CPT CODE **SERVICE** | **ICD–9–CM**

42802 Biopsy; hypopharynx

CPT NOTES

- For laryngoscopic biopsy, see 31510, 31535, 31536.

148.0	M-Neoplasm, Postcricoid hypopharynx
148.1	M-Neoplasm, Pyriform sinus
148.2	M-Neoplasm, Aryepiglottic fold
148.3	M-Neoplasm, Posterior hypopharynx
148.8	M-Neoplasm, Hypopharynx NEC
148.9	M-Neoplasm, Hypopharynx NOS
210.8	B-Neoplasm, Hypopharynx
478.26	Cyst of pharynx/nasopharynx

REIMBURSEMENT INFORMATION

Medicare

- Follow–up Days — 10
- Assistant Surgeon — not paid
- Supply Charges — not allowed
- Outpatient Limit — does not apply
- Minor Surgery Rules Apply

42804 Biopsy; nasopharynx, visible lesion, simple

CPT NOTES

- For laryngoscopic biopsy, see 31510, 31535, 31536.

147.0	M-Neoplasm, Nasopharynx superior
147.1	M-Neoplasm, Nasopharynx posterior
147.2	M-Neoplasm, Nasopharynx lateral
147.3	M-Neoplasm, Nasopharynx anterior
147.8	M-Neoplasm, Nasopharynx NEC
210.7	B-Neoplasm, Nasopharynx
239.8	Neoplasm NOS, site NEC
289.1	Chronic lymphadenitis
474.0	Chronic tonsillitis

REIMBURSEMENT INFORMATION

Medicare

- Follow–up Days — 10
- Assistant Surgeon — not paid
- Supply Charges — not allowed
- Outpatient Limit — does not apply
- Minor Surgery Rules Apply

42806 Biopsy; nasopharynx, survey for unknown primary lesion

CPT NOTES

- For laryngoscopic biopsy, see 31510, 31535, 31536.

147.0	M-Neoplasm, Nasopharynx superior
147.1	M-Neoplasm, Nasopharynx posterior
147.2	M-Neoplasm, Nasopharynx lateral
147.3	M-Neoplasm, Nasopharynx anterior
147.8	M-Neoplasm, Nasopharynx NEC
195.0	M-Neoplasm, Head/face/neck

REIMBURSEMENT INFORMATION

Medicare

- Follow–up Days — 10
- Assistant Surgeon — not paid
- Supply Charges — not allowed
- Outpatient Limit — does not apply
- Minor Surgery Rules Apply

CPT CODE	SERVICE	ICD–9–CM
42808	Excision or destruction of lesion of pharynx, any method	148.9 M-Neoplasm, Hypopharynx NOS 149.0 M-Neoplasm, Pharynx NOS 161.3 M-Neoplasm, Laryngeal cartilages 161.8 M-Neoplasm, Larynx NEC 210.4 B-Neoplasm, Mouth NEC/NOS 210.5 B-Neoplasm, Tonsil 210.6 B-Neoplasm, Oropharynx NEC 210.7 B-Neoplasm, Nasopharynx 210.8 B-Neoplasm, Hypopharynx 230.0 CA in situ, Oral cavity/pharynx 235.1 UB-Neoplasm, Oral cavity/pharynx 289.1 Chronic lymphadenitis **REIMBURSEMENT INFORMATION** Medicare ♦ Follow–up Days — 10 ♦ Assistant Surgeon — not paid ♦ Supply Charges — not allowed ♦ Outpatient Limit — does not apply ♦ Minor Surgery Rules Apply
42809	Removal of foreign body from pharynx	933.0 Foreign body in pharynx 938 Foreign body, digestive system NOS **REIMBURSEMENT INFORMATION** Medicare ♦ Follow–up Days — 10 ♦ Assistant Surgeon — not paid ♦ Supply Charges — not allowed ♦ Outpatient Limit — does not apply ♦ Minor Surgery Rules Apply
42810	Excision branchial cleft cyst or vestige, confined to skin and subcutaneous tissues	744.41 Branchial cleft sinus/fistula 744.42 Branchial cleft cyst **REIMBURSEMENT INFORMATION** Medicare ♦ Follow–up Days — 90 ♦ Assistant Surgeon — paid ♦ Supply Charges — not allowed ♦ Outpatient Limit — does not apply ♦ Major Surgery Rules Apply

CPT CODE	SERVICE	ICD–9–CM
42810	Excision branchial cleft cyst, vestige, or fistula, extending beneath subcutaneous tissues and/or into pharynx	744.41 Branchial cleft sinus/fistula 744.42 Branchial cleft cyst

REIMBURSEMENT INFORMATION

Medicare

- Follow–up Days — 90
- Assistant Surgeon — paid
- Supply Charges — not allowed
- Outpatient Limit — does not apply
- Major Surgery Rules Apply

42820 Tonsillectomy and adenoidectomy; under age 12

034.0	Streptococcal sore throat
463	Acute tonsillitis
474.0	Chronic tonsillitis
474.10	Hypertrophy of tonsils/adenoids
474.11	Hypertrophy of tonsils
474.12	Hypertrophy of adenoids
474.2	Adenoid vegetations
474.9	Chronic tonsil/adenoid disease NOS
475	Peritonsillar abscess
780.57	Sleep apnea NOS

REIMBURSEMENT INFORMATION

Medicare

- Follow–up Days — 90
- Assistant Surgeon — by report
- Supply Charges — not allowed
- Outpatient Limit — does not apply
- Major Surgery Rules Apply

42821 Tonsillectomy and adenoidectomy; age 12 or over

463	Acute tonsillitis
474.0	Chronic tonsillitis
474.10	Hypertrophy of tonsils/adenoids
474.11	Hypertrophy of tonsils
474.12	Hypertrophy of adenoids
474.9	Chronic tonsil/adenoid disease NOS
475	Peritonsillar abscess

REIMBURSEMENT INFORMATION

Medicare

- Follow–up Days — 90
- Assistant Surgeon — not paid
- Supply Charges — not allowed
- Outpatient Limit — does not apply
- Major Surgery Rules Apply

CPT CODE	SERVICE	ICD–9–CM
42825	Tonsillectomy, primary or secondary; under age 12	034.0 Streptococcal sore throat 463 Acute tonsillitis 474.0 Chronic tonsillitis 474.10 Hypertrophy of tonsils/adenoids 474.11 Hypertrophy of tonsils 474.12 Hypertrophy of adenoids 475 Peritonsillar abscess **REIMBURSEMENT INFORMATION** Medicare ♦ Follow–up Days — 90 ♦ Assistant Surgeon — by report ♦ Supply Charges — not allowed ♦ Outpatient Limit — does not apply ♦ Major Surgery Rules Apply
42826	Tonsillectomy, primary or secondary; age 12 or over	141.6 M-Neoplasm, Lingual tonsil 210.5 B-Neoplasm, Tonsil 235.1 UB-Neoplasm, Oral cavity/pharynx 463 Acute tonsillitis 474.0 Chronic tonsillitis 474.10 Hypertrophy of tonsils/adenoids 474.11 Hypertrophy of tonsils 474.12 Hypertrophy of adenoids 475 Peritonsillar abscess **REIMBURSEMENT INFORMATION** Medicare ♦ Follow–up Days — 90 ♦ Assistant Surgeon — not paid ♦ Supply Charges — not allowed ♦ Outpatient Limit — does not apply ♦ Major Surgery Rules Apply
42830	Adenoidectomy, primary; under age 12	474.12 Hypertrophy of adenoids 474.8 Chronic tonsil/adenoid disease NEC 474.9 Chronic tonsil/adenoid disease NOS **REIMBURSEMENT INFORMATION** Medicare ♦ Follow–up Days — 90 ♦ Assistant Surgeon — by report ♦ Supply Charges — not allowed ♦ Outpatient Limit — does not apply ♦ Major Surgery Rules Apply

CPT CODE	SERVICE	ICD–9–CM
42831	Adenoidectomy, primary; age 12 or over	474.12 Hypertrophy of adenoids 474.8 Chronic tonsil/adenoid disease NEC 474.9 Chronic tonsil/adenoid disease NOS **REIMBURSEMENT INFORMATION** Medicare ♦ Follow–up Days — 90 ♦ Assistant Surgeon — by report ♦ Supply Charges — not allowed ♦ Outpatient Limit — does not apply ♦ Major Surgery Rules Apply
42835	Adenoidectomy, secondary; under age 12	474.12 Hypertrophy of adenoids 474.9 Chronic tonsil/adenoid disease NOS **REIMBURSEMENT INFORMATION** Medicare ♦ Follow–up Days — 90 ♦ Assistant Surgeon — by report ♦ Supply Charges — not allowed ♦ Outpatient Limit — does not apply ♦ Major Surgery Rules Apply
42836	Adenoidectomy, secondary; age 12 or over	474.12 Hypertrophy of adenoids 474.9 Chronic tonsil/adenoid disease NOS **REIMBURSEMENT INFORMATION** Medicare ♦ Follow–up Days — 90 ♦ Assistant Surgeon — by report ♦ Supply Charges — not allowed ♦ Outpatient Limit — does not apply ♦ Major Surgery Rules Apply

CPT CODE **SERVICE**

42842 Radical resection of tonsil, tonsillar pillars, and/or retromolar trigone; without closure

CPT NOTES

- For closure with other flap(s), use appropriate number for flap(s).
- When combined with radical neck dissection, use also 38720.

ICD–9–CM

141.6	M-Neoplasm, Lingual tonsil
210.5	B-Neoplasm, Tonsil
235.1	UB-Neoplasm, Oral cavity/pharynx
463	Acute tonsillitis
474.0	Chronic tonsillitis
474.10	Hypertrophy of tonsils/adenoids
474.11	Hypertrophy of tonsils
474.12	Hypertrophy of adenoids
475	Peritonsillar abscess
478.26	Cyst of pharynx/nasopharynx

REIMBURSEMENT INFORMATION

Medicare

- Follow–up Days — 90
- Assistant Surgeon — not paid
- Supply Charges — not allowed
- Outpatient Limit — does not apply
- Major Surgery Rules Apply

42844 Radical resection of tonsil, tonsillar pillars, and/or retromolar trigone; closure with local flap (eg, tongue, buccal)

CPT NOTES

- For closure with other flap(s), use appropriate number for flap(s).
- When combined with radical neck dissection, use also 38720.

141.6	M-Neoplasm, Lingual tonsil
210.5	B-Neoplasm, Tonsil
235.1	UB-Neoplasm, Oral cavity/pharynx
463	Acute tonsillitis
474.0	Chronic tonsillitis
474.10	Hypertrophy of tonsils/adenoids
474.11	Hypertrophy of tonsils
474.12	Hypertrophy of adenoids
475	Peritonsillar abscess
478.26	Cyst of pharynx/nasopharynx

REIMBURSEMENT INFORMATION

Medicare

- Follow–up Days — 90
- Assistant Surgeon — paid
- Supply Charges — not allowed
- Outpatient Limit — does not apply
- Major Surgery Rules Apply

CPT CODE	SERVICE	ICD–9–CM
42845	Radical resection of tonsil, tonsillar pillars, and/or retromolar trigone; closure with other flap **CPT NOTES** ♦ For closure with other flap(s), use appropriate number for flap(s). ♦ When combined with radical neck dissection, use also 38720.	141.6 M-Neoplasm, Lingual tonsil 210.5 B-Neoplasm, Tonsil 235.1 UB-Neoplasm, Oral cavity/pharynx 463 Acute tonsillitis 474.0 Chronic tonsillitis 474.10 Hypertrophy of tonsils/adenoids 474.11 Hypertrophy of tonsils 474.12 Hypertrophy of adenoids 475 Peritonsillar abscess 478.26 Cyst of pharynx/nasopharynx **REIMBURSEMENT INFORMATION** <u>Medicare</u> ♦ Follow–up Days — 90 ♦ Assistant Surgeon — paid ♦ Supply Charges — not allowed ♦ Outpatient Limit — does not apply ♦ Major Surgery Rules Apply
42860	Excision of tonsil tags	474.0 Chronic tonsillitis **REIMBURSEMENT INFORMATION** <u>Medicare</u> ♦ Follow–up Days — 90 ♦ Assistant Surgeon — not paid ♦ Supply Charges — not allowed ♦ Outpatient Limit — does not apply ♦ Major Surgery Rules Apply
42870	Excision or destruction lingual tonsil, any method (separate procedure)	141.6 M-Neoplasm, Lingual tonsil 198.89 M2-Neoplasm NEC 210.1 B-Neoplasm, Tongue 235.1 UB-Neoplasm, Oral cavity/pharynx 463 Acute tonsillitis 474.0 Chronic tonsillitis **REIMBURSEMENT INFORMATION** <u>General</u> ♦ Separate procedure rules apply. <u>Medicare</u> ♦ Follow–up Days — 90 ♦ Assistant Surgeon — not paid ♦ Supply Charges — not allowed ♦ Outpatient Limit — does not apply ♦ Major Surgery Rules Apply

CPT CODE	SERVICE	ICD-9-CM
42880	Excision nasopharyngeal lesion (eg, fibroma) **CPT NOTES** ♦ For excision and repair of hypophanryngeal diverticulum, cervical approach, see 43130.	147.0 M-Neoplasm, Nasopharynx superior 147.1 M-Neoplasm, Nasopharynx posterior 147.2 M-Neoplasm, Nasopharynx lateral 147.3 M-Neoplasm, Nasopharynx anterior 147.8 M-Neoplasm, Nasopharynx NEC 210.7 B-Neoplasm, Nasopharynx 230.0 CA in situ, Oral cavity/pharynx 235.1 UB-Neoplasm, Oral cavity/pharynx **REIMBURSEMENT INFORMATION** Medicare ♦ Follow-up Days — 90 ♦ Assistant Surgeon — not paid ♦ Supply Charges — not allowed ♦ Outpatient Limit — does not apply ♦ Major Surgery Rules Apply
42890	Limited pharyngectomy	141.0 M-Neoplasm, Tongue base 149.0 M-Neoplasm, Pharynx NOS 210.7 B-Neoplasm, Nasopharynx **REIMBURSEMENT INFORMATION** Medicare ♦ Follow-up Days — 90 ♦ Assistant Surgeon — paid ♦ Supply Charges — not allowed ♦ Outpatient Limit — does not apply ♦ Major Surgery Rules Apply
42892	Resection of lateral pharyngeal wall or pyriform sinus, direct closure by advancement of lateral and posterior pharyngeal walls **CPT NOTES** ♦ When combined with radical neck dissection, use also 38720.	141.0 M-Neoplasm, Tongue base 148.8 M-Neoplasm, Hypopharynx NEC 149.0 M-Neoplasm, Pharynx NOS 210.1 B-Neoplasm, Tongue 210.7 B-Neoplasm, Nasopharynx 210.8 B-Neoplasm, Hypopharynx **REIMBURSEMENT INFORMATION** Medicare ♦ Follow-up Days — 90 ♦ Assistant Surgeon — paid ♦ Supply Charges — not allowed ♦ Outpatient Limit — does not apply ♦ Major Surgery Rules Apply

CPT CODE	SERVICE	ICD–9–CM
42894	Resection of pharyngeal wall requiring closure with myocutaneous flap **CPT NOTES** ♦ When combined with radical neck dissection, use also 38720.	141.0 M-Neoplasm, Tongue base 149.0 M-Neoplasm, Pharynx NOS 210.7 B-Neoplasm, Nasopharynx 478.29 Disease of pharynx NEC **REIMBURSEMENT INFORMATION** Medicare ♦ Follow–up Days — 90 ♦ Assistant Surgeon — paid ♦ Supply Charges — not allowed ♦ Outpatient Limit — does not apply ♦ Major Surgery Rules Apply
42900	Suture pharynx for wound or injury	874.4 Open wound of pharynx 874.5 Open wound of pharynx, complicated **REIMBURSEMENT INFORMATION** Medicare ♦ Follow–up Days — 10 ♦ Assistant Surgeon — by report ♦ Supply Charges — not allowed ♦ Outpatient Limit — does not apply ♦ Minor Surgery Rules Apply
42950	Pharyngoplasty (plastic or reconstructive operation on pharynx) **CPT NOTES** ♦ For pharyngeal flap, see 42225.	149.0 M-Neoplasm, Pharynx NOS 210.7 B-Neoplasm, Nasopharynx 478.29 Disease of pharynx NEC 787.2 Dysphagia 874.4 Open wound of pharynx 874.5 Open wound of pharynx, complicated **REIMBURSEMENT INFORMATION** Medicare ♦ Follow–up Days — 90 ♦ Assistant Surgeon — paid ♦ Supply Charges — not allowed ♦ Outpatient Limit — does not apply ♦ Major Surgery Rules Apply

CPT CODE	SERVICE	ICD–9–CM
42953	Pharyngoesophageal repair **CPT NOTES** ♦ For closure with myocutaneous or other flap, use appropriate number in addition.	148.8 M-Neoplasm, Hypopharynx NEC 149.0 M-Neoplasm, Pharynx NOS 210.7 B-Neoplasm, Nasopharynx 210.8 B-Neoplasm, Hypopharynx 874.4 Open wound of pharynx 874.5 Open wound of pharynx, complicated **REIMBURSEMENT INFORMATION** Medicare ♦ Follow–up Days — 90 ♦ Assistant Surgeon — paid ♦ Supply Charges — not allowed ♦ Outpatient Limit — does not apply ♦ Major Surgery Rules Apply
42960	Control oropharyngeal hemorrhage (primary or secondary, eg, posttonsillectomy); simple	474.8 Chronic tonsil/adenoid disease NEC 528.9 Oral soft tissue disease NEC 784.8 Hemorrhage from throat 874.4 Open wound of pharynx 874.5 Open wound of pharynx, complicated 998.1 Hemorrhage complicating a procedure **REIMBURSEMENT INFORMATION** Medicare ♦ Follow–up Days — 10 ♦ Assistant Surgeon — not paid ♦ Supply Charges — not allowed ♦ Outpatient Limit — does not apply ♦ Minor Surgery Rules Apply
42961	Control oropharyngeal hemorrhage (primary or secondary, eg, posttonsillectomy); complicated, requiring hospitalization	474.8 Chronic tonsil/adenoid disease NEC 528.9 Oral soft tissue disease NEC 784.8 Hemorrhage from throat 874.4 Open wound of pharynx 874.5 Open wound of pharynx, complicated 998.1 Hemorrhage complicating a procedure **REIMBURSEMENT INFORMATION** Medicare ♦ Follow–up Days — 90 ♦ Assistant Surgeon — paid ♦ Supply Charges — not allowed ♦ Outpatient Limit — does not apply ♦ Major Surgery Rules Apply

CPT CODE	SERVICE	ICD–9–CM
42962	Control oropharyngeal hemorrhage (primary or secondary, eg, posttonsillectomy); with secondary surgical intervention	474.8 Chronic tonsil/adenoid disease NEC 528.9 Oral soft tissue disease NEC 784.8 Hemorrhage from throat 874.4 Open wound of pharynx 874.5 Open wound of pharynx, complicated 998.1 Hemorrhage complicating a procedure **REIMBURSEMENT INFORMATION** Medicare ♦ Follow–up Days — 90 ♦ Assistant Surgeon — paid ♦ Supply Charges — not allowed ♦ Outpatient Limit — does not apply ♦ Major Surgery Rules Apply
42970	Control of nasopharyngeal hemorrhage (primary or secondary, eg, postadenoidectomy); simple, with posterior nasal packs, with or without anterior packs and/or cauterization	210.7 B-Neoplasm, Nasopharynx 474.8 Chronic tonsil/adenoid disease NEC 478.29 Disease of pharynx NEC 784.7 Epistaxis 784.8 Hemorrhage from throat 959.0 Face and neck injury NOS 998.1 Hemorrhage complicating a procedure **REIMBURSEMENT INFORMATION** Medicare ♦ Follow–up Days — 90 ♦ Assistant Surgeon — not paid ♦ Supply Charges — not allowed ♦ Outpatient Limit — does not apply ♦ Major Surgery Rules Apply
42971	Control of nasopharyngeal hemorrhage (primary or secondary, eg, postadenoidectomy); complicated, requiring hospitalization	210.7 B-Neoplasm, Nasopharynx 784.7 Epistaxis 784.8 Hemorrhage from throat 959.0 Face and neck injury NOS 998.1 Hemorrhage complicating a procedure **REIMBURSEMENT INFORMATION** Medicare ♦ Follow–up Days — 90 ♦ Assistant Surgeon — paid ♦ Supply Charges — not allowed ♦ Outpatient Limit — does not apply ♦ Major Surgery Rules Apply

CPT CODE	SERVICE	ICD–9–CM
42972	Control of nasopharyngeal hemorrhage (primary or secondary, eg, postadenoidectomy); with secondary surgical intervention	210.7 B-Neoplasm, Nasopharynx 784.7 Epistaxis 784.8 Hemorrhage from throat 959.0 Face and neck injury NOS 998.1 Hemorrhage complicating a procedure **REIMBURSEMENT INFORMATION** Medicare ♦ Follow–up Days — 90 ♦ Assistant Surgeon — paid ♦ Supply Charges — not allowed ♦ Outpatient Limit — does not apply ♦ Major Surgery Rules Apply
42999	Unlisted procedure, pharynx, adenoids, or tonsils	210.5 B-Neoplasm, Tonsil 474.10 Hypertrophy of tonsils/adenoids 474.11 Hypertrophy of tonsils 478.29 Disease of pharynx NEC **REIMBURSEMENT INFORMATION** Medicare ♦ Follow–up Days — determined by local carrier ♦ Assistant Surgeon — determined by local carrier ♦ Supply Charges — determined by local carrier ♦ Outpatient Limit — determined by local carrier
43020	Esophagotomy, cervical approach; with removal of foreign body **CPT NOTES** ♦ For esophageal intubation with laparotomy, see 43510.	935.1 Foreign body in esophagus **REIMBURSEMENT INFORMATION** Medicare ♦ Follow–up Days — 90 ♦ Assistant Surgeon — paid ♦ Supply Charges — not allowed ♦ Outpatient Limit — does not apply ♦ Major Surgery Rules Apply

CPT CODE SERVICE	ICD–9–CM
43030 Cricopharyngeal myotomy **CPT NOTES** ♦ For esophageal intubation with laparotomy, see 43510.	210.8 B-Neoplasm, Hypopharynx 530.0 Achalasia and cardiospasm 787.2 Dysphagia **REIMBURSEMENT INFORMATION** Medicare ♦ Follow–up Days — 90 ♦ Assistant Surgeon — paid ♦ Supply Charges — not allowed ♦ Outpatient Limit — does not apply ♦ Major Surgery Rules Apply
▲ **43100** Excision of lesion, esophagus, with primary repair; cervical approach **CPT NOTES** ♦ For gastrointestinal reconstruction for previous esophagectomy, see 43360, 43361.	150.0 M-Neoplasm, Cervical esophagus 211.0 B-Neoplasm, Esophagus 230.1 CA in situ, Esophagus **REIMBURSEMENT INFORMATION** General ♦ Description changed in 1995 CPT. Medicare ♦ Follow–up Days — 90 ♦ Assistant Surgeon — paid ♦ Supply Charges — not allowed ♦ Outpatient Limit — does not apply ♦ Major Surgery Rules Apply
43130 Diverticulectomy of hypopharynx or esophagus, with or without myotomy; cervical approach **CPT NOTES** ♦ For gastrointestinal reconstruction for previous esophagectomy, see 43360, 43361.	530.6 Acquired esophageal diverticulum 787.2 Dysphagia **REIMBURSEMENT INFORMATION** Medicare ♦ Follow–up Days — 90 ♦ Assistant Surgeon — paid ♦ Supply Charges — not allowed ♦ Outpatient Limit — does not apply ♦ Major Surgery Rules Apply

CPT CODE **SERVICE**

43200 Esophagoscopy, rigid or flexible; diagnostic, with or without collection of specimen(s) by brushing or washing (separate procedure)

CPT NOTES

- For endoscopic procedures, code appropriate endoscopy of each anatomic site examined.
- Surgical endoscopy always includes diagnostic endoscopy.
- For radiological supervision and interpretation, see 74235.

ICD–9–CM

148.8	M-Neoplasm, Hypopharynx NEC
150.0	M-Neoplasm, Cervical esophagus
150.3	M-Neoplasm, Upper 1/3 of esophagus
150.4	M-Neoplasm, Middle 1/3 of esophagus
150.5	M-Neoplasm, Lower 1/3 of esophagus
210.8	B-Neoplasm, Hypopharynx
211.0	B-Neoplasm, Esophagus
530.3	Esophageal stricture
530.6	Acquired esophageal diverticulum
558.9	Noninfect gastroenteritis NEC
750.3	Congen esophageal fistula/atresia
787.2	Dysphagia
935.1	Foreign body in esophagus
947.2	Burn of Esophagus

REIMBURSEMENT INFORMATION

General

- Separate procedure rules apply.

Medicare

- Follow–up Days — 0
- Assistant Surgeon — not paid
- Supply Charges — allowed
- Outpatient Limit — does not apply
- Minor Surgery Rules Apply

CPT CODE	SERVICE

43202 Esophagoscopy, rigid or flexible; with biopsy, single or multiple

CPT NOTES

- For endoscopic procedures, code appropriate endoscopy of each anatomic site examined.
- Surgical endoscopy always includes diagnostic endoscopy.
- For radiological supervision and interpretation, see 74235.

ICD–9–CM

140.0	M-Neoplasm, Hypopharynx NEC
150.0	M-Neoplasm, Cervical esophagus
150.3	M-Neoplasm, Upper 1/3 of esophagus
150.4	M-Neoplasm, Middle 1/3 of esophagus
150.5	M-Neoplasm, Lower 1/3 of esophagus
210.8	B-Neoplasm, Hypopharynx
211.8	B-Neoplasm, Peritoneum
530.3	Esophageal stricture
530.6	Acquired esophageal diverticulum
558.9	Noninfect gastroenteritis NEC
750.3	Congen esophageal fistula/atresia
787.2	Dysphagia
935.1	Foreign body in esophagus
947.2	Burn of Esophagus

REIMBURSEMENT INFORMATION

Medicare

- Follow–up Days — 0
- Assistant Surgeon — not paid
- Supply Charges — allowed
- Outpatient Limit — does not apply
- Minor Surgery Rules Apply

43215 Esophagoscopy, rigid or flexible; with removal of foreign body

CPT NOTES

- For endoscopic procedures, code appropriate endoscopy of each anatomic site examined.
- Surgical endoscopy always includes diagnostic endoscopy.
- For radiological supervision and interpretation, see 74235.

933.0	Foreign body in pharynx
935.1	Foreign body in esophagus

REIMBURSEMENT INFORMATION

Medicare

- Follow–up Days — 0
- Assistant Surgeon — not paid
- Supply Charges — not allowed
- Outpatient Limit — does not apply
- Minor Surgery Rules Apply

CPT CODE **SERVICE**

43219 Esophagoscopy, rigid or flexible; with insertion of plastic tube or stent

CPT NOTES

- For endoscopic procedures, code appropriate endoscopy of each anatomic site examined.
- Surgical endoscopy always includes diagnostic endoscopy.

ICD–9–CM

150.4	M-Neoplasm, Middle 1/3 of esophagus
211.0	B-Neoplasm, Esophagus
530.3	Esophageal stricture
750.3	Congen esophageal fistula/atresia
787.2	Dysphagia
947.2	Burn of Esophagus

REIMBURSEMENT INFORMATION

Medicare

- Follow–up Days — 0
- Assistant Surgeon — not paid
- Supply Charges — not allowed
- Outpatient Limit — does not apply
- Minor Surgery Rules Apply

43220 Esophagoscopy, rigid or flexible; with balloon dilation (less than 30 mm diameter):

CPT NOTES

- For endoscopic procedures, code appropriate endoscopy of each anatomic site examined.
- Surgical endoscopy always includes diagnostic endoscopy.
- For endoscopic dilation with balloon 30 mm diameter or larger, use 43458.
- For dilation without visualization, see 43450–43453.

150.4	M-Neoplasm, Middle 1/3 of esophagus
150.5	M-Neoplasm, Lower 1/3 of esophagus
211.0	B-Neoplasm, Esophagus
530.0	Achalasia and cardiospasm
750.3	Congen esophageal fistula/atresia
787.2	Dysphagia
947.2	Burn of Esophagus

REIMBURSEMENT INFORMATION

Medicare

- Follow–up Days — 0
- Assistant Surgeon — not paid
- Supply Charges — allowed
- Outpatient Limit — does not apply
- Minor Surgery Rules Apply

CPT CODE **SERVICE** | **ICD–9–CM**

43226 Esophagoscopy, rigid or flexible, with insertion of guide wire followed by dilation over guide wire

CPT NOTES

- For endoscopic procedures, code appropriate endoscopy of each anatomic site examined.
- Surgical endoscopy always includes diagnostic endoscopy.
- For radiological supervision and interpretation, see 74360.

ICD–9–CM

150.4 M-Neoplasm, Middle 1/3 of esophagus
150.5 M-Neoplasm, Lower 1/3 of esophagus
211.0 B-Neoplasm, Esophagus
530.0 Achalasia and cardiospasm
750.3 Congen esophageal fistula/atresia
787.2 Dysphagia
947.2 Burn of Esophagus

REIMBURSEMENT INFORMATION

Medicare

- Follow–up Days — 0
- Assistant Surgeon — not paid
- Supply Charges — allowed
- Outpatient Limit — does not apply
- Minor Surgery Rules Apply

43450* Dilation of esophagus, by unguided sound or bougie, single or multiple passes

CPT NOTES

- For associated esophagogram, use 74220.

530.0 Achalasia and cardiospasm
750.3 Congen esophageal fistula/atresia
787.2 Dysphagia
935.1 Foreign body in esophagus
947.2 Burn of Esophagus

REIMBURSEMENT INFORMATION

General

- Starred procedure.

Medicare

- Follow–up Days — 0
- Assistant Surgeon — not paid
- Supply Charges — not allowed
- Outpatient Limit — does not apply
- Minor Surgery Rules Apply

43458 Dilation of esophagus with balloon (30 mm diameter or larger) for achalasia

CPT NOTES

- For associated esophagogram, use 74220.
- For dilation with balloon less than 30 mm diameter, use 43220.
- For radiological supervision and interpretation, see 74360.

530.0 Achalasia and cardiospasm
787.2 Dysphagia
935.1 Foreign body in esophagus

REIMBURSEMENT INFORMATION

Medicare

- Follow–up Days — 0
- Assistant Surgeon — not paid
- Supply Charges — allowed
- Outpatient Limit — does not apply
- Minor Surgery Rules Apply

CPT CODE SERVICE	ICD–9–CM
60000* Incision and drainage of thyroglossal cyst, infected **CPT NOTES** ♦ For pituitary and pineal gland surgery, see Nervous System.	683 Acute lymphadenitis 759.2 Endocrine gland anomaly NEC **REIMBURSEMENT INFORMATION** General ♦ Starred procedure. Medicare ♦ Follow–up Days — 10 ♦ Assistant Surgeon — not paid ♦ Supply Charges — not allowed ♦ Outpatient Limit — does not apply ♦ Minor Surgery Rules Apply
● **60001** Aspiration and/or injection, thyroid cyst **CPT NOTES** ♦ For pituitary and pineal gland surgery, see Nervous System. ♦ For fine needle aspiration, see 88170, 88171.	193 M-Neoplasm, Thyroid gland 226 B-Neoplasm, Thyroid gland 240.0 Simple goiter 240.9 Goiter NOS 241.0 Nontoxic uninodular goiter 241.1 Nontoxic multinodular goiter 241.9 Nontoxic nodular goiter NOS 242.10 Toxic uninodular goiter, no crisis 244 Acquired hypothyroidism 246.2 Cyst of thyroid 759.2 Endocrine gland anomaly NEC 784.2 Swelling in head/neck **REIMBURSEMENT INFORMATION** General ♦ New procedure, 1995 CPT. Medicare ♦ Follow–up Days — 10 ♦ Assistant Surgeon — not paid ♦ Supply Charges — not allowed ♦ Outpatient Limit — does not apply ♦ Minor Surgery Rules Apply

CPT CODE **SERVICE**

▲ **60100*** Biopsy thyroid, percutaneous core needle

CPT NOTES

- For pituitary and pineal surgery, see Nervous System.
- For radiological supervision and interpretation, see 76360, 76942.
- For fine needle aspiration, preparation, and interpretation of smears, see 88170–88173.

ICD–9–CM

193	M-Neoplasm, Thyroid gland
226	B-Neoplasm, Thyroid gland
240.0	Simple goiter
240.9	Goiter NOS
241.0	Nontoxic uninodular goiter
241.1	Nontoxic multinodular goiter
241.9	Nontoxic nodular goiter NOS
242.10	Toxic uninodular goiter, no crisis
245.3	Chronic fibrous thyroiditis
246.2	Cyst of thyroid
759.2	Endocrine gland anomaly NEC
784.2	Swelling in head/neck

REIMBURSEMENT INFORMATION

General

- Starred procedure.
- Description changed in 1995 CPT.

Medicare

- Follow–up Days — 0
- Assistant Surgeon — not paid
- Supply Charges — not allowed
- Outpatient Limit — applies
- Minor Surgery Rules Apply

60200 Excision of cyst or adenoma of thyroid, or transection of isthmus

CPT NOTES

- For pituitary and pineal surgery, see Nervous System.

226	B-Neoplasm, Thyroid gland
239.7	Endocrine/CNS neoplasm NOS
240.9	Goiter NOS
241.0	Nontoxic uninodular goiter
241.1	Nontoxic multinodular goiter
246.2	Cyst of thyroid

REIMBURSEMENT INFORMATION

Medicare

- Follow–up Days — 90
- Assistant Surgeon — paid
- Supply Charges — not allowed
- Outpatient Limit — does not apply
- Major Surgery Rules Apply

CPT CODE **SERVICE**

● **60210** Partial thyroid lobectomy, unilateral; with or without isthmusectomy

CPT NOTES

- For pituitary and pineal gland surgery, see Nervous System.
- For fine needle aspiration, see 88170, 88171.

ICD–9–CM

193	M-Neoplasm, Thyroid gland
194.1	M-Neoplasm, Parathyroid gland
226	B-Neoplasm, Thyroid gland
237.4	UB-Neoplasm, Endocrine gland NEC
239.7	Endocrine/CNS neoplasm NOS
240.9	Goiter NOS
241.0	Nontoxic uninodular goiter
241.1	Nontoxic multinodular goiter
241.9	Nontoxic nodular goiter NOS
242.1	Thyrotoxicosis
242.2	Thyrotoxicosis
242.3	Thyrotoxicosis
245.0	Acute thyroiditis
245.1	Subacute thyroiditis
245.2	Chronic lymphocytic thyroiditis
245.3	Chronic fibrous thyroiditis
246.2	Cyst of thyroid
246.9	Disorder of thyroid NOS
759.2	Endocrine gland anomaly NEC

REIMBURSEMENT INFORMATION

General

- New procedure, 1995 CPT.

Medicare

- Follow–up Days — 10
- Assistant Surgeon — not paid
- Supply Charges — not allowed
- Outpatient Limit — does not apply
- Minor Surgery Rules Apply

CPT CODE **SERVICE**

● **60212** Partial thyroid lobectomy, unilateral; with contralateral subtotal lobectomy, including isthmusectomy

CPT NOTES

- For pituitary and pineal gland surgery, see Nervous System.
- For fine needle aspiration, see 88170, 88171.

ICD–9–CM

193	M-Neoplasm, Thyroid gland
194.1	M-Neoplasm, Parathyroid gland
226	B-Neoplasm, Thyroid gland
237.4	UB-Neoplasm, Endocrine gland NEC
239.7	Endocrine/CNS neoplasm NOS
240.9	Goiter NOS
241.0	Nontoxic uninodular goiter
241.1	Nontoxic multinodular goiter
241.9	Nontoxic nodular goiter NOS
242.1	Thyrotoxicosis
242.2	Thyrotoxicosis
242.3	Thyrotoxicosis
245.0	Acute thyroiditis
245.1	Subacute thyroiditis
245.2	Chronic lymphocytic thyroiditis
245.3	Chronic fibrous thyroiditis
246.2	Cyst of thyroid
246.9	Disorder of thyroid NOS
759.2	Endocrine gland anomaly NEC

REIMBURSEMENT INFORMATION

General

- New procedure, 1995 CPT.

Medicare

- Follow–up Days — 10
- Assistant Surgeon — not paid
- Supply Charges — not allowed
- Outpatient Limit — does not apply
- Minor Surgery Rules Apply

CPT CODE **SERVICE**

▲ **60220** Total thyroid lobectomy, unilateral; with or without isthmusectomy

CPT NOTES

- For pituitary and pineal surgery, see Nervous System.

ICD–9–CM

193	M-Neoplasm, Thyroid gland
226	B-Neoplasm, Thyroid gland
237.4	UB-Neoplasm, Endocrine gland NEC
239.7	Endocrine/CNS neoplasm NOS
240.9	Goiter NOS
241.0	Nontoxic uninodular goiter
241.1	Nontoxic multinodular goiter
241.9	Nontoxic nodular goiter NOS
242.10	Toxic uninodular goiter, no crisis
242.11	Toxic uninodular goiter, w/crisis
242.20	Toxic multinodul goiter, no crisis
242.21	Toxic multinodular goiter, w/crisis
245.0	Acute thyroiditis
245.1	Subacute thyroiditis
245.2	Chronic lymphocytic thyroiditis
245.3	Chronic fibrous thyroiditis
246.2	Cyst of thyroid
246.9	Disorder of thyroid NOS
759.2	Endocrine gland anomaly NEC

REIMBURSEMENT INFORMATION

General

- Description changed in 1995 CPT.

Medicare

- Follow–up Days — 90
- Assistant Surgeon — paid
- Supply Charges — not allowed
- Outpatient Limit — does not apply
- Major Surgery Rules Apply

CPT CODE **SERVICE**

▲ [illegible] Total thyroid lobectomy, unilateral; with contralateral subtotal lobectomy, including isthmusectomy

CPT NOTES

- For pituitary and pineal surgery, see Nervous System.

ICD–9–CM

193	M-Neoplasm, Thyroid gland
226	B-Neoplasm, Thyroid gland
237.4	UB-Neoplasm, Endocrine gland NEC
239.7	Endocrine/CNS neoplasm NOS
240.9	Goiter NOS
241.0	Nontoxic uninodular goiter
241.1	Nontoxic multinodular goiter
241.9	Nontoxic nodular goiter NOS
242.10	Toxic uninodular goiter, no crisis
242.11	Toxic uninodular goiter, w/crisis
242.20	Toxic multinodul goiter, no crisis
242.21	Toxic multinodular goiter, w/crisis
242.30	Toxic nodular goiter, no crisis
242.31	Toxic nodular goiter, w/crisis
246.2	Cyst of thyroid
246.9	Disorder of thyroid NOS
759.2	Endocrine gland anomaly NEC

REIMBURSEMENT INFORMATION

General

- Description changed in 1995 CPT.

Medicare

- Follow–up Days — 90
- Assistant Surgeon — paid
- Supply Charges — not allowed
- Outpatient Limit — does not apply
- Major Surgery Rules Apply

CPT CODE	SERVICE	ICD–9–CM

60240 Thyroidectomy, total or complete

CPT NOTES

- For pituitary and pineal surgery, see Nervous System.

ICD–9–CM	
193	M-Neoplasm, Thyroid gland
226	B-Neoplasm, Thyroid gland
237.4	UB-Neoplasm, Endocrine gland NEC
241.0	Nontoxic uninodular goiter
241.1	Nontoxic multinodular goiter
242.00	Toxic diffuse goiter, no crisis
242.01	Toxic diffuse goiter, w/crisis
242.10	Toxic uninodular goiter, no crisis
242.11	Toxic uninodular goiter, w/crisis
242.20	Toxic multinodul goiter, no crisis
242.21	Toxic multinodular goiter, w/crisis
242.80	Thyrotoxicosis orig NEC, no crisis
242.9	Thyrotoxicosis NOS
245.2	Chronic lymphocytic thyroiditis
245.3	Chronic fibrous thyroiditis
759.2	Endocrine gland anomaly NEC

REIMBURSEMENT INFORMATION

Medicare

- Follow–up Days — 90
- Assistant Surgeon — paid
- Supply Charges — not allowed
- Outpatient Limit — does not apply
- Major Surgery Rules Apply

60252 Thyroidectomy, total or subtotal for malignancy; with limited neck dissection

CPT NOTES

- For pituitary and pineal surgery, see Nervous System.

ICD–9–CM	
193	M-Neoplasm, Thyroid gland
198.89	M2-Neoplasm NEC
200.11	Lymphosarcoma, head/neck/face
200.81	Mixed lymphosarcoma, head/neck/face
202.8	Lymphoma

REIMBURSEMENT INFORMATION

Medicare

- Follow–up Days — 90
- Assistant Surgeon — paid
- Supply Charges — not allowed
- Outpatient Limit — does not apply
- Major Surgery Rules Apply

CPT CODE	SERVICE	ICD–9–CM

60254 Thyroidectomy, total or subtotal for malignancy; with radical neck dissection

CPT NOTES

- For pituitary and pineal surgery, see Nervous System.

ICD–9–CM

193	M-Neoplasm, Thyroid gland
200.11	Lymphosarcoma, head/neck/face
200.81	Mixed lymphosarcoma, head/neck/face
202.8	Lymphoma

REIMBURSEMENT INFORMATION

Medicare

- Follow–up Days — 90
- Assistant Surgeon — paid
- Supply Charges — not allowed
- Outpatient Limit — does not apply
- Major Surgery Rules Apply

▲ **60260** Thyroidectomy, removal of all remaining thyroid tissue following previous removal of a portion of thyroid

CPT NOTES

- For pituitary and pineal surgery, see Nervous System.

ICD–9–CM

193	M-Neoplasm, Thyroid gland
202.8	Lymphoma
226	B-Neoplasm, Thyroid gland
237.4	UB-Neoplasm, Endocrine gland NEC
240.9	Goiter NOS
241.0	Nontoxic uninodular goiter
242.00	Toxic diffuse goiter, no crisis
242.01	Toxic diffuse goiter, w/crisis
242.10	Toxic uninodular goiter, no crisis
242.11	Toxic uninodular goiter, w/crisis
242.20	Toxic multinodul goiter, no crisis
242.21	Toxic multinodular goiter, w/crisis
242.9	Thyrotoxicosis NOS
245.2	Chronic lymphocytic thyroiditis
759.2	Endocrine gland anomaly NEC

REIMBURSEMENT INFORMATION

General

- Description changed in 1995 CPT.

Medicare

- Follow–up Days — 90
- Assistant Surgeon — paid
- Supply Charges — not allowed
- Outpatient Limit — does not apply
- Major Surgery Rules Apply

CPT CODE	SERVICE
60270	Thyroidectomy, including substernal thyroid gland; sternal split or transthoracic approach

CPT NOTES

- For pituitary and pineal surgery, see Nervous System.

ICD–9–CM

193	M-Neoplasm, Thyroid gland
202.8	Lymphoma
226	B-Neoplasm, Thyroid gland
237.4	UB-Neoplasm, Endocrine gland NEC
240.9	Goiter NOS
241.0	Nontoxic uninodular goiter
242.00	Toxic diffuse goiter, no crisis
242.01	Toxic diffuse goiter, w/crisis
242.10	Toxic uninodular goiter, no crisis
242.11	Toxic uninodular goiter, w/crisis
242.20	Toxic multinodul goiter, no crisis
242.21	Toxic multinodular goiter, w/crisis
242.9	Thyrotoxicosis NOS
245.2	Chronic lymphocytic thyroiditis
759.2	Endocrine gland anomaly NEC

REIMBURSEMENT INFORMATION

Medicare

- Follow–up Days — 90
- Assistant Surgeon — paid
- Supply Charges — not allowed
- Outpatient Limit — does not apply
- Major Surgery Rules Apply

CPT CODE **SERVICE**

● **60271** Thyroidectomy, including substernal thyroid gland; cervical approach

CPT NOTES

- For pituitary and pineal surgery, see Nervous System.

ICD-9-CM

193	M-Neoplasm, Thyroid gland
194.1	M-Neoplasm, Parathyroid gland
202.8	Lymphoma
226	B-Neoplasm, Thyroid gland
237.4	UB-Neoplasm, Endocrine gland NEC
240.9	Goiter NOS
241.0	Nontoxic uninodular goiter
242.00	Toxic diffuse goiter, no crisis
242.10	Toxic uninodular goiter, no crisis
242.11	Toxic uninodular goiter, w/crisis
242.20	Toxic multinodul goiter, no crisis
242.21	Toxic multinodular goiter, w/crisis
242.9	Thyrotoxicosis NOS
245.2	Chronic lymphocytic thyroiditis
478.34	Vocal cord paralysis, bilat, total
496	Chronic airway obstruction NEC
759.2	Endocrine gland anomaly NEC
787.2	Dysphagia

REIMBURSEMENT INFORMATION

General

- New procedure, 1995 CPT.

Medicare

- Follow–up Days — 90
- Assistant Surgeon — paid
- Supply Charges — not allowed
- Outpatient Limit — does not apply
- Major Surgery Rules Apply

60280 Excision of thyroglossal duct cyst or sinus

CPT NOTES

- For pituitary and pineal surgery, see Nervous System.
- For thyroid ultrasonography, see 76536.

683	Acute lymphadenitis
759.2	Endocrine gland anomaly NEC

REIMBURSEMENT INFORMATION

Medicare

- Follow–up Days — 90
- Assistant Surgeon — paid
- Supply Charges — not allowed
- Outpatient Limit — does not apply
- Major Surgery Rules Apply

CPT CODE	SERVICE	ICD–9–CM
60281	Excision of thyroglossal duct cyst or sinus; recurrent **CPT NOTES** ♦ For pituitary and pineal surgery, see Nervous System. ♦ For thyroid ultrasonography, see 76536.	759.2 Endocrine gland anomaly NEC **REIMBURSEMENT INFORMATION** Medicare ♦ Follow–up Days — 90 ♦ Assistant Surgeon — paid ♦ Supply Charges — not allowed ♦ Outpatient Limit — does not apply ♦ Major Surgery Rules Apply
60500	Parathyroidectomy or exploration of parathyroid(s) **CPT NOTES** ♦ For pituitary and pineal surgery, see Nervous System.	194.1 M-Neoplasm, Parathyroid gland 227.1 B-Neoplasm, Parathyroid gland 252.0 Hyperparathyroidism 252.1 Hypoparathyroidism **REIMBURSEMENT INFORMATION** Medicare ♦ Follow–up Days — 90 ♦ Assistant Surgeon — paid ♦ Supply Charges — not allowed ♦ Outpatient Limit — does not apply ♦ Major Surgery Rules Apply
60502	Parathyroidectomy or exploration of parathyroid(s); re- exploration **CPT NOTES** ♦ For pituitary and pineal surgery, see Nervous System.	194.1 M-Neoplasm, Parathyroid gland 227.1 B-Neoplasm, Parathyroid gland 252.0 Hyperparathyroidism 252.1 Hypoparathyroidism 275.4 Disorders of calcium metabolism **REIMBURSEMENT INFORMATION** Medicare ♦ Follow–up Days — 90 ♦ Assistant Surgeon — paid ♦ Supply Charges — not allowed ♦ Outpatient Limit — does not apply ♦ Major Surgery Rules Apply

CPT CODE	SERVICE	ICD–9–CM

60505 Parathyroidectomy or exploration of parathyroid(s); with mediastinal exploration, sternal split or transthoracic approach

CPT NOTES

- For pituitary and pineal surgery, see Nervous System.

194.1 M-Neoplasm, Parathyroid gland
227.1 B-Neoplasm, Parathyroid gland

REIMBURSEMENT INFORMATION

Medicare

- Follow–up Days — 90
- Assistant Surgeon — paid
- Supply Charges — not allowed
- Outpatient Limit — does not apply
- Major Surgery Rules Apply

● **60512** Parathyroid autotransplantation

CPT NOTES

- For pituitary and pineal surgery, see Nervous System.

193 M-Neoplasm, Thyroid gland
240.9 Goiter NOS
242 Thyrotoxicosis

REIMBURSEMENT INFORMATION

General

- New procedure, 1995 CPT.

Medicare

- Follow–up Days — 90
- Assistant Surgeon — paid
- Supply Charges — not allowed
- Outpatient Limit — does not apply
- Major Surgery Rules Apply

▲ **60520** Thymectomy, partial or total; transcervical approach (separate procedure)

CPT NOTES

- For pituitary and pineal surgery, see Nervous System.

164.0 M-Neoplasm, Thymus
212.6 B-Neoplasm, Thymus
254.0 Persistent hyperplasia of thymus

REIMBURSEMENT INFORMATION

General

- Separate procedure rules apply.
- Description changed in 1995 CPT.

Medicare

- Follow–up Days — 90
- Assistant Surgeon — paid
- Supply Charges — not allowed
- Outpatient Limit — does not apply
- Major Surgery Rules Apply

CPT CODE SERVICE	ICD–9–CM
64400* Injection, anesthetic agent; trigeminal nerve, any division or branch **CPT NOTES** ♦ For intracranial surgery on cranial nerves, see 61450, 61460, 61790. ♦ For phenol destruction, see 64600–64640. ♦ For subarachnoid or subdural injection, see 62274–62277. ♦ For epidural or caudal injection, see 62278, 62279.	239.8 Neoplasm NOS, site NEC 350.1 Trigeminal neuralgia **REIMBURSEMENT INFORMATION** General ♦ Starred procedure. Medicare ♦ Follow–up Days — 0 ♦ Assistant Surgeon — not paid ♦ Supply Charges — not allowed ♦ Outpatient Limit — applies ♦ Minor Surgery Rules Apply
68720 Dacryocystorhinostomy (fistulization of lacrimal sac to nasal cavity) **CPT NOTES** ♦ For removal of foreign body, see 62505 et. seq. ♦ For diagnostic and treatment ophthalmological services, see medicine, ophthalmology, and 92002 et seq.	375.20 Epiphora NOS 375.5 Stenosis/insufficiency, lacrimal **REIMBURSEMENT INFORMATION** Medicare ♦ Follow–up Days — 90 ♦ Assistant Surgeon — paid ♦ Supply Charges — not allowed ♦ Outpatient Limit — does not apply ♦ Major Surgery Rules Apply
68745 Conjunctivorhinostomy (fistulization of conjunctiva to nasal cavity; without tube **CPT NOTES** ♦ For removal of foreign body, see 62505 et. seq. ♦ For diagnostic and treatment ophthalmological services, see medicine, ophthalmology, and 92002 et seq.	375.56 Acquired nasolacrimal duct stenosis **REIMBURSEMENT INFORMATION** Medicare ♦ Follow–up Days — 90 ♦ Assistant Surgeon — paid ♦ Supply Charges — not allowed ♦ Outpatient Limit — does not apply ♦ Major Surgery Rules Apply

CPT CODE	SERVICE	ICD–9–CM

68750 Conjunctivorhinostomy (fistulization of conjunctiva to nasal cavity; with insertion of tube or stent

CPT NOTES

- For removal of foreign body, see 62505 et. seq.
- For diagnostic and treatment ophthalmological services, see medicine, ophthalmology, and 92002 et seq.

375.20 Epiphora NOS
375.56 Acquired nasolacrimal duct stenosis

REIMBURSEMENT INFORMATION

Medicare

- Follow–up Days — 90
- Assistant Surgeon — paid
- Supply Charges — not allowed
- Outpatient Limit — does not apply
- Major Surgery Rules Apply

69000* Drainage external ear, abscess or hematoma; simple

CPT NOTES

- For diagnostic services, (e.g., audiometry, vestibular tests), see 92502 et seq).

380.10 Infective otitis externa NOS
380.31 Hematoma of auricle/pinna
738.7 Cauliflower ear
959.0 Face and neck injury NOS

REIMBURSEMENT INFORMATION

General

- Starred procedure.

Medicare

- Follow–up Days — 10
- Assistant Surgeon — not paid
- Supply Charges — not allowed
- Outpatient Limit — applies
- Minor Surgery Rules Apply

69005 Drainage external ear, abscess or hematoma; complicated

CPT NOTES

- For diagnostic services, (e.g., audiometry, vestibular tests), see 92502 et seq).

380.10 Infective otitis externa NOS
380.31 Hematoma of auricle/pinna
738.7 Cauliflower ear
959.0 Face and neck injury NOS

REIMBURSEMENT INFORMATION

Medicare

- Follow–up Days — 10
- Assistant Surgeon — not paid
- Supply Charges — not allowed
- Outpatient Limit — does not apply
- Minor Surgery Rules Apply

CPT CODE	SERVICE	ICD–9–CM

69020* Drainage external auditory canal, abscess

CPT NOTES

- For diagnostic services, (e.g., audiometry, vestibular tests), see 92502 et seq).

380.10 Infective otitis externa NOS
380.31 Hematoma of auricle/pinna
738.7 Cauliflower ear
959.0 Face and neck injury NOS

REIMBURSEMENT INFORMATION

General

- Starred procedure.

Medicare

- Follow–up Days — 10
- Assistant Surgeon — not paid
- Supply Charges — not allowed
- Outpatient Limit — applies
- Minor Surgery Rules Apply

69090 Ear piercing

CPT NOTES

- For diagnostic services, (e.g., audiometry, vestibular tests), see 92502 et seq).

V50.3 Ear piercing

REIMBURSEMENT INFORMATION

Medicare

- Follow–up Days — global concept does not apply
- Assistant Surgeon — not paid
- Supply Charges — not allowed
- Outpatient Limit — does not apply

69100 Biopsy external ear

CPT NOTES

- For diagnostic services, (e.g., audiometry, vestibular tests), see 92502 et seq).

173.2 M-Neoplasm, Skin of ear
216.2 B-Neoplasm, Skin of ear
232.2 CA in situ, Skin of ear
238.2 UB-Neoplasm, Skin
385.30 Cholesteatoma NOS

REIMBURSEMENT INFORMATION

Medicare

- Follow–up Days — 10
- Assistant Surgeon — not paid
- Supply Charges — not allowed
- Outpatient Limit — applies
- Minor Surgery Rules Apply

CPT CODE **SERVICE**

ICD–9–CM

69105 Biopsy external auditory canal

CPT NOTES

- For diagnostic services, (e.g., audiometry, vestibular tests), see 92502 et seq).

173.2	M-Neoplasm, Skin of ear
216.2	B-Neoplasm, Skin of ear
380.23	Chronic otitis externa NEC

REIMBURSEMENT INFORMATION

Medicare

- Follow–up Days — 0
- Assistant Surgeon — not paid
- Supply Charges — not allowed
- Outpatient Limit — does not apply
- Minor Surgery Rules Apply

69110 Excision external ear; partial, simple repair

CPT NOTES

- For diagnostic services, (e.g., audiometry, vestibular tests), see 92502 et seq).
- For reconstruction of ear, see 15120 et seq.

173.2	M-Neoplasm, Skin of ear
216.2	B-Neoplasm, Skin of ear
232.2	CA in situ, Skin of ear

REIMBURSEMENT INFORMATION

Medicare

- Follow–up Days — 90
- Assistant Surgeon — not paid
- Supply Charges — not allowed
- Outpatient Limit — does not apply
- Major Surgery Rules Apply

69120 Excision external ear; complete amputation

CPT NOTES

- For diagnostic services, (e.g., audiometry, vestibular tests), see 92502 et seq).
- For reconstruction of ear, see 15120 et seq.

173.2	M-Neoplasm, Skin of ear
232.2	CA in situ, Skin of ear
872.01	Open wound of auricle
872.11	Open wound of auricle, complicated

REIMBURSEMENT INFORMATION

Medicare

- Follow–up Days — 90
- Assistant Surgeon — not paid
- Supply Charges — not allowed
- Outpatient Limit — does not apply
- Major Surgery Rules Apply

CPT CODE / SERVICE	ICD–9–CM
69140 Excision exostosis(es), external auditory canal **CPT NOTES** ♦ For diagnostic services, (e.g., audiometry, vestibular tests), see 92502 et seq).	380.50 Acquired stenosis ear canal NOS 380.51 Stenosis ext ear canal d/t trauma 380.52 Stenosis ext ear canal d/t surgery 380.53 Stenosis ext ear canal d/t inflam 380.81 Exostosis of external ear canal 389.01 Conductive hearing loss, extern ear **REIMBURSEMENT INFORMATION** Medicare ♦ Follow–up Days — 90 ♦ Assistant Surgeon — not paid ♦ Supply Charges — not allowed ♦ Outpatient Limit — does not apply ♦ Major Surgery Rules Apply
69145 Excision soft tissue lesion, external auditory canal **CPT NOTES** ♦ For diagnostic services, (e.g., audiometry, vestibular tests), see 92502 et seq).	380.89 External ear disorder NEC **REIMBURSEMENT INFORMATION** Medicare ♦ Follow–up Days — 90 ♦ Assistant Surgeon — not paid ♦ Supply Charges — not allowed ♦ Outpatient Limit — does not apply ♦ Major Surgery Rules Apply
69150 Radical excision external auditory canal lesion; without neck dissection **CPT NOTES** ♦ For diagnostic services, (e.g., audiometry, vestibular tests), see 92502 et seq). ♦ For resection of temporal bone, see 69535. ♦ For skin grafting, see 15000–15261.	171.0 M-Neoplasm, Soft tissue, head 173.2 M-Neoplasm, Skin of ear 195.0 M-Neoplasm, Head/face/neck 198.2 M2-Neoplasm, Skin 215.0 B-Neoplasm, Soft tissue, head 216.2 B-Neoplasm, Skin of ear 380.89 External ear disorder NEC **REIMBURSEMENT INFORMATION** Medicare ♦ Follow–up Days — 90 ♦ Assistant Surgeon — paid ♦ Supply Charges — not allowed ♦ Outpatient Limit — does not apply ♦ Major Surgery Rules Apply

CPT CODE **SERVICE**

69155 Radical excision external auditory canal lesion; with neck dissection

CPT NOTES

- For diagnostic services, (e.g., audiometry, vestibular tests), see 92502 et seq).
- For resection of temporal bone, see 69535.
- For skin grafting, see 15000–15261.

ICD–9–CM

171.0 M-Neoplasm, Soft tissue, head
173.2 M-Neoplasm, Skin of ear
195.0 M-Neoplasm, Head/face/neck
198.2 M2-Neoplasm, Skin

REIMBURSEMENT INFORMATION

Medicare

- Follow–up Days — 90
- Assistant Surgeon — paid
- Supply Charges — not allowed
- Outpatient Limit — does not apply
- Major Surgery Rules Apply

69200 Removal foreign body from external auditory canal; without general anesthesia

CPT NOTES

- For diagnostic services, (e.g., audiometry, vestibular tests), see 92502 et seq).

931 Foreign body in ear

REIMBURSEMENT INFORMATION

Medicare

- Follow–up Days — 0
- Assistant Surgeon — not paid
- Supply Charges — not allowed
- Outpatient Limit — applies
- Minor Surgery Rules Apply

69205 Removal foreign body from external auditory canal; with general anesthesia

CPT NOTES

- For diagnostic services, (e.g., audiometry, vestibular tests), see 92502 et seq).

931 Foreign body in ear

REIMBURSEMENT INFORMATION

Medicare

- Follow–up Days — 10
- Assistant Surgeon — not paid
- Supply Charges — not allowed
- Outpatient Limit — does not apply
- Minor Surgery Rules Apply

CPT CODE SERVICE	ICD-9-CM
69210 Removal impacted cerumen (separate procedure), one or both ears **CPT NOTES** ♦ For diagnostic services, (e.g., audiometry, vestibular tests), see 92502 et seq).	380.4 Impacted cerumen **REIMBURSEMENT INFORMATION** General ♦ Separate procedure rules apply. Medicare ♦ Follow-up Days — 0 ♦ Assistant Surgeon — not paid ♦ Supply Charges — not allowed ♦ Outpatient Limit — applies ♦ Minor Surgery Rules Apply
69220 Debridement, mastoidectomy cavity, simple (eg, routine cleaning) **CPT NOTES** ♦ For diagnostic services, (e.g., audiometry, vestibular tests), see 92502 et seq).	382.3 Chronic suppurativ otitis media NOS 383.30 Postmastoidectomy complication NOS 383.32 Postmastoidectomy cholesteatoma 383.33 Postmastoidectomy granulations **REIMBURSEMENT INFORMATION** Medicare ♦ Follow-up Days — 0 ♦ Assistant Surgeon — not paid ♦ Supply Charges — not allowed ♦ Outpatient Limit — applies ♦ Minor Surgery Rules Apply
69222 Debridement, mastoidectomy cavity, complex (eg, with anesthesia or more than routine cleaning) **CPT NOTES** ♦ For diagnostic services, (e.g., audiometry, vestibular tests), see 92502 et seq).	382.3 Chronic suppurativ otitis media NOS 383.30 Postmastoidectomy complication NOS 383.32 Postmastoidectomy cholesteatoma 383.33 Postmastoidectomy granulations **REIMBURSEMENT INFORMATION** Medicare ♦ Follow-up Days — 10 ♦ Assistant Surgeon — not paid ♦ Supply Charges — not allowed ♦ Outpatient Limit — applies ♦ Minor Surgery Rules Apply

CPT CODE **SERVICE**

ICD–9–CM

69300 Otoplasty, protruding ear, with or without size reduction

CPT NOTES

- For diagnostic services, (e.g., audiometry, vestibular tests), see 92502 et seq).
- For suture of wound or injury of external ear, see 12011–14300.

380.32 Acquired deformity auricle/pinna
744.22 Macrotia
744.29 Ear anomalies NEC
744.3 Ear anomaly NOS

REIMBURSEMENT INFORMATION

Medicare

- Follow–up Days — determined by local carrier
- Assistant Surgeon — determined by local carrier
- Supply Charges — determined by local carrier
- Outpatient Limit — determined by local carrier

69310 Reconstruction of external auditory canal (meatoplasty) (eg, for stenosis due to trauma, infection), (separate procedure)

CPT NOTES

- For diagnostic services, (e.g., audiometry, vestibular tests), see 92502 et seq).
- For suture of wound or injury of external ear, see 12011–14300.

380.32 Acquired deformity auricle/pinna
380.51 Stenosis ext ear canal d/t trauma
385.30 Cholesteatoma NOS
385.32 Cholesteatoma of middle ear
744.02 Ext ear anomaly NEC, hearing impair

REIMBURSEMENT INFORMATION

General

- Separate procedure rules apply.

Medicare

- Follow–up Days — 90
- Assistant Surgeon — not paid
- Supply Charges — not allowed
- Outpatient Limit — does not apply
- Major Surgery Rules Apply

69320 Reconstruction external auditory canal for congenital atresia, single stage

CPT NOTES

- For diagnostic services, (e.g., audiometry, vestibular tests), see 92502 et seq).
- For suture of wound or injury of external ear, see 12011–14300.
- For combination with middle ear reconstruction, see 69631, 69641.
- For other reconstructive procedures with grafts (e.g., skin, cartilage, bone), see 13150–15760, 21230–21235.

744.02 Ext ear anomaly NEC, hearing impair

REIMBURSEMENT INFORMATION

Medicare

- Follow–up Days — 90
- Assistant Surgeon — paid
- Supply Charges — not allowed
- Outpatient Limit — does not apply
- Major Surgery Rules Apply

CPT CODE **SERVICE**

69399 Unlisted procedure, external ear

CPT NOTES

- For diagnostic services, (e.g., audiometry, vestibular tests), see 92502 et seq).
- For otoscopy under general anesthesia, see 92502.

ICD–9–CM

385.30 Cholesteatoma NOS
389.18 Sensorineural hear loss comb type
744.3 Ear anomaly NOS

REIMBURSEMENT INFORMATION

General

- Separate procedure rules apply.

Medicare

- Follow–up Days — determined by local carrier
- Assistant Surgeon — determined by local carrier
- Supply Charges — determined by local carrier
- Outpatient Limit — determined by local carrier

69400 Eustachian tube inflation, transnasal; with catheterization

CPT NOTES

- For diagnostic services, (e.g., audiometry, vestibular tests), see 92502 et seq).

381.4 Chron nonsup otitis media NOS
381.81 Dysfunction of Eustachian tube
389.03 Conductive hearing loss, middle ear

REIMBURSEMENT INFORMATION

Medicare

- Follow–up Days — 0
- Assistant Surgeon — not paid
- Supply Charges — not allowed
- Outpatient Limit — applies
- Minor Surgery Rules Apply

69401 Eustachian tube inflation, transnasal; without catheterization

CPT NOTES

- For diagnostic services, (e.g., audiometry, vestibular tests), see 92502 et seq).

381.4 Chron nonsup otitis media NOS

REIMBURSEMENT INFORMATION

Medicare

- Follow–up Days — 0
- Assistant Surgeon — not paid
- Supply Charges — not allowed
- Outpatient Limit — applies
- Minor Surgery Rules Apply

CPT CODE / SERVICE	ICD-9-CM
69405 Eustachian tube catheterization, transtympanic **CPT NOTES** ♦ For diagnostic services, (e.g., audiometry, vestibular tests), see 92502 et seq).	381.4 Chron nonsup otitis media NOS **REIMBURSEMENT INFORMATION** Medicare ♦ Follow–up Days — 10 ♦ Assistant Surgeon — not paid ♦ Supply Charges — not allowed ♦ Outpatient Limit — does not apply ♦ Minor Surgery Rules Apply
69410 Focal application of phase control substance, middle ear (baffle technique) **CPT NOTES** ♦ For diagnostic services, (e.g., audiometry, vestibular tests), see 92502 et seq).	381.4 Chron nonsup otitis media NOS 384.21 Cent perforate tympanic membrane 389.03 Conductive hearing loss, middle ear **REIMBURSEMENT INFORMATION** Medicare ♦ Follow–up Days — 0 ♦ Assistant Surgeon — not paid ♦ Supply Charges — not allowed ♦ Outpatient Limit — does not apply ♦ Minor Surgery Rules Apply
69420* Myringotomy including aspiration and/or eustachian tube inflation **CPT NOTES** ♦ For diagnostic services, (e.g., audiometry, vestibular tests), see 92502 et seq).	381.00 Acute nonsup otitis media NOS 381.01 Acute serous otitis media 381.04 Acute allergic serous otitis media 381.10 Chron serous otitis media simp/NOS 381.4 Chron nonsup otitis media NOS 381.81 Dysfunction of Eustachian tube 382.3 Chronic suppurativ otitis media NOS 382.4 Suppurative otitis media NOS 382.9 Otitis media NOS 385.32 Cholesteatoma of middle ear 386.50 Labyrinthine dysfunction NOS 388.71 Otogenic pain 389.00 Conductive hearing loss NOS 389.2 Mixed hearing loss **REIMBURSEMENT INFORMATION** General ♦ Starred procedure. Medicare ♦ Follow–up Days — 10 ♦ Assistant Surgeon — not paid ♦ Supply Charges — not allowed ♦ Outpatient Limit — applies ♦ Minor Surgery Rules Apply

CPT CODE	SERVICE	ICD–9–CM

69421* Myringotomy including aspiration and/or eustachian tube inflation requiring general anesthesia

CPT NOTES

- For diagnostic services, (e.g., audiometry, vestibular tests), see 92502 et seq).

381.00	Acute nonsup otitis media NOS
381.01	Acute serous otitis media
381.04	Acute allergic serous otitis media
381.10	Chron serous otitis media simp/NOS
381.4	Chron nonsup otitis media NOS
381.81	Dysfunction of Eustachian tube
382.3	Chronic suppurativ otitis media NOS
382.9	Otitis media NOS
385.32	Cholesteatoma of middle ear
386.50	Labyrinthine dysfunction NOS
388.71	Otogenic pain
389.00	Conductive hearing loss NOS
389.2	Mixed hearing loss

REIMBURSEMENT INFORMATION

General

- Starred procedure.

Medicare

- Follow–up Days — 10
- Assistant Surgeon — not paid
- Supply Charges — not allowed
- Outpatient Limit — does not apply
- Minor Surgery Rules Apply

69424 Ventilating tube removal when originally inserted by another physician

CPT NOTES

- For diagnostic services, (e.g., audiometry, vestibular tests), see 92502 et seq).

381.00	Acute nonsup otitis media NOS
381.01	Acute serous otitis media
381.10	Chron serous otitis media simp/NOS
381.4	Chron nonsup otitis media NOS
381.81	Dysfunction of Eustachian tube
382.9	Otitis media NOS
388.60	Otorrhea NOS
701.5	Abnormal granulation tissue NEC
931	Foreign body in ear

REIMBURSEMENT INFORMATION

Medicare

- Follow–up Days — 0
- Assistant Surgeon — not paid
- Supply Charges — not allowed
- Outpatient Limit — does not apply
- Minor Surgery Rules Apply

CPT CODE **SERVICE**

60433* Tympanostomy (requiring insertion of ventilating tube), local or topical anesthesia

CPT NOTES

- For diagnostic services, (e.g., audiometry, vestibular tests), see 92502 et seq).

ICD–9–CM

380.10	Infective otitis externa NOS
381.00	Acute nonsup otitis media NOS
381.01	Acute serous otitis media
381.04	Acute allergic serous otitis media
381.10	Chron serous otitis media simp/NOS
381.19	Chronic serous otitis media NEC
381.20	Chron mucoid otitis media simp/NOS
381.3	Chronic nonsuppurative otitis media
381.4	Chron nonsup otitis media NOS
381.60	Obstruction of Eustachian tube NOS
381.81	Dysfunction of Eustachian tube
382.00	Acute suppurative otitis media NOS
382.3	Chronic suppurativ otitis media NOS
382.4	Suppurative otitis media NOS
382.9	Otitis media NOS
385.10	Adhesive middle ear disease NOS
385.30	Cholesteatoma NOS
749.01	Unilateral cleft palate, complete
749.02	Unilateral cleft palate, incomplete
749.03	Bilateral cleft palate, complete
749.04	Bilateral cleft palate, incomplete

REIMBURSEMENT INFORMATION

General

- Starred procedure.

Medicare

- Follow–up Days — 10
- Assistant Surgeon — not paid
- Supply Charges — not allowed
- Outpatient Limit — does not apply
- Minor Surgery Rules Apply

CPT CODE **SERVICE**

69436 Tympanostomy (requiring insertion of ventilating tube), general anesthesia

CPT NOTES

- For diagnostic services, (e.g., audiometry, vestibular tests), see 92502 et seq).

ICD–9–CM

380.10	Infective otitis externa NOS
380.16	Chron infective otitis externa NEC
381.00	Acute nonsup otitis media NOS
381.01	Acute serous otitis media
381.02	Acute mucoid otitis media
381.04	Acute allergic serous otitis media
381.05	Acute allergic mucoid otitis media
381.10	Chron serous otitis media simp/NOS
381.3	Chronic nonsuppurative otitis media
381.4	Chron nonsup otitis media NOS
381.81	Dysfunction of Eustachian tube
382.00	Acute suppurative otitis media NOS
382.3	Chronic suppurativ otitis media NOS
382.4	Suppurative otitis media NOS
382.9	Otitis media NOS
384.9	Tympanic membrane disorder NOS
385.10	Adhesive middle ear disease NOS
385.30	Cholesteatoma NOS
389.00	Conductive hearing loss NOS
389.03	Conductive hearing loss, middle ear
749.01	Unilateral cleft palate, complete
749.02	Unilateral cleft palate, incomplete
749.03	Bilateral cleft palate, complete
749.04	Bilateral cleft palate, incomplete

REIMBURSEMENT INFORMATION

Medicare

- Follow–up Days — 10
- Assistant Surgeon — not paid
- Supply Charges — not allowed
- Outpatient Limit — does not apply
- Minor Surgery Rules Apply

CPT CODE	SERVICE	ICD–9–CM

69440 Middle ear exploration through postauricular or ear canal incision

CPT NOTES

- For diagnostic services, (e.g., audiometry, vestibular tests), see 92502 et seq).
- For atticotomy, see 69601 et seq.

160.1	M-Neoplasm, Middle ear
212.0	B-Neoplasm, Nasal cavity/sinus
381.00	Acute nonsup otitis media NOS
382.00	Acute suppurative otitis media NOS
382.3	Chronic suppurativ otitis media NOS
382.9	Otitis media NOS
383.9	Mastoiditis NOS
384.20	Perforation tympanic membrane NOS
385.30	Cholesteatoma NOS
385.82	Cholesterin granuloma
386.41	Labyrinthine, round window fistula
386.42	Labyrinthine, oval window fistula
387.0	Otosclerosis, oval window, nonoblit
389.00	Conductive hearing loss NOS
389.9	Hearing loss NOS
767.5	Facial nerve injury at birth

REIMBURSEMENT INFORMATION

Medicare

- Follow–up Days — 90
- Assistant Surgeon — not paid
- Supply Charges — not allowed
- Outpatient Limit — does not apply
- Major Surgery Rules Apply

69450 Tympanolysis, transcanal

CPT NOTES

- For diagnostic services, (e.g., audiometry, vestibular tests), see 92502 et seq).

381.00	Acute nonsup otitis media NOS
382.00	Acute suppurative otitis media NOS
382.3	Chronic suppurativ otitis media NOS
382.9	Otitis media NOS
383.9	Mastoiditis NOS
384.20	Perforation tympanic membrane NOS
385.00	Tympanosclerosis NOS
385.30	Cholesteatoma NOS
385.82	Cholesterin granuloma
387.0	Otosclerosis, oval window, nonoblit
389.00	Conductive hearing loss NOS
389.9	Hearing loss NOS

REIMBURSEMENT INFORMATION

Medicare

- Follow–up Days — 90
- Assistant Surgeon — not paid
- Supply Charges — not allowed
- Outpatient Limit — does not apply
- Major Surgery Rules Apply

CPT CODE **SERVICE**

ICD–9–CM

69501 Transmastoid antrotomy ("simple" mastoidectomy)

CPT NOTES

- For diagnostic services, (e.g., audiometry, vestibular tests), see 92502 et seq).

212.0	B-Neoplasm, Nasal cavity/sinus
381.00	Acute nonsup otitis media NOS
382.00	Acute suppurative otitis media NOS
382.3	Chronic suppurativ otitis media NOS
382.9	Otitis media NOS
383.9	Mastoiditis NOS
384.20	Perforation tympanic membrane NOS
385.33	Cholesteatoma, middle ear/mastoid
385.82	Cholesterin granuloma
386.41	Labyrinthine, round window fistula
386.42	Labyrinthine, oval window fistula
387.0	Otosclerosis, oval window, nonoblit
389.00	Conductive hearing loss NOS
389.9	Hearing loss NOS

REIMBURSEMENT INFORMATION

Medicare

- Follow–up Days — 90
- Assistant Surgeon — paid
- Supply Charges — not allowed
- Outpatient Limit — does not apply
- Major Surgery Rules Apply

69502 Mastoidectomy; complete

CPT NOTES

- For diagnostic services, (e.g., audiometry, vestibular tests), see 92502 et seq).
- For skin graft, see 15000 et seq.
- For mastoidectomy cavity debridement, see 69220, 69222.

160.1	M-Neoplasm, Middle Ear
212.0	B-Neoplasm, Nasal cavity/sinus
381.00	Acute nonsup otitis media NOS
382.00	Acute suppurative otitis media NOS
382.3	Chronic suppurativ otitis media NOS
382.9	Otitis media NOS
383.00	Acute mastoiditis w/o complications
383.9	Mastoiditis NOS
384.20	Perforation tympanic membrane NOS
385.33	Cholesteatoma, middle ear/mastoid
385.82	Cholesterin granuloma
386.41	Labyrinthine, round window fistula
386.42	Labyrinthine, oval window fistula
387.0	Otosclerosis, oval window, nonoblit
389.00	Conductive hearing loss NOS
389.9	Hearing loss NOS

REIMBURSEMENT INFORMATION

Medicare

- Follow–up Days — 90
- Assistant Surgeon — not paid
- Supply Charges — not allowed
- Outpatient Limit — does not apply
- Major Surgery Rules Apply

CPT CODE **SERVICE**

69505 Mastoidectomy; modified radical

CPT NOTES

- For diagnostic services, (e.g., audiometry, vestibular tests), see 92502 et seq).
- For skin graft, see 15000 et seq.
- For mastoidectomy cavity debridement, see 69220, 69222.

ICD–9–CM

160.1	M-Neoplasm, Middle Ear
212.0	B-Neoplasm, Nasal cavity/sinus
381.00	Acute nonsup otitis media NOS
382.00	Acute suppurative otitis media NOS
382.3	Chronic suppurativ otitis media NOS
382.9	Otitis media NOS
383.9	Mastoiditis NOS
384.20	Perforation tympanic membrane NOS
385.33	Cholesteatoma, middle ear/mastoid
385.82	Cholesterin granuloma
386.41	Labyrinthine, round window fistula
386.42	Labyrinthine, oval window fistula
387.0	Otosclerosis, oval window, nonoblit
389.00	Conductive hearing loss NOS
389.9	Hearing loss NOS

REIMBURSEMENT INFORMATION

Medicare

- Follow–up Days — 90
- Assistant Surgeon — not paid
- Supply Charges — not allowed
- Outpatient Limit — does not apply
- Major Surgery Rules Apply

69511 Mastoidectomy; radical

CPT NOTES

- For diagnostic services, (e.g., audiometry, vestibular tests), see 92502 et seq).
- For skin graft, see 15000 et seq.
- for mastoidectomy cavity debridement, see 69220, 69222.

160.1	M-Neoplasm, Middle Ear
212.0	B-Neoplasm, Nasal cavity/sinus
381.00	Acute nonsup otitis media NOS
382.00	Acute suppurative otitis media NOS
382.3	Chronic suppurativ otitis media NOS
382.9	Otitis media NOS
383.9	Mastoiditis NOS
384.20	Perforation tympanic membrane NOS
385.33	Cholesteatoma, middle ear/mastoid
385.82	Cholesterin granuloma
386.41	Labyrinthine, round window fistula
386.42	Labyrinthine, oval window fistula
387.0	Otosclerosis, oval window, nonoblit
389.00	Conductive hearing loss NOS
389.9	Hearing loss NOS
526.2	Jaw cysts NEC

REIMBURSEMENT INFORMATION

Medicare

- Follow–up Days — 90
- Assistant Surgeon — not paid
- Supply Charges — not allowed
- Outpatient Limit — does not apply
- Major Surgery Rules Apply

CPT CODE **SERVICE**

69530 Petrous apicectomy including radical mastoidectomy

CPT NOTES

- For diagnostic services, (e.g., audiometry, vestibular tests), see 92502 et seq).

ICD–9–CM

170.0	M-Neoplasm, Skull/Face bone
213.0	B-Neoplasm, Skull/Face bone
381.00	Acute nonsup otitis media NOS
382.00	Acute suppurative otitis media NOS
382.3	Chronic suppurativ otitis media NOS
382.9	Otitis media NOS
383.21	Acute petrositis
383.22	Chronic petrositis
383.9	Mastoiditis NOS
385.33	Cholesteatoma, middle ear/mastoid
385.82	Cholesterin granuloma
387.0	Otosclerosis, oval window, nonoblit
389.00	Conductive hearing loss NOS
389.9	Hearing loss NOS

REIMBURSEMENT INFORMATION

Medicare

- Follow–up Days — 90
- Assistant Surgeon — paid
- Supply Charges — not allowed
- Outpatient Limit — does not apply
- Major Surgery Rules Apply

69535 Resection temporal bone, external approach

CPT NOTES

- For diagnostic services, (e.g., audiometry, vestibular tests), see 92502 et seq).
- For middle fossa approach, see 69950–69970.

170.0	M-Neoplasm, Skull/Face bone
213.0	B-Neoplasm, Skull/Face bone
383.21	Acute petrositis
383.22	Chronic petrositis
383.30	Postmastoidectomy complication NOS
385.33	Cholesteatoma, middle ear/mastoid
385.82	Cholesterin granuloma
387.0	Otosclerosis, oval window, nonoblit
389.00	Conductive hearing loss NOS
389.9	Hearing loss NOS

REIMBURSEMENT INFORMATION

Medicare

- Follow–up Days — 90
- Assistant Surgeon — paid
- Supply Charges — not allowed
- Outpatient Limit — does not apply
- Major Surgery Rules Apply

CPT CODE	SERVICE	ICD–9–CM
69540	Excision aural polyp **CPT NOTES** ♦ For diagnostic services, (e.g., audiometry, vestibular tests), see 92502 et seq).	381.00 Acute nonsup otitis media NOS 382.00 Acute suppurative otitis media NOS 382.3 Chronic suppurativ otitis media NOS 382.9 Otitis media NOS 383.9 Mastoiditis NOS 385.30 Cholesteatoma NOS 385.82 Cholesterin granuloma 387.0 Otosclerosis, oval window, nonoblit 389.00 Conductive hearing loss NOS 389.9 Hearing loss NOS **REIMBURSEMENT INFORMATION** Medicare ♦ Follow–up Days — 10 ♦ Assistant Surgeon — not paid ♦ Supply Charges — not allowed ♦ Outpatient Limit — does not apply ♦ Minor Surgery Rules Apply
69550	Excision aural glomus tumor; transcanal **CPT NOTES** ♦ For diagnostic services, (e.g., audiometry, vestibular tests), see 92502 et seq).	192.0 M-Neoplasm, Cranial nerves 194.6 M-Neoplasm, Paraganglia NEC 198.4 M2-Neoplasm, Nervous system NEC 225.1 B-Neoplasm, Cranial nerve 227.6 B-Neoplasm, Paraganglia NEC 237.9 UB-Neoplasm, Nervous system NEC 388.32 Objective tinnitus 389.00 Conductive hearing loss NOS 389.9 Hearing loss NOS **REIMBURSEMENT INFORMATION** Medicare ♦ Follow–up Days — 90 ♦ Assistant Surgeon — paid ♦ Supply Charges — not allowed ♦ Outpatient Limit — does not apply ♦ Major Surgery Rules Apply

CPT CODE	SERVICE	ICD–9–CM
69552	Excision aural glomus tumor; transmastoid **CPT NOTES** ♦ For diagnostic services, (e.g., audiometry, vestibular tests), see 92502 et seq).	192.0 M-Neoplasm, Cranial nerves 194.6 M-Neoplasm, Paraganglia NEC 198.4 M2-Neoplasm, Nervous system NEC 225.1 B-Neoplasm, Cranial nerve 227.6 B-Neoplasm, Paraganglia NEC 237.9 UB-Neoplasm, Nervous system NEC 388.32 Objective tinnitus 389.00 Conductive hearing loss NOS 389.9 Hearing loss NOS **REIMBURSEMENT INFORMATION** Medicare ♦ Follow–up Days — 90 ♦ Assistant Surgeon — paid ♦ Supply Charges — not allowed ♦ Outpatient Limit — does not apply ♦ Major Surgery Rules Apply
69554	Excision aural glomus tumor; extended (extratemporal) **CPT NOTES** ♦ For diagnostic services, (e.g., audiometry, vestibular tests), see 92502 et seq).	192.0 M-Neoplasm, Cranial nerves 194.6 M-Neoplasm, Paraganglia NEC 198.4 M2-Neoplasm, Nervous system NEC 225.1 B-Neoplasm, Cranial nerve 227.6 B-Neoplasm, Paraganglia NEC 237.9 UB-Neoplasm, Nervous system NEC 388.32 Objective tinnitus 389.00 Conductive hearing loss NOS 389.9 Hearing loss NOS **REIMBURSEMENT INFORMATION** Medicare ♦ Follow–up Days — 90 ♦ Assistant Surgeon — paid ♦ Supply Charges — not allowed ♦ Outpatient Limit — does not apply ♦ Major Surgery Rules Apply

CPT CODE	SERVICE	ICD–9–CM

69601 Revision mastoidectomy; resulting in complete mastoidectomy

CPT NOTES

- For diagnostic services, (e.g., audiometry, vestibular tests), see 92502 et seq).
- For planned secondary tympanoplasty after mastoidectomy, see 69631, 69632.
- For skin graft see 15120, 15121, 15260, 15261.

ICD–9–CM

381.00	Acute nonsup otitis media NOS
382.00	Acute suppurative otitis media NOS
382.3	Chronic suppurativ otitis media NOS
382.9	Otitis media NOS
383.1	Chronic mastoiditis
383.31	Postmastoidectomy mucosal cyst
383.32	Postmastoidectomy cholesteatoma
383.33	Postmastoidectomy granulations
383.9	Mastoiditis NOS
385.33	Cholesteatoma, middle ear/mastoid
385.82	Cholesterin granuloma
387.0	Otosclerosis, oval window, nonoblit
389.00	Conductive hearing loss NOS
389.9	Hearing loss NOS

REIMBURSEMENT INFORMATION

Medicare

- Follow–up Days — 90
- Assistant Surgeon — not paid
- Supply Charges — not allowed
- Outpatient Limit — does not apply
- Major Surgery Rules Apply

69602 Revision mastoidectomy; resulting in modified radical mastoidectomy

CPT NOTES

- For diagnostic services, (e.g., audiometry, vestibular tests), see 92502 et seq).
- For planned secondary tympanoplasty after mastoidectomy, see 69631, 69632.
- For skin graft see 15120, 15121, 15260, 15261.

ICD–9–CM

381.00	Acute nonsup otitis media NOS
382.00	Acute suppurative otitis media NOS
382.3	Chronic suppurativ otitis media NOS
382.9	Otitis media NOS
383.1	Chronic mastoiditis
383.31	Postmastoidectomy mucosal cyst
383.32	Postmastoidectomy cholesteatoma
383.33	Postmastoidectomy granulations
383.9	Mastoiditis NOS
385.33	Cholesteatoma, middle ear/mastoid
385.82	Cholesterin granuloma
387.0	Otosclerosis, oval window, nonoblit
389.00	Conductive hearing loss NOS
389.9	Hearing loss NOS

REIMBURSEMENT INFORMATION

Medicare

- Follow–up Days — 90
- Assistant Surgeon — paid
- Supply Charges — not allowed
- Outpatient Limit — does not apply
- Major Surgery Rules Apply

CPT CODE	SERVICE	ICD–9–CM

69603 Revision mastoidectomy; resulting in radical mastoidectomy

CPT NOTES

- For diagnostic services, (e.g., audiometry, vestibular tests), see 92502 et seq).
- For planned secondary tympanoplasty after mastoidectomy, see 69631, 69632.
- For skin graft see 15120, 15121, 15260, 15261.

381.00 Acute nonsup otitis media NOS
382.00 Acute suppurative otitis media NOS
382.3 Chronic suppurativ otitis media NOS
382.9 Otitis media NOS
383.1 Chronic mastoiditis
383.31 Postmastoidectomy mucosal cyst
383.32 Postmastoidectomy cholesteatoma
383.33 Postmastoidectomy granulations
383.9 Mastoiditis NOS
385.33 Cholesteatoma, middle ear/mastoid
385.82 Cholesterin granuloma
387.0 Otosclerosis, oval window, nonoblit
389.00 Conductive hearing loss NOS

REIMBURSEMENT INFORMATION

Medicare

- Follow–up Days — 90
- Assistant Surgeon — not paid
- Supply Charges — not allowed
- Outpatient Limit — does not apply
- Major Surgery Rules Apply

69604 Revision mastoidectomy; resulting in tympanoplasty

CPT NOTES

- For diagnostic services, (e.g., audiometry, vestibular tests), see 92502 et seq).
- For planned secondary tympanoplasty after mastoidectomy, see 69631, 69632.
- For skin graft see 15120, 15121, 15260, 15261.

381.00 Acute nonsup otitis media NOS
382.00 Acute suppurative otitis media NOS
382.3 Chronic suppurativ otitis media NOS
382.9 Otitis media NOS
383.1 Chronic mastoiditis
383.31 Postmastoidectomy mucosal cyst
383.32 Postmastoidectomy cholesteatoma
383.33 Postmastoidectomy granulations
383.9 Mastoiditis NOS
384.20 Perforation tympanic membrane NOS
385.32 Cholesteatoma of middle ear
385.33 Cholesteatoma, middle ear/mastoid
385.82 Cholesterin granuloma
387.0 Otosclerosis, oval window, nonoblit
389.00 Conductive hearing loss NOS

REIMBURSEMENT INFORMATION

Medicare

- Follow–up Days — 90
- Assistant Surgeon — paid
- Supply Charges — not allowed
- Outpatient Limit — does not apply
- Major Surgery Rules Apply

CPT CODE	SERVICE	ICD–9–CM

69605 Revision mastoidectomy, with apicectomy

CPT NOTES

- For diagnostic services, (e.g., audiometry, vestibular tests), see 92502 et seq).
- For skin graft see 15120, 15121, 15260, 15261.

381.00	Acute nonsup otitis media NOS
382.00	Acute suppurative otitis media NOS
382.3	Chronic suppurativ otitis media NOS
382.9	Otitis media NOS
383.1	Chronic mastoiditis
383.21	Acute petrositis
383.22	Chronic petrositis
383.31	Postmastoidectomy mucosal cyst
383.32	Postmastoidectomy cholesteatoma
383.33	Postmastoidectomy granulations
383.9	Mastoiditis NOS
384.20	Perforation tympanic membrane NOS
385.32	Cholesteatoma of middle ear
385.33	Cholesteatoma, middle ear/mastoid
385.82	Cholesterin granuloma
387.0	Otosclerosis, oval window, nonoblit
389.00	Conductive hearing loss NOS

REIMBURSEMENT INFORMATION

<u>Medicare</u>

- Follow–up Days — 90
- Assistant Surgeon — paid
- Supply Charges — not allowed
- Outpatient Limit — does not apply
- Major Surgery Rules Apply

69610 Tympanic membrane repair, with or without site preparation or perforation preparation for closure with or without patch

CPT NOTES

- For diagnostic services, (e.g., audiometry, vestibular tests), see 92502 et seq).

381.00	Acute nonsup otitis media NOS
381.81	Dysfunction of Eustachian tube
382.00	Acute suppurative otitis media NOS
382.3	Chronic suppurativ otitis media NOS
382.9	Otitis media NOS
383.02	Acute mastoiditis w/complic NEC
384.21	Cent perforate tympanic membrane
384.22	Attic perforate tympanic membrane
384.23	Marginal perf tympanic membrane NEC
384.24	Multiple perfs tympanic membrane
384.25	Total perforate tympanic membrane
385.00	Tympanosclerosis NOS
385.33	Cholesteatoma, middle ear/mastoid
389.02	Conductive hearing loss, tympanic
389.03	Conductive hearing loss, middle ear
872.61	Open wound of eardrum

REIMBURSEMENT INFORMATION

<u>Medicare</u>

- Follow–up Days — 10
- Assistant Surgeon — not paid
- Supply Charges — not allowed
- Outpatient Limit — applies
- Minor Surgery Rules Apply

CPT CODE	SERVICE	ICD–9–CM

69620 Myringoplasty (surgery confined to drumhead and donor area)

CPT NOTES

- For diagnostic services, (e.g., audiometry, vestibular tests), see 92502 et seq).

ICD–9–CM

381.00	Acute nonsup otitis media NOS
381.4	Chron nonsup otitis media NOS
381.81	Dysfunction of Eustachian tube
382.00	Acute suppurative otitis media NOS
382.3	Chronic suppurativ otitis media NOS
382.9	Otitis media NOS
383.02	Acute mastoiditis w/complic NEC
384.21	Cent perforate tympanic membrane
384.22	Attic perforate tympanic membrane
384.23	Marginal perf tympanic membrane NEC
384.24	Multiple perfs tympanic membrane
384.25	Total perforate tympanic membrane
385.00	Tympanosclerosis NOS
385.33	Cholesteatoma, middle ear/mastoid
389.02	Conductive hearing loss, tympanic
389.03	Conductive hearing loss, middle ear
872.61	Open wound of eardrum

REIMBURSEMENT INFORMATION

Medicare

- Follow–up Days — 90
- Assistant Surgeon — not paid
- Supply Charges — not allowed
- Outpatient Limit — does not apply
- Major Surgery Rules Apply

69631 Tympanoplasty without mastoidectomy (including canalplasty, atticotomy and/or middle ear surgery), initial or revision; without ossicular chain reconstruction

CPT NOTES

- For diagnostic services, (e.g., audiometry, vestibular tests), see 92502 et seq).

381.00	Acute nonsup otitis media NOS
381.81	Dysfunction of Eustachian tube
382.00	Acute suppurative otitis media NOS
382.3	Chronic suppurativ otitis media NOS
382.9	Otitis media NOS
383.02	Acute mastoiditis w/complic NEC
384.20	Perforation tympanic membrane NOS
384.21	Cent perforate tympanic membrane
384.23	Marginal perf tympanic membrane NEC
385.00	Tympanosclerosis NOS
385.30	Cholesteatoma NOS
385.33	Cholesteatoma, middle ear/mastoid
389.02	Conductive hearing loss, tympanic
389.03	Conductive hearing loss, middle ear
872.61	Open wound of eardrum

REIMBURSEMENT INFORMATION

Medicare

- Follow–up Days — 90
- Assistant Surgeon — not paid
- Supply Charges — not allowed
- Outpatient Limit — does not apply
- Major Surgery Rules Apply

CPT CODE **SERVICE**

69632 Tympanoplasty without mastoidectomy (including canalplasty, atticotomy and/or middle ear surgery), initial or revision; with ossicular chain reconstruction

CPT NOTES

- For diagnostic services, (e.g., audiometry, vestibular tests), see 92502 et seq).

ICD–9–CM

381.00	Acute nonsup otitis media NOS
381.81	Dysfunction of Eustachian tube
382.00	Acute suppurative otitis media NOS
382.3	Chronic suppurativ otitis media NOS
382.9	Otitis media NOS
383.02	Acute mastoiditis w/complic NEC
383.33	Postmastoidectomy granulations
384.20	Perforation tympanic membrane NOS
384.21	Cent perforate tympanic membrane
384.23	Marginal perf tympanic membrane NEC
385.00	Tympanosclerosis NOS
385.10	Adhesive middle ear disease NOS
385.23	Dislocation of ear ossicles
385.30	Cholesteatoma NOS
385.33	Cholesteatoma, middle ear/mastoid
387.2	Cochlear otosclerosis
389.00	Conductive hearing loss NOS
389.02	Conductive hearing loss, tympanic
389.03	Conductive hearing loss, middle ear
389.9	Hearing loss NOS
872.61	Open wound of eardrum

REIMBURSEMENT INFORMATION

Medicare

- Follow–up Days — 90
- Assistant Surgeon — not paid
- Supply Charges — not allowed
- Outpatient Limit — does not apply
- Major Surgery Rules Apply

CPT CODE **SERVICE**

69633 Tympanoplasty without mastoidectomy (including canalplasty, atticotomy and/or middle ear surgery), initial or revision; with ossicular chain reconstruction and synthetic prosthesis (eg, partial ossicular replacement prosthesis, (PORP), total ossicular replacement prosthesis (TORP))

CPT NOTES

- For diagnostic services, (e.g., audiometry, vestibular tests), see 92502 et seq).

ICD–9–CM

381.00	Acute nonsup otitis media NOS
381.81	Dysfunction of Eustachian tube
382.00	Acute suppurative otitis media NOS
382.3	Chronic suppurativ otitis media NOS
382.9	Otitis media NOS
383.02	Acute mastoiditis w/complic NEC
383.33	Postmastoidectomy granulations
384.20	Perforation tympanic membrane NOS
384.21	Cent perforate tympanic membrane
384.22	Attic perforate tympanic membrane
384.23	Marginal perf tympanic membrane NEC
384.25	Total perforate tympanic membrane
385.00	Tympanosclerosis NOS
385.10	Adhesive middle ear disease NOS
385.23	Dislocation of ear ossicles
385.30	Cholesteatoma NOS
385.33	Cholesteatoma, middle ear/mastoid
385.89	Middle Ear/Mastoid disorder NEC
387.2	Cochlear otosclerosis
389.00	Conductive hearing loss NOS
389.02	Conductive hearing loss, tympanic
389.03	Conductive hearing loss, middle ear
389.9	Hearing loss NOS

REIMBURSEMENT INFORMATION

Medicare

- Follow–up Days — 90
- Assistant Surgeon — not paid
- Supply Charges — not allowed
- Outpatient Limit — does not apply
- Major Surgery Rules Apply

CPT CODE	SERVICE
69635	Tympanoplasty with antrotomy or mastoidotomy (including canalplasty, atticotomy, middle ear surgery, and/or tympanic membrane repair); without ossicular chain reconstruction

CPT NOTES

- For diagnostic services, (e.g., audiometry, vestibular tests), see 92502 et seq).

ICD-9-CM

381.00	Acute nonsup otitis media NOS
381.81	Dysfunction of Eustachian tube
382.00	Acute suppurative otitis media NOS
382.3	Chronic suppurativ otitis media NOS
382.9	Otitis media NOS
383.02	Acute mastoiditis w/complic NEC
383.1	Chronic mastoiditis
383.33	Postmastoidectomy granulations
384.20	Perforation tympanic membrane NOS
384.21	Cent perforate tympanic membrane
384.22	Attic perforate tympanic membrane
384.23	Marginal perf tympanic membrane NEC
384.25	Total perforate tympanic membrane
385.00	Tympanosclerosis NOS
385.10	Adhesive middle ear disease NOS
385.23	Dislocation of ear ossicles
385.30	Cholesteatoma NOS
385.32	Cholesteatoma of middle ear
385.33	Cholesteatoma, middle ear/mastoid
385.89	Middle Ear/Mastoid disorder NEC
387.2	Cochlear otosclerosis
389.00	Conductive hearing loss NOS
389.02	Conductive hearing loss, tympanic
389.03	Conductive hearing loss, middle ear
389.9	Hearing loss NOS

REIMBURSEMENT INFORMATION

Medicare

- Follow–up Days — 90
- Assistant Surgeon — not paid
- Supply Charges — not allowed
- Outpatient Limit — does not apply
- Major Surgery Rules Apply

CPT CODE **SERVICE**

69636 Tympanoplasty with antrotomy or mastoidotomy (including canalplasty, atticotomy, middle ear surgery, and/or tympanic membrane repair); with ossicular chain reconstruction

CPT NOTES

- For diagnostic services, (e.g., audiometry, vestibular tests), see 92502 et seq).

ICD–9–CM

381.00	Acute nonsup otitis media NOS
381.81	Dysfunction of Eustachian tube
382.00	Acute suppurative otitis media NOS
382.3	Chronic suppurativ otitis media NOS
382.9	Otitis media NOS
383.02	Acute mastoiditis w/complic NEC
383.1	Chronic mastoiditis
383.33	Postmastoidectomy granulations
384.20	Perforation tympanic membrane NOS
384.21	Cent perforate tympanic membrane
384.22	Attic perforate tympanic membrane
384.23	Marginal perf tympanic membrane NEC
384.25	Total perforate tympanic membrane
385.10	Adhesive middle ear disease NOS
385.23	Dislocation of ear ossicles
385.30	Cholesteatoma NOS
385.32	Cholesteatoma of middle ear
385.33	Cholesteatoma, middle ear/mastoid
385.89	Middle Ear/Mastoid disorder NEC
387.2	Cochlear otosclerosis
389.00	Conductive hearing loss NOS
389.02	Conductive hearing loss, tympanic
389.03	Conductive hearing loss, middle ear
389.9	Hearing loss NOS

REIMBURSEMENT INFORMATION

Medicare

- Follow–up Days — 90
- Assistant Surgeon — not paid
- Supply Charges — not allowed
- Outpatient Limit — does not apply
- Major Surgery Rules Apply

CPT CODE	SERVICE
69637	Tympanoplasty with antrotomy or mastoidotomy (including canalplasty, atticotomy, middle ear surgery, and/or tympanic membrane repair); with ossicular chain reconstruction and synthetic prosthesis (eg, partial ossicular replacement prosthesis, (PORP), total ossicular replacement prosthesis (TORP))

CPT NOTES

- For diagnostic services, (e.g., audiometry, vestibular tests), see 92502 et seq).

ICD–9–CM

381.00	Acute nonsup otitis media NOS
381.81	Dysfunction of Eustachian tube
382.00	Acute suppurative otitis media NOS
382.3	Chronic suppurativ otitis media NOS
382.9	Otitis media NOS
383.02	Acute mastoiditis w/complic NEC
383.1	Chronic mastoiditis
383.33	Postmastoidectomy granulations
384.20	Perforation tympanic membrane NOS
384.21	Cent perforate tympanic membrane
384.22	Attic perforate tympanic membrane
384.23	Marginal perf tympanic membrane NEC
384.25	Total perforate tympanic membrane
385.00	Tympanosclerosis NOS
385.10	Adhesive middle ear disease NOS
385.23	Dislocation of ear ossicles
385.30	Cholesteatoma NOS
385.32	Cholesteatoma of middle ear
385.33	Cholesteatoma, middle ear/mastoid
385.89	Middle Ear/Mastoid disorder NEC
387.2	Cochlear otosclerosis
389.00	Conductive hearing loss NOS
389.02	Conductive hearing loss, tympanic
389.03	Conductive hearing loss, middle ear
389.9	Hearing loss NOS

REIMBURSEMENT INFORMATION

Medicare

- Follow–up Days — 90
- Assistant Surgeon — not paid
- Supply Charges — not allowed
- Outpatient Limit — does not apply
- Major Surgery Rules Apply

CPT CODE **SERVICE**

69641 Tympanoplasty with mastoidectomy (including canalplasty, middle ear surgery, tympanic membrane repair); without ossicular chain reconstruction

CPT NOTES

- For diagnostic services, (e.g., audiometry, vestibular tests), see 92502 et seq).

ICD–9–CM

381.00	Acute nonsup otitis media NOS
381.10	Chron serous otitis media simp/NOS
381.81	Dysfunction of Eustachian tube
382.00	Acute suppurative otitis media NOS
382.2	Chronic atticoantral suppurative OM
382.3	Chronic suppurativ otitis media NOS
382.9	Otitis media NOS
383.02	Acute mastoiditis w/complic NEC
383.1	Chronic mastoiditis
383.33	Postmastoidectomy granulations
383.9	Mastoiditis NOS
384.20	Perforation tympanic membrane NOS
384.21	Cent perforate tympanic membrane
384.22	Attic perforate tympanic membrane
384.23	Marginal perf tympanic membrane NEC
384.25	Total perforate tympanic membrane
385.00	Tympanosclerosis NOS
385.10	Adhesive middle ear disease NOS
385.23	Dislocation of ear ossicles
385.30	Cholesteatoma NOS
385.32	Cholesteatoma of middle ear
385.33	Cholesteatoma, middle ear/mastoid
385.89	Middle Ear/Mastoid disorder NEC
387.2	Cochlear otosclerosis
389.00	Conductive hearing loss NOS
389.02	Conductive hearing loss, tympanic
389.03	Conductive hearing loss, middle ear
389.9	Hearing loss NOS

REIMBURSEMENT INFORMATION

Medicare

- Follow–up Days — 90
- Assistant Surgeon — not paid
- Supply Charges — not allowed
- Outpatient Limit — does not apply
- Major Surgery Rules Apply

CPT CODE	SERVICE
69642	Tympanoplasty with mastoidectomy (including canalplasty, middle ear surgery, tympanic membrane repair); with ossicular chain reconstruction

CPT NOTES

- For diagnostic services, (e.g., audiometry, vestibular tests), see 92502 et seq).

ICD–9–CM

381.00	Acute nonsup otitis media NOS
381.10	Chron serous otitis media simp/NOS
381.81	Dysfunction of Eustachian tube
382.00	Acute suppurative otitis media NOS
382.2	Chronic atticoantral suppurative OM
382.3	Chronic suppurativ otitis media NOS
382.9	Otitis media NOS
383.02	Acute mastoiditis w/complic NEC
383.1	Chronic mastoiditis
383.33	Postmastoidectomy granulations
383.9	Mastoiditis NOS
384.20	Perforation tympanic membrane NOS
384.21	Cent perforate tympanic membrane
384.22	Attic perforate tympanic membrane
384.23	Marginal perf tympanic membrane NEC
384.25	Total perforate tympanic membrane
385.00	Tympanosclerosis NOS
385.10	Adhesive middle ear disease NOS
385.23	Dislocation of ear ossicles
385.30	Cholesteatoma NOS
385.32	Cholesteatoma of middle ear
385.33	Cholesteatoma, middle ear/mastoid
385.89	Middle Ear/Mastoid disorder NEC
387.2	Cochlear otosclerosis
389.00	Conductive hearing loss NOS
389.02	Conductive hearing loss, tympanic
389.03	Conductive hearing loss, middle ear
389.9	Hearing loss NOS

REIMBURSEMENT INFORMATION

<u>Medicare</u>

- Follow–up Days — 90
- Assistant Surgeon — not paid
- Supply Charges — not allowed
- Outpatient Limit — does not apply
- Major Surgery Rules Apply

CPT CODE **SERVICE**

69643 Tympanoplasty with mastoidectomy (including canalplasty, middle ear surgery, tympanic membrane repair); with intact or reconstructed wall, without ossicular chain reconstruction

CPT NOTES

- For diagnostic services, (e.g., audiometry, vestibular tests), see 92502 et seq).

ICD–9–CM

381.00	Acute nonsup otitis media NOS
381.10	Chron serous otitis media simp/NOS
381.81	Dysfunction of Eustachian tube
382.00	Acute suppurative otitis media NOS
382.2	Chronic atticoantral suppurative OM
382.3	Chronic suppurativ otitis media NOS
382.9	Otitis media NOS
383.02	Acute mastoiditis w/complic NEC
383.1	Chronic mastoiditis
383.33	Postmastoidectomy granulations
383.9	Mastoiditis NOS
384.20	Perforation tympanic membrane NOS
384.21	Cent perforate tympanic membrane
384.22	Attic perforate tympanic membrane
384.23	Marginal perf tympanic membrane NEC
384.25	Total perforate tympanic membrane
385.00	Tympanosclerosis NOS
385.10	Adhesive middle ear disease NOS
385.23	Dislocation of ear ossicles
385.30	Cholesteatoma NOS
385.32	Cholesteatoma of middle ear
385.33	Cholesteatoma, middle ear/mastoid
385.89	Middle Ear/Mastoid disorder NEC
387.2	Cochlear otosclerosis
389.00	Conductive hearing loss NOS
389.02	Conductive hearing loss, tympanic
389.03	Conductive hearing loss, middle ear
389.9	Hearing loss NOS

REIMBURSEMENT INFORMATION

Medicare

- Follow–up Days — 90
- Assistant Surgeon — not paid
- Supply Charges — not allowed
- Outpatient Limit — does not apply
- Major Surgery Rules Apply

CPT CODE **SERVICE**

69644 Tympanoplasty with mastoidectomy (including canalplasty, middle ear surgery, tympanic membrane repair); with intact or reconstructed canal wall, with ossicular chain reconstruction

CPT NOTES

- For diagnostic services, (e.g., audiometry, vestibular tests), see 92502 et seq).

ICD–9–CM

381.00	Acute nonsup otitis media NOS
381.10	Chron serous otitis media simp/NOS
381.81	Dysfunction of Eustachian tube
382.00	Acute suppurative otitis media NOS
382.2	Chronic atticoantral suppurative OM
382.3	Chronic suppurativ otitis media NOS
382.9	Otitis media NOS
383.02	Acute mastoiditis w/complic NEC
383.1	Chronic mastoiditis
383.33	Postmastoidectomy granulations
383.9	Mastoiditis NOS
384.20	Perforation tympanic membrane NOS
384.21	Cent perforate tympanic membrane
384.22	Attic perforate tympanic membrane
384.23	Marginal perf tympanic membrane NEC
384.25	Total perforate tympanic membrane
385.00	Tympanosclerosis NOS
385.10	Adhesive middle ear disease NOS
385.23	Dislocation of ear ossicles
385.30	Cholesteatoma NOS
385.32	Cholesteatoma of middle ear
385.33	Cholesteatoma, middle ear/mastoid
385.89	Middle Ear/Mastoid disorder NEC
387.2	Cochlear otosclerosis
389.00	Conductive hearing loss NOS
389.02	Conductive hearing loss, tympanic
389.03	Conductive hearing loss, middle ear
389.9	Hearing loss NOS

REIMBURSEMENT INFORMATION

Medicare

- Follow–up Days — 90
- Assistant Surgeon — not paid
- Supply Charges — not allowed
- Outpatient Limit — does not apply
- Major Surgery Rules Apply

CPT CODE **SERVICE**

69645 Tympanoplasty with mastoidectomy (including canalplasty, middle ear surgery, tympanic membrane repair); radical or complete, without ossicular chain reconstruction

CPT NOTES

- For diagnostic services, (e.g., audiometry, vestibular tests), see 92502 et seq).

ICD–9–CM

381.00	Acute nonsup otitis media NOS
381.10	Chron serous otitis media simp/NOS
381.81	Dysfunction of Eustachian tube
382.00	Acute suppurative otitis media NOS
382.2	Chronic atticoantral suppurative OM
382.3	Chronic suppurativ otitis media NOS
382.9	Otitis media NOS
383.02	Acute mastoiditis w/complic NEC
383.1	Chronic mastoiditis
383.33	Postmastoidectomy granulations
383.9	Mastoiditis NOS
384.20	Perforation tympanic membrane NOS
384.21	Cent perforate tympanic membrane
384.22	Attic perforate tympanic membrane
384.23	Marginal perf tympanic membrane NEC
384.25	Total perforate tympanic membrane
385.00	Tympanosclerosis NOS
385.10	Adhesive middle ear disease NOS
385.23	Dislocation of ear ossicles
385.30	Cholesteatoma NOS
385.32	Cholesteatoma of middle ear
385.33	Cholesteatoma, middle ear/mastoid
385.89	Middle Ear/Mastoid disorder NEC
387.2	Cochlear otosclerosis
389.00	Conductive hearing loss NOS
389.02	Conductive hearing loss, tympanic
389.03	Conductive hearing loss, middle ear
389.9	Hearing loss NOS

REIMBURSEMENT INFORMATION

Medicare

- Follow–up Days — 90
- Assistant Surgeon — not paid
- Supply Charges — not allowed
- Outpatient Limit — does not apply
- Major Surgery Rules Apply

CPT CODE **SERVICE**

69646 Tympanoplasty with mastoidectomy (including canalplasty, middle ear surgery, tympanic membrane repair); radical or complete, with ossicular chain reconstruction

CPT NOTES

- For diagnostic services, (e.g., audiometry, vestibular tests), see 92502 et seq).

ICD–9–CM

381.00	Acute nonsupp otitis media NOS
381.10	Chron serous otitis media simp/NOS
381.81	Dysfunction of Eustachian tube
382.00	Acute suppurative otitis media NOS
382.2	Chronic atticoantral suppurative OM
382.3	Chronic suppurativ otitis media NOS
382.9	Otitis media NOS
383.02	Acute mastoiditis w/complic NEC
383.1	Chronic mastoiditis
383.33	Postmastoidectomy granulations
383.9	Mastoiditis NOS
385.00	Tympanosclerosis NOS
385.10	Adhesive middle ear disease NOS
385.23	Dislocation of ear ossicles
385.30	Cholesteatoma NOS
385.32	Cholesteatoma of middle ear
385.33	Cholesteatoma, middle ear/mastoid
385.89	Middle Ear/Mastoid disorder NEC
387.2	Cochlear otosclerosis
389.00	Conductive hearing loss NOS
389.02	Conductive hearing loss, tympanic
389.03	Conductive hearing loss, middle ear
389.9	Hearing loss NOS

REIMBURSEMENT INFORMATION

Medicare

- Follow–up Days — 90
- Assistant Surgeon — not paid
- Supply Charges — not allowed
- Outpatient Limit — does not apply
- Major Surgery Rules Apply

CPT CODE SERVICE	ICD–9–CM
69650 Stapes mobilization **CPT NOTES** ♦ For diagnostic services, (e.g., audiometry, vestibular tests), see 92502 et seq).	385.22 Ankylosis ear ossicle NEC 385.23 Dislocation of ear ossicles 387.0 Otosclerosis, oval window, nonoblit 387.2 Cochlear otosclerosis 387.8 Otosclerosis NEC 387.9 Otosclerosis NOS 389.00 Conductive hearing loss NOS 389.02 Conductive hearing loss, tympanic 389.03 Conductive hearing loss, middle ear 389.9 Hearing loss NOS 872.62 Open wound of ossicles 872.72 Open wound of ossicles, complicated **REIMBURSEMENT INFORMATION** Medicare ♦ Follow–up Days — 90 ♦ Assistant Surgeon — paid ♦ Supply Charges — not allowed ♦ Outpatient Limit — does not apply ♦ Major Surgery Rules Apply
69660 Stapedectomy or stapedotomy with reestablishment of ossicular continuity, with or without use of foreign material **CPT NOTES** ♦ For diagnostic services, (e.g., audiometry, vestibular tests), see 92502 et seq).	385.23 Dislocation of ear ossicles 387.0 Otosclerosis, oval window, nonoblit 387.2 Cochlear otosclerosis 387.8 Otosclerosis NEC 387.9 Otosclerosis NOS 389.00 Conductive hearing loss NOS 389.02 Conductive hearing loss, tympanic 389.9 Hearing loss NOS 872.62 Open wound of ossicles 872.72 Open wound of ossicles, complicated **REIMBURSEMENT INFORMATION** Medicare ♦ Follow–up Days — 90 ♦ Assistant Surgeon — not paid ♦ Supply Charges — not allowed ♦ Outpatient Limit — does not apply ♦ Major Surgery Rules Apply

CPT CODE	SERVICE	ICD–9–CM

69661 Stapedectomy or stapedotomy with reestablishment of ossicular continuity, with or without use of foreign material; with footplate drill out

CPT NOTES

- For diagnostic services, (e.g., audiometry, vestibular tests), see 92502 et seq).

385.23	Dislocation of ear ossicles
387.0	Otosclerosis, oval window, nonoblit
387.2	Cochlear otosclerosis
387.8	Otosclerosis NEC
387.9	Otosclerosis NOS
389.00	Conductive hearing loss NOS
389.02	Conductive hearing loss, tympanic
389.9	Hearing loss NOS
872.62	Open wound of ossicles
872.72	Open wound of ossicles, complicated

REIMBURSEMENT INFORMATION

Medicare

- Follow–up Days — 90
- Assistant Surgeon — not paid
- Supply Charges — not allowed
- Outpatient Limit — does not apply
- Major Surgery Rules Apply

69662 Revision of stapedectomy or stapedotomy

CPT NOTES

- For diagnostic services, (e.g., audiometry, vestibular tests), see 92502 et seq).

385.23	Dislocation of ear ossicles
387.0	Otosclerosis, oval window, nonoblit
387.2	Cochlear otosclerosis
387.8	Otosclerosis NEC
387.9	Otosclerosis NOS
389.00	Conductive hearing loss NOS
389.02	Conductive hearing loss, tympanic
389.9	Hearing loss NOS
872.62	Open wound of ossicles
872.72	Open wound of ossicles, complicated

REIMBURSEMENT INFORMATION

Medicare

- Follow–up Days — 90
- Assistant Surgeon — not paid
- Supply Charges — not allowed
- Outpatient Limit — does not apply
- Major Surgery Rules Apply

CPT CODE SERVICE	ICD–9–CM
69666 Repair oval window fistula **CPT NOTES** ♦ For diagnostic services, (e.g., audiometry, vestibular tests), see 92502 et seq).	386.10 Peripheral vertigo NOS 386.40 Labyrinthine fistula NOS 386.42 Labyrinthine, oval window fistula 801.00 Closed skull base fracture **REIMBURSEMENT INFORMATION** Medicare ♦ Follow–up Days — 90 ♦ Assistant Surgeon — not paid ♦ Supply Charges — not allowed ♦ Outpatient Limit — does not apply ♦ Major Surgery Rules Apply
69667 Repair round window fistula **CPT NOTES** ♦ For diagnostic services, (e.g., audiometry, vestibular tests), see 92502 et seq).	386.10 Peripheral vertigo NOS 386.41 Labyrinthine, round window fistula **REIMBURSEMENT INFORMATION** Medicare ♦ Follow–up Days — 90 ♦ Assistant Surgeon — not paid ♦ Supply Charges — not allowed ♦ Outpatient Limit — does not apply ♦ Major Surgery Rules Apply
69670 Mastoid obliteration (separate procedure) **CPT NOTES** ♦ For diagnostic services, (e.g., audiometry, vestibular tests), see 92502 et seq).	383.1 Chronic mastoiditis 383.31 Postmastoidectomy mucosal cyst 383.32 Postmastoidectomy cholesteatoma 383.33 Postmastoidectomy granulations 385.33 Cholesteatoma, middle ear/mastoid **REIMBURSEMENT INFORMATION** Medicare ♦ Follow–up Days — 90 ♦ Assistant Surgeon — paid ♦ Supply Charges — not allowed ♦ Outpatient Limit — does not apply ♦ Major Surgery Rules Apply

CPT CODE **SERVICE** | **ICD–9–CM**

69700 Closure postauricular fistula, mastoid (separate procedure)

CPT NOTES

- For diagnostic services, (e.g., audiometry, vestibular tests), see 92502 et seq).

383.81 Postauricular fistula

REIMBURSEMENT INFORMATION

Medicare

- Follow–up Days — 90
- Assistant Surgeon — paid
- Supply Charges — not allowed
- Outpatient Limit — does not apply
- Major Surgery Rules Apply

69710 Implantation or replacement of electromagnetic bone conduction hearing device in temporal bone

CPT NOTES

- For diagnostic services, (e.g., audiometry, vestibular tests), see 92502 et seq).
- Replacement procedure includes removal of old device.

385.03 Tympanosclerosis, all parts
387.0 Otosclerosis, oval window, nonoblit
387.1 Otosclerosis, oval window, obliter
387.8 Otosclerosis NEC
389.01 Conductive hearing loss, extern ear
389.02 Conductive hearing loss, tympanic
389.03 Conductive hearing loss, middle ear
389.04 Conductive hearing loss, inner ear
389.08 Conductive hearing loss, comb type
744.03 Middle ear anomaly NEC

REIMBURSEMENT INFORMATION

Medicare

- Follow–up Days — global concept does not apply
- Assistant Surgeon — not paid
- Supply Charges — not allowed
- Outpatient Limit — does not apply

69711 Removal or repair of electromagnetic bone conduction hearing device in temporal bone

CPT NOTES

- For diagnostic services, (e.g., audiometry, vestibular tests), see 92502 et seq).

385.03 Tympanosclerosis, all parts
387.0 Otosclerosis, oval window, nonoblit
387.1 Otosclerosis, oval window, obliter
387.8 Otosclerosis NEC
389.01 Conductive hearing loss, extern ear
389.02 Conductive hearing loss, tympanic
389.03 Conductive hearing loss, middle ear
389.04 Conductive hearing loss, inner ear
389.08 Conductive hearing loss, comb type
744.03 Middle ear anomaly NEC

REIMBURSEMENT INFORMATION

Medicare

- Follow–up Days — 90
- Assistant Surgeon — paid
- Supply Charges — not allowed
- Outpatient Limit — does not apply
- Major Surgery Rules Apply

CPT CODE	SERVICE	ICD–9–CM

69720 Decompression facial nerve, intratemporal; lateral to geniculate ganglion

CPT NOTES

- For diagnostic services, (e.g., audiometry, vestibular tests), see 92502 et seq).

142.0	M-Neoplasm, Parotid gland
160.1	M-Neoplasm, Middle Ear
170.0	M-Neoplasm, Skull/Face bone
210.2	B-Neoplasm, Major salivary glands
212.0	B-Neoplasm, Nasal cavity/sinus
213.0	B-Neoplasm, Skull/Face bone
351.0	Bell's palsy
767.5	Facial nerve injury at birth
951.5	Injury to acoustic nerve
998.2	Accidental op laceration/puncture

REIMBURSEMENT INFORMATION

Medicare

- Follow–up Days — 90
- Assistant Surgeon — paid
- Supply Charges — not allowed
- Outpatient Limit — does not apply
- Major Surgery Rules Apply

69725 Decompression facial nerve, intratemporal; including medial to geniculate ganglion

CPT NOTES

- For diagnostic services, (e.g., audiometry, vestibular tests), see 92502 et seq).

142.0	M-Neoplasm, Parotid gland
160.1	M-Neoplasm, Middle Ear
170.0	M-Neoplasm, Skull/Face bone
210.2	B-Neoplasm, Major salivary glands
212.0	B-Neoplasm, Nasal cavity/sinus
213.0	B-Neoplasm, Skull/Face bone
351.0	Bell's palsy
767.5	Facial nerve injury at birth
951.5	Injury to acoustic nerve
998.2	Accidental op laceration/puncture

REIMBURSEMENT INFORMATION

Medicare

- Follow–up Days — 90
- Assistant Surgeon — paid
- Supply Charges — not allowed
- Outpatient Limit — does not apply
- Major Surgery Rules Apply

CPT CODE **SERVICE**

ICD–9–CM

69740 Suture facial nerve, intratemporal, with or without graft or decompression; lateral to geniculate ganglion

CPT NOTES

- For diagnostic services, (e.g., audiometry, vestibular tests), see 92502 et seq).
- For extracranial suture of facial nerve, see 64864.

142.0	M-Neoplasm, Parotid gland
160.1	M-Neoplasm, Middle Ear
170.0	M-Neoplasm, Skull/Face bone
210.2	B-Neoplasm, Major salivary glands
212.0	B-Neoplasm, Nasal cavity/sinus
213.0	B-Neoplasm, Skull/Face bone
351.0	Bell's palsy
767.5	Facial nerve injury at birth
951.5	Injury to acoustic nerve
998.2	Accidental op laceration/puncture

REIMBURSEMENT INFORMATION

Medicare

- Follow–up Days — 90
- Assistant Surgeon — paid
- Supply Charges — not allowed
- Outpatient Limit — does not apply
- Major Surgery Rules Apply

69745 Suture facial nerve, intratemporal, with or without graft or decompression; including medial to geniculate ganglion

CPT NOTES

- For diagnostic services, (e.g., audiometry, vestibular tests), see 92502 et seq).
- For extracranial suture of facial nerve, see 64864.

142.0	M-Neoplasm, Parotid gland
160.1	M-Neoplasm, Middle Ear
170.0	M-Neoplasm, Skull/Face bone
210.2	B-Neoplasm, Major salivary glands
212.0	B-Neoplasm, Nasal cavity/sinus
213.0	B-Neoplasm, Skull/Face bone
351.0	Bell's palsy
767.5	Facial nerve injury at birth
951.5	Injury to acoustic nerve
998.2	Accidental op laceration/puncture

REIMBURSEMENT INFORMATION

Medicare

- Follow–up Days — 90
- Assistant Surgeon — paid
- Supply Charges — not allowed
- Outpatient Limit — does not apply
- Major Surgery Rules Apply

CPT CODE	SERVICE	ICD–9–CM

69799 Unlisted procedure, middle ear

CPT NOTES

- For diagnostic services, (e.g., audiometry, vestibular tests), see 92502 et seq).

380.4	Impacted cerumen
381.00	Acute nonsup otitis media NOS
381.10	Chron serous otitis media simp/NOS
382.9	Otitis media NOS
384.20	Perforation tympanic membrane NOS
385.30	Cholesteatoma NOS
385.32	Cholesteatoma of middle ear
385.83	Old foreign body of middle ear
387.9	Otosclerosis NOS
388.8	Ear disorders NEC
389.00	Conductive hearing loss NOS
389.2	Mixed hearing loss
931	Foreign body in ear

REIMBURSEMENT INFORMATION

Medicare

- Follow–up Days — determined by local carrier
- Assistant Surgeon — determined by local carrier
- Supply Charges — determined by local carrier
- Outpatient Limit — determined by local carrier

69801 Labyrinthotomy, with or without cryosurgery or other nonexcisional destructive procedures or tack procedure; transcanal

CPT NOTES

- For diagnostic services, (e.g., audiometry, vestibular tests), see 92502 et seq).

386.00	Meniere's disease NOS
386.01	Meniere's disease cochleovestibular
386.02	Meniere's disease, cochlear
386.03	Meniere's disease, vestibular
386.04	Inactive Meniere's disease
386.30	Labyrinthitis NOS
386.31	Serous labyrinthitis
386.33	Suppurative labyrinthitis
386.34	Toxic labyrinthitis
386.35	Viral labyrinthitis

REIMBURSEMENT INFORMATION

Medicare

- Follow–up Days — 90
- Assistant Surgeon — paid
- Supply Charges — not allowed
- Outpatient Limit — does not apply
- Major Surgery Rules Apply

CPT CODE **SERVICE**

69802 Labyrinthotomy, with or without cryosurgery or other nonexcisional destructive procedures or tack procedure; with mastoidectomy

CPT NOTES

- For diagnostic services, (e.g., audiometry, vestibular tests), see 92502 et seq).

ICD–9–CM

386.00 Meniere's disease NOS
386.01 Meniere's disease cochleovestibular
386.02 Meniere's disease, cochlear
386.03 Meniere's disease, vestibular
386.04 Inactive Meniere's disease
386.30 Labyrinthitis NOS
386.31 Serous labyrinthitis
386.33 Suppurative labyrinthitis
386.34 Toxic labyrinthitis
386.35 Viral labyrinthitis

REIMBURSEMENT INFORMATION

Medicare

- Follow–up Days — 90
- Assistant Surgeon — paid
- Supply Charges — not allowed
- Outpatient Limit — does not apply
- Major Surgery Rules Apply

69805 Endolymphatic sac operation; without shunt

CPT NOTES

- For diagnostic services, (e.g., audiometry, vestibular tests), see 92502 et seq).

386.00 Meniere's disease NOS
386.01 Meniere's disease cochleovestibular
386.02 Meniere's disease, cochlear
386.03 Meniere's disease, vestibular
386.04 Inactive Meniere's disease
386.30 Labyrinthitis NOS
386.31 Serous labyrinthitis
386.33 Suppurative labyrinthitis
386.34 Toxic labyrinthitis
386.35 Viral labyrinthitis

REIMBURSEMENT INFORMATION

Medicare

- Follow–up Days — 90
- Assistant Surgeon — paid
- Supply Charges — not allowed
- Outpatient Limit — does not apply
- Major Surgery Rules Apply

CPT CODE / SERVICE	ICD–9–CM
69806 Endolymphatic sac operation; with shunt **CPT NOTES** ♦ For diagnostic services, (e.g., audiometry, vestibular tests), see 92502 et seq).	386.00 Meniere's disease NOS 386.01 Meniere's disease cochleovestibular 386.02 Meniere's disease, cochlear 386.03 Meniere's disease, vestibular 386.04 Inactive Meniere's disease 386.30 Labyrinthitis NOS 386.31 Serous labyrinthitis 386.33 Suppurative labyrinthitis 386.34 Toxic labyrinthitis 386.35 Viral labyrinthitis **REIMBURSEMENT INFORMATION** <u>Medicare</u> ♦ Follow–up Days — 90 ♦ Assistant Surgeon — not paid ♦ Supply Charges — not allowed ♦ Outpatient Limit — does not apply ♦ Major Surgery Rules Apply
69820 Fenestration semicircular canal **CPT NOTES** ♦ For diagnostic services, (e.g., audiometry, vestibular tests), see 92502 et seq).	386.43 Semicircular canal fistula **REIMBURSEMENT INFORMATION** <u>Medicare</u> ♦ Follow–up Days — 90 ♦ Assistant Surgeon — paid ♦ Supply Charges — not allowed ♦ Outpatient Limit — does not apply ♦ Major Surgery Rules Apply
69840 Revision fenestration operation **CPT NOTES** ♦ For diagnostic services, (e.g., audiometry, vestibular tests), see 92502 et seq).	386.43 Semicircular canal fistula **REIMBURSEMENT INFORMATION** <u>Medicare</u> ♦ Follow–up Days — 90 ♦ Assistant Surgeon — paid ♦ Supply Charges — not allowed ♦ Outpatient Limit — does not apply ♦ Major Surgery Rules Apply

CPT CODE	SERVICE	ICD–9–CM

69905 Labyrinthectomy, transcanal

CPT NOTES

- For diagnostic services, (e.g., audiometry, vestibular tests), see 92502 et seq).

386.00 Meniere's disease NOS
386.01 Meniere's disease cochleovestibular
386.02 Meniere's disease, cochlear
386.03 Meniere's disease, vestibular
386.04 Inactive Meniere's disease
386.30 Labyrinthitis NOS
386.31 Serous labyrinthitis
386.33 Suppurative labyrinthitis
386.34 Toxic labyrinthitis
386.35 Viral labyrinthitis

REIMBURSEMENT INFORMATION

Medicare

- Follow–up Days — 90
- Assistant Surgeon — paid
- Supply Charges — not allowed
- Outpatient Limit — does not apply
- Major Surgery Rules Apply

69910 Labyrinthectomy; with mastoidectomy

CPT NOTES

- For diagnostic services, (e.g., audiometry, vestibular tests), see 92502 et seq).

386.00 Meniere's disease NOS
386.01 Meniere's disease cochleovestibular
386.02 Meniere's disease, cochlear
386.03 Meniere's disease, vestibular
386.04 Inactive Meniere's disease
386.30 Labyrinthitis NOS
386.31 Serous labyrinthitis
386.33 Suppurative labyrinthitis
386.34 Toxic labyrinthitis
386.35 Viral labyrinthitis

REIMBURSEMENT INFORMATION

Medicare

- Follow–up Days — 90
- Assistant Surgeon — not paid
- Supply Charges — not allowed
- Outpatient Limit — does not apply
- Major Surgery Rules Apply

CPT CODE / SERVICE	ICD-9-CM
69915 Vestibular nerve section, translabyrinthine approach **CPT NOTES** ♦ For diagnostic services, (e.g., audiometry, vestibular tests), see 92502 et seq). ♦ For transcranial approach, see 69950.	386.00 Meniere's disease NOS 386.01 Meniere's disease cochleovestibular 386.02 Meniere's disease, cochlear 386.03 Meniere's disease, vestibular 386.04 Inactive Meniere's disease **REIMBURSEMENT INFORMATION** Medicare ♦ Follow-up Days — 90 ♦ Assistant Surgeon — paid ♦ Supply Charges — not allowed ♦ Outpatient Limit — does not apply ♦ Major Surgery Rules Apply
69930 Cochlear device implantation, with or without mastoidectomy **CPT NOTES** ♦ For diagnostic services, (e.g., audiometry, vestibular tests), see 92502 et seq).	389.04 Conductive hearing loss, inner ear 389.10 Sensorineural hearing loss NOS 389.2 Mixed hearing loss **REIMBURSEMENT INFORMATION** Medicare ♦ Follow-up Days — 90 ♦ Assistant Surgeon — not paid ♦ Supply Charges — not allowed ♦ Outpatient Limit — does not apply ♦ Major Surgery Rules Apply
69949 Unlisted procedure, inner ear **CPT NOTES** ♦ For diagnostic services, (e.g., audiometry, vestibular tests), see 92502 et seq).	238.0 UB-Neoplasm, Bone **REIMBURSEMENT INFORMATION** Medicare ♦ Follow-up Days — determined by local carrier ♦ Assistant Surgeon — determined by local carrier ♦ Supply Charges — determined by local carrier ♦ Outpatient Limit — determined by local carrier

CPT CODE **SERVICE** | **ICD–9–CM**

69950 Vestibular nerve section, transcranial approach

CPT NOTES

- For diagnostic services, (e.g., audiometry, vestibular tests), see 92502 et seq).
- For external approach, see 69535.

386.00	Meniere's disease NOS
386.01	Meniere's disease cochleovestibular
386.02	Meniere's disease, cochlear
386.03	Meniere's disease, vestibular
386.04	Inactive Meniere's disease

REIMBURSEMENT INFORMATION

Medicare

- Follow–up Days — 90
- Assistant Surgeon — paid
- Supply Charges — not allowed
- Outpatient Limit — does not apply
- Major Surgery Rules Apply

69955 Total facial nerve decompression and/or repair (may include graft)

CPT NOTES

- For diagnostic services, (e.g., audiometry, vestibular tests), see 92502 et seq).
- For external approach, see 69535.

142.0	M-Neoplasm, Parotid gland
160.1	M-Neoplasm, Middle Ear
170.0	M-Neoplasm, Skull/Face bone
210.2	B-Neoplasm, Major salivary glands
212.0	B-Neoplasm, Nasal cavity/sinus
213.0	B-Neoplasm, Skull/Face bone
351.0	Bell's palsy
767.5	Facial nerve injury at birth
951.5	Injury to acoustic nerve
998.2	Accidental op laceration/puncture

REIMBURSEMENT INFORMATION

Medicare

- Follow–up Days — 90
- Assistant Surgeon — paid
- Supply Charges — not allowed
- Outpatient Limit — does not apply
- Major Surgery Rules Apply

69960 Decompression internal auditory canal

CPT NOTES

- For diagnostic services, (e.g., audiometry, vestibular tests), see 92502 et seq).
- For external approach, see 69535.

170.0	M-Neoplasm, Skull/Face bone
198.5	M2-Neoplasm, Bone and bone marrow
213.0	B-Neoplasm, Skull/Face bone
238.0	UB-Neoplasm, Bone
872.8	Open wound of ear NOS
872.9	Open wound of ear NOS, complicated

REIMBURSEMENT INFORMATION

Medicare

- Follow–up Days — 90
- Assistant Surgeon — paid
- Supply Charges — not allowed
- Outpatient Limit — does not apply
- Major Surgery Rules Apply

CPT CODE **SERVICE**

69970 Removal of tumor, temporal bone

CPT NOTES

- For diagnostic services, (e.g., audiometry, vestibular tests), see 92502 et seq).
- For external approach, see 69535.

ICD–9–CM

170.0	M-Neoplasm, Skull/Face bone
198.5	M2-Neoplasm, Bone and bone marrow
213.0	B-Neoplasm, Skull/Face bone
238.0	UB-Neoplasm, Bone

REIMBURSEMENT INFORMATION

Medicare

- Follow–up Days — 90
- Assistant Surgeon — paid
- Supply Charges — not allowed
- Outpatient Limit — does not apply
- Major Surgery Rules Apply

RADIOLOGY

CPT CODE	SERVICE	ICD-9-CM	
70100	Radiologic examination, mandible; partial, less than four views	171.9	M-Neoplasm, Soft tissue NOS
		524.6x	Temporomandibular joint disorder
		526.0	Developmental odontogenic cysts
		526.1	Fissural cysts of jaw
		526.2	Jaw cysts NEC
		527.5	Sialolithiasis
		784.2	Swelling in head/neck
		802.2x	Fracture, Mandible, closed
		802.3x	Fracture, Mandible, open
		959.0	Face and neck injury NOS
70110	Radiologic examination, mandible; complete, minimum of four views	171.9	M-Neoplasm, Soft tissue NOS
		527.5	Sialolithiasis
		784.2	Swelling in head/neck
		802.2x	Fracture, Mandible, closed
		802.3x	Fracture, Mandible, open
		959.0	Face and neck injury NOS
		REIMBURSEMENT INFORMATION	
		Medicare	
		♦ Fragments — 70100	
70120	Radiologic examination, mastoids; less than three views per side	195.0	M-Neoplasm, Head/face/neck
		382.3	Chronic suppurativ otitis media NOS
		383.1	Chronic mastoiditis
		383.9	Mastoiditis NOS
		384.2x	Perforation of tympanic membrane
		385.3x	Cholesteatoma, middle ear/mastoid
		386.1x	Peripheral vertigo
		388.71	Otogenic pain
		389.0x	Conductive hearing loss
		389.9	Hearing loss NOS

CPT CODE	SERVICE	ICD–9–CM
70130	Radiologic examination, mastoids; complete, minimum of three views per side	195.0 M-Neoplasm, Head/face/neck 382.3 Chronic suppurativ otitis media NOS 383.1 Chronic mastoiditis 383.9 Mastoiditis NOS 384.2x Perforation of tympanic membrane 385.3x Cholesteatoma, middle ear/mastoid 386.1x Peripheral vertigo 388.71 Otogenic pain 389.0x Conductive hearing loss 389.9 Hearing loss NOS **REIMBURSEMENT INFORMATION** <u>Medicare</u> ♦ Fragments — 70120
70134	Radiologic examination, internal auditory meati, complete	195.0 M-Neoplasm, Head/face/neck 225.1 B-Neoplasm, Cranial nerve 386.3x Labyrinthitis 386.9 Vertiginous syndromes NOS 388.11 Acoustic trauma 388.2 Sudden hearing loss NOS 389.1x Sensorineural hearing loss
70160	Radiologic examination, nasal bones, complete, minimum of three views	738.0 Acquired nose deformity 748.1 Congenital nose anomaly NEC 749.0x Cleft palate 784.7 Epistaxis 802.0 Nasal bone Fx, closed 802.1 Nasal bone Fx, open 920 Contusion face/scalp/neck
70200	Radiologic examination; orbits, complete, minimum of four views	160.2 M-Neoplasm, Maxillary sinus 195.0 M-Neoplasm, Head/face/neck 802.6 Fx orbital floor, closed 870.3 Penetrating orbit wound w/o FB

CPT CODE	SERVICE	ICD–9–CM	
70210	Radiologic examination, sinuses, paranasal, less than three views	350.2	Atypical face pain
		461.0	Acute maxillary sinusitis
		461.1	Acute frontal sinusitis
		461.2	Acute ethmoidal sinusitis
		461.8	Other acute sinusitis
		461.9	Acute sinusitis NOS
		470	Deviated nasal septum
		471.8	Nasal sinus polyp NEC
		472.0	Chronic rhinitis
		473.0	Chronic maxillary sinusitis
		473.1	Chronic frontal sinusitis
		473.2	Chronic ethmoidal sinusitis
		473.8	Chronic sinusitis NEC
		473.9	Chronic sinusitis NOS
		477.0	Allergic rhinitis d/t pollen
		477.9	Allergic rhinitis NOS
		478.1	Nasal and sinus disease NEC
		754.0	Congen skull/face/jaw deformity
		784.2	Swelling in head/neck
		802.8	Fx facial bone NEC, closed
		802.9	Fx facial bone NEC, open
		959.0	Face and neck injury NOS
70220	Radiologic examination, sinuses, paranasal, complete, minimum of three views	350.2	Atypical face pain
		461.0	Acute maxillary sinusitis
		461.1	Acute frontal sinusitis
		461.2	Acute ethmoidal sinusitis
		461.8	Other acute sinusitis
		461.9	Acute sinusitis NOS
		470	Deviated nasal septum
		471.8	Nasal sinus polyp NEC
		472.0	Chronic rhinitis
		473.0	Chronic maxillary sinusitis
		473.1	Chronic frontal sinusitis
		473.2	Chronic ethmoidal sinusitis
		473.8	Chronic sinusitis NEC
		473.9	Chronic sinusitis NOS
		477.0	Allergic rhinitis d/t pollen
		477.9	Allergic rhinitis NOS
		478.1	Nasal and sinus disease NEC
		754.0	Congen skull/face/jaw deformity
		784.2	Swelling in head/neck
		802.8	Fx facial bone NEC, closed
		802.9	Fx facial bone NEC, open
		959.0	Face and neck injury NOS

REIMBURSEMENT INFORMATION

Medicare

- Fragments — 70210

CPT CODE	SERVICE	ICD–9–CM
[illegible]	Radiologic examination, skull; complete, minimum of four views, with or without stereo	[illegible] M-Neoplasm, Pituitary gland 227.3 B-Neoplasm, Pituitary gland 348.2 Benign intracranial hypertension 873.8 Open wound of head NEC

REIMBURSEMENT INFORMATION

Medicare

- Fragments — 70250

CPT CODE	SERVICE	ICD–9–CM
70330	Radiologic examination, temporomandibular joint, open and closed mouth; bilateral	350.2 Atypical face pain 524.6x Temporomandibular joint disorder 714.0 Rheumatoid arthritis 729.1 Myalgia and myositis NOS 784.0 Headache 830.0 Dislocation jaw, closed 830.1 Dislocation jaw, open 848.1 Sprain of jaw

REIMBURSEMENT INFORMATION

Medicare

- Fragments — 70328

CPT CODE	SERVICE	ICD–9–CM
70332	Temporomandibular joint arthrography, radiological supervision and interpretation	350.2 Atypical face pain 524.6x Temporomandibular joint disorder 714.0 Rheumatoid arthritis 729.1 Myalgia and myositis NOS 784.0 Headache 830.0 Dislocation jaw, closed 830.1 Dislocation jaw, open 848.1 Sprain of jaw

CPT CODE	SERVICE	ICD–9–CM
70360	Radiologic examination; neck, soft tissue	464.30 Acute epiglottitis, no obstruction 478.24 Retropharyngeal abscess 723.1 Cervicalgia 729.6 Old foreign body in soft tissue 787.2 Dysphagia
70371	Complex dynamic pharyngeal and speech evaluation by cine or video recording	161.9 M-Neoplasm, Larynx NOS 476.0 Chronic laryngitis 478.2x Diseases of pharynx 478.3x Paralysis of vocal cords or larynx 478.4 Polyp of vocal cord/larynx 478.5 Vocal cord disease NEC 478.7x Disease of larynx 784.49 Voice disturbance NEC
70380	Radiologic examination, salivary gland for calculus	527.2 Sialoadenitis 527.5 Sialolithiasis 527.7 Salivary secretion disturbance 784.2 Swelling in head/neck
70460	Computerized axial tomography, head or brain; with contrast material(s) **CPT NOTES** ♦ For coronal, sagittal, and/or oblique sections, see 76375.	215.0 B-Neoplasm, Soft tissue, head 225.1 B-Neoplasm, Cranial nerve 237.72 Neurofibromatosis, type 2 386.1x Peripheral vertigo 388.3x Tinnitus 389.1x Sensorineural hearing loss
70480	Computerized axial tomography, orbit, sella, or posterior fossa or outer, middle, or inner ear; without contrast material **CPT NOTES** ♦ For coronal, sagittal, and/or oblique sections, see 76375.	160.2 M-Neoplasm, Maxillary sinus 195.0 M-Neoplasm, Head/face/neck 382.9 Otitis media NOS 386.1x Peripheral vertigo 387.9 Otosclerosis NOS 388.71 Otogenic pain 388.9 Ear disorder NOS 473.8 Chronic sinusitis NEC

CPT CODE	SERVICE	ICD–9–CM	
70486	Computerized axial tomography, maxillofacial area; without contrast material **CPT NOTES** ♦ For coronal, sagittal, and/or oblique sections, see 76375.	160.2 212.0 472.0 473.0 473.8 473.9 744.9 784.0 784.7 959.0	M-Neoplasm, Maxillary sinus B-Neoplasm, Nasal cavity/sinus Chronic rhinitis Chronic maxillary sinusitis Chronic sinusitis NEC Chronic sinusitis NOS Congenital face/neck anomaly NOS Headache Epistaxis Face and neck injury NOS
70488	Computerized axial tomography, maxillofacial area; without contrast material, followed by contrast material(s) and further sections **CPT NOTES** ♦ For coronal, sagittal, and/or oblique sections, see 76375.	473x 784.0 784.7 **REIMBURSEMENT INFORMATION** Medicare ♦ Fragments — 70486, 70487	Chronic sinusitis Headache Epistaxis
70491	Computerized axial tomography, soft tissue neck; with contrast material(s) **CPT NOTES** ♦ For coronal, sagittal, and/or oblique sections, see 76375. ♦ For cervical spine, see 72125, 72126.	464.3x 478.24 723.1 787.2	Acute epiglottitis Retropharyngeal abscess Cervicalgia Dysphagia
71020	Radiologic examination, chest, two views, frontal and lateral	478.6 486 487.1 490 934.0 934.1	Edema of larynx Pneumonia, organism NOS Flu w/respiratory manifestation NEC Bronchitis NOS Foreign body, trachea Foreign body, main bronchus
74220	Radiologic examination; esophagus **CPT NOTES** ♦ For percutaneous placement of gastrostomy tube, see 43750.	461.9 530.1x 784.5 787.2 935.0	Acute sinusitis NOS Esophagitis Speech disturbance NEC Dysphagia Foreign body in mouth

CPT CODE	SERVICE	ICD–9–CM	
74230	Swallowing function, pharynx and/or esophagus, with cineradiography and/or video	478.2x	Diseases of pharynx NEC
		530.0	Achalasia and cardiospasm
		530.1x	Esophagitis
		530.3	Esophageal stricture
		530.5	Dyskinesia of esophagus
		787.2	Dysphagia

CPT NOTES

- For percutaneous placement of gastrostomy tube, see 43750.

CPT CODE	SERVICE	ICD–9–CM	
76140	Consultation on x-ray examination made elsewhere, written report	381.0x	Acute nonsuppurative otitis media
		383.1	Chronic mastoiditis
		384.2x	Perforation of tympanic membrane
		386.0x	Meniere's disease
		473.9	Chronic sinusitis NOS

CPT NOTES

- For arthrography of shoulder, see 73040; elbow, see 73085; wrist, see 73115; hip, see 73525; knee, see 73580; ankle, see 73615.

CPT CODE	SERVICE	ICD–9–CM	
76536	Echography, soft tissues of head and neck (eg, thyroid, parathyroid, parotid), B-scan and/or real time with image documentation	246.2	Cyst of thyroid
		252.8	Parathyroid gland disorder NEC
		464.3x	Acute epiglottitis
		478.24	Retropharyngeal abscess
		527.6	Salivary gland mucocele
		723.1	Cervicalgia
		759.2	Endocrine gland anomaly NEC
		787.2	Dysphagia

CPT NOTES

- ***A-mode:*** Implies a one–dimensional ultrasonic measurement procedure.
- ***M-mode:*** Implies a one–dimensional ultrasonic measurement procedure with movement of the trace to record amplitude and velocity of moving echo–producing structures.
- ***B-scan:*** Implies a two–dimensional ultrasonic scanning procedure with a two–dimensional display.
- ***Real-time scan:*** Implies a two–dimensional ultrasonic scanning procedure with display of both two–dimensional structure and motion with time.

RADIATION ONCOLOGY
77261–77799

Listings for Radiation Oncology provide for teletherapy and brachytherapy to include initial consultation, clinical treatment planning, simulation, medical radiation physics, dosimetry, treatment devices, special services, and clinical treatment management procedures. They include normal follow–up care during course of treatment and for three months following its completion.

When a service or procedure is provided that is not listed in this edition of CPT it should be identified by a Special Report (see Special Services and Reports in your CPT book) and one of the unlisted procedure codes listed below:

77299 Unlisted procedure, therapeutic radiology clinical treatment planning

77399 Unlisted procedure, medical radiation physics, dosimetry and treatment devices

77499 Unlisted procedure, therapeutic radiology clinical treatment management

77799 Unlisted procedure, clinical brachytherapy

(For treatment by injectable or ingestible isotopes, see subsection NUCLEAR MEDICINE.)

Consultation: Clinical Management

Preliminary consultation, evaluation of patient prior to decision to treat, or full medical care (in addition to treatment management) when provided by the therapeutic radiologist may be identified by the appropriate procedure codes from Evaluation and Management, Medicine or Surgery sections.

Radiation Treatment Delivery
77401–77417

Radiation treatment delivery (77401-77417) recognizes the technical component and the various energy levels.

Clinical Treatment Management
77419–77499

Weekly clinical management is based on five fractions delivered comprising one week regardless of the time interval separating the delivery of treatments.

Definitions:

Simple — single treatment area, single port or parallel opposed ports, simple blocks.

Intermediate — two separate treatment areas, three or more ports on a single treatment area, use of special blocks.

Complex — three or more separate treatment areas, highly complex blocking (mantle, inverted Y), tangential ports, wedges, rotational compensators or other special beam considerations.

Conformal — multiple custom megavoltage treatment beams focused on a large 3-dimensional reconstructed target.

CPT CODE	SERVICE	ICD–9–CM

77407 Radiation treatment delivery, two separate treatment areas, three or more ports on a single treatment area, use of multiple blocks; up to 5 MeV

CPT NOTES

- Radiation treatment delivery (77401-77416) recognizes the technical component and the various energy levels.

141x	Malignant neoplasm of tongue
142x	Malignant neoplasm, salivary glands
146x	Malignant neoplasm, Oropharynx
147x	Malignant neoplasm, Nasopharynx
148x	Malignant neoplasm, Hypopharynx
149x	M-Neoplasm, Lip/Oral cavity/Pharynx
150.0	M-Neoplasm, Cervical esophagus
160x	M-Neoplasm, Ear/Sinus/Nasal cavity
161x	Malignant neoplasm, Larynx
173.2	M-Neoplasm, Skin of ear
173.3	M-Neoplasm, Skin of face NEC
195.0	M-Neoplasm, Head/face/neck
V58.0	Radiotherapy encounter

REIMBURSEMENT INFORMATION

General

- See notes on page 342.

77412 Radiation treatment delivery, three or more separate treatment areas, custom blocking, tangential ports, wedges, rotational beam, compensators, special particle beam (eg, electron or neutrons); up to 5 MeV

CPT NOTES

- Radiation treatment delivery (77401-77416) recognizes the technical component and the various energy levels.

141x	Malignant neoplasm of tongue
142x	Malignant neoplasm, salivary glands
146x	Malignant neoplasm, Oropharynx
147x	Malignant neoplasm, Nasopharynx
148x	Malignant neoplasm, Hypopharynx
149x	M-Neoplasm, Lip/Oral cavity/Pharynx
150.0	M-Neoplasm, Cervical esophagus
160x	M-Neoplasm, Ear/Sinus/Nasal cavity
161x	Malignant neoplasm, Larynx
173.2	M-Neoplasm, Skin of ear
173.3	M-Neoplasm, Skin of face NEC
195.0	M-Neoplasm, Head/face/neck
V58.0	Radiotherapy encounter

REIMBURSEMENT INFORMATION

General

- See notes on page 342.

CPT CODE **SERVICE**

77418 Radiation treatment delivery, three or more separate treatment areas, custom blocking, tangential ports, wedges, rotational beam, compensators, special particle beam (eg, electron or neutrons); 6-10 MeV

CPT NOTES

- Radiation treatment delivery (77401-77416) recognizes the technical component and the various energy levels.

ICD–9–CM

141x	Malignant neoplasm of tongue
142x	Malignant neoplasm, salivary glands
146x	Malignant neoplasm, Oropharynx
147x	Malignant neoplasm, Nasopharynx
148x	Malignant neoplasm, Hypopharynx
149x	M-Neoplasm, Lip/Oral cavity/Pharynx
150.0	M-Neoplasm, Cervical esophagus
160x	M-Neoplasm, Ear/Sinus/Nasal cavity
161x	Malignant neoplasm, Larynx
173.2	M-Neoplasm, Skin of ear
173.3	M-Neoplasm, Skin of face NEC
195.0	M-Neoplasm, Head/face/neck
V58.0	Radiotherapy encounter

REIMBURSEMENT INFORMATION

General

- See notes on page 342.

77420 Weekly radiology therapy management; simple

141x	Malignant neoplasm of tongue
142x	Malignant neoplasm, salivary glands
146x	Malignant neoplasm, Oropharynx
147x	Malignant neoplasm, Nasopharynx
148x	Malignant neoplasm, Hypopharynx
149x	M-Neoplasm, Lip/Oral cavity/Pharynx
150.0	M-Neoplasm, Cervical esophagus
160x	M-Neoplasm, Ear/Sinus/Nasal cavity
161x	Malignant neoplasm, Larynx
173.2	M-Neoplasm, Skin of ear
173.3	M-Neoplasm, Skin of face NEC
195.0	M-Neoplasm, Head/face/neck
V58.0	Radiotherapy encounter

REIMBURSEMENT INFORMATION

General

- See notes on page 342.

CPT CODE	SERVICE	ICD–9–CM

77425 Weekly radiology therapy management; intermediate

141x	Malignant neoplasm of tongue
142x	Malignant neoplasm, salivary glands
146x	Malignant neoplasm, Oropharynx
147x	Malignant neoplasm, Nasopharynx
148x	Malignant neoplasm, Hypopharynx
149x	M-Neoplasm, Lip/Oral cavity/Pharynx
150.0	M-Neoplasm, Cervical esophagus
160x	M-Neoplasm, Ear/Sinus/Nasal cavity
161x	Malignant neoplasm, Larynx
173.2	M-Neoplasm, Skin of ear
173.3	M-Neoplasm, Skin of face NEC
195.0	M-Neoplasm, Head/face/neck
V58.0	Radiotherapy encounter

REIMBURSEMENT INFORMATION

General

- ♦ See notes on page 342.

Medicare

- ♦ Fragments — 77420

77430 Weekly radiology therapy management; complex

141x	Malignant neoplasm of tongue
142x	Malignant neoplasm, salivary glands
146x	Malignant neoplasm, Oropharynx
147x	Malignant neoplasm, Nasopharynx
148x	Malignant neoplasm, Hypopharynx
149x	M-Neoplasm, Lip/Oral cavity/Pharynx
150.0	M-Neoplasm, Cervical esophagus
160x	M-Neoplasm, Ear/Sinus/Nasal cavity
161x	Malignant neoplasm, Larynx
173.2	M-Neoplasm, Skin of ear
173.3	M-Neoplasm, Skin of face NEC
195.0	M-Neoplasm, Head/face/neck
V58.0	Radiotherapy encounter

REIMBURSEMENT INFORMATION

General

- ♦ See notes on page 342.

Medicare

- ♦ Fragments — 77420

PATHOLOGY AND LABORATORY

CPT CODE	SERVICE
80002	Automated multichannel test; 1 or 2 clinical chemistry test(s)

CPT NOTES

- The following list contains those tests that can be and are frequently done as groups and combinations ("profiles") on automated multichannel equipment. For any combination of tests among those listed immediately below, use the appropriate number 80002–80019. Groups of the tests listed here are distinguished from multiple tests performed individually for immediate or "stat" reporting. (For handling of specimen, see 99000 and 99001.)

Alanine aminotransferase (ALT, SGPT)
Albumin
Aspartate aminotransferase (AST, SGOT)
Bilirubin, direct
Bilirubin, total
Calcium
Carbon dioxide content
Chloride
Cholesterol
Creatinine
Glucose
Lactate dehydrogenase (LD)
Phosphatase, alkaline
Phosphorus (inorganic phosphate)
Potassium
Protein, total
Sodium
Urea Nitrogen (BUN)
Uric acid

ICD–9–CM

173.3	M-Neoplasm, Skin of face NEC
241.0	Nontoxic uninodular goiter
386.0x	Meniere's disease
386.1x	Peripheral vertigo
477.9	Allergic rhinitis NOS
780.4	Dizziness and giddiness
780.7	Malaise and fatigue
784.49	Voice disturbance NEC

CPT CODE	SERVICE
80003	Automated multichannel test, 3 clinical chemistry tests

CPT NOTES

- The following list contains those tests that can be and are frequently done as groups and combinations ("profiles") on automated multichannel equipment. For any combination of tests among those listed immediately below, use the appropriate number 80002–80019. Groups of the tests listed here are distinguished from multiple tests performed individually for immediate or "stat" reporting. (For handling of specimen, see 99000 and 99001.)

Alanine aminotransferase (ALT, SGPT)
Albumin
Aspartate aminotransferase (AST, SGOT)
Bilirubin, direct
Bilirubin, total
Calcium
Carbon dioxide content
Chloride
Cholesterol
Creatinine
Glucose
Lactate dehydrogenase (LD)
Phosphatase, alkaline
Phosphorus (inorganic phosphate)
Potassium
Protein, total
Sodium
Urea Nitrogen (BUN)
Uric acid

ICD–9–CM	
173.3	M Neoplasm, skin of face NEC
241.0	Nontoxic uninodular goiter
386.0x	Meniere's disease
386.1x	Peripheral vertigo
477.9	Allergic rhinitis NOS
780.4	Dizziness and giddiness
780.7	Malaise and fatigue
784.49	Voice disturbance NEC

CPT CODE **SERVICE**

80004 Automated multichannel test; 4 clinical chemistry tests

CPT NOTES

- The following list contains those tests that can be and are frequently done as groups and combinations ("profiles") on automated multichannel equipment. For any combination of tests among those listed immediately below, use the appropriate number 80002–80019. Groups of the tests listed here are distinguished from multiple tests performed individually for immediate or "stat" reporting. (For handling of specimen, see 99000 and 99001.)

Alanine aminotransferase (ALT, SGPT)
Albumin
Aspartate aminotransferase (AST, SGOT)
Bilirubin, direct
Bilirubin, total
Calcium
Carbon dioxide content
Chloride
Cholesterol
Creatinine
Glucose
Lactate dehydrogenase (LD)
Phosphatase, alkaline
Phosphorus (inorganic phosphate)
Potassium
Protein, total
Sodium
Urea Nitrogen (BUN)
Uric acid

ICD–9–CM

173.3	M-Neoplasm, Skin of face NEC
241.0	Nontoxic uninodular goiter
386.0x	Meniere's disease
386.1x	Peripheral vertigo
477.9	Allergic rhinitis NOS
780.4	Dizziness and giddiness
780.7	Malaise and fatigue
784.49	Voice disturbance NEC

CPT CODE **SERVICE**

80007 Automated multichannel test; 7 clinical chemistry tests

CPT NOTES

- The following list contains those tests that can be and are frequently done as groups and combinations ("profiles") on automated multichannel equipment. For any combination of tests among those listed immediately below, use the appropriate number 80002–80019. Groups of the tests listed here are distinguished from multiple tests performed individually for immediate or "stat" reporting. (For handling of specimen, see 99000 and 99001.)

Alanine aminotransferase (ALT, SGPT)
Albumin
Aspartate aminotransferase (AST, SGOT)
Bilirubin, direct
Bilirubin, total
Calcium
Carbon dioxide content
Chloride
Cholesterol
Creatinine
Glucose
Lactate dehydrogenase (LD)
Phosphatase, alkaline
Phosphorus (inorganic phosphate)
Potassium
Protein, total
Sodium
Urea Nitrogen (BUN)
Uric acid

ICD–9–CM

173.3 M Neoplasm, skin of face NEC
241.0 Nontoxic uninodular goiter
386.0x Meniere's disease
386.1x Peripheral vertigo
477.9 Allergic rhinitis NOS
780.4 Dizziness and giddiness
780.7 Malaise and fatigue
784.49 Voice disturbance NEC

CPT CODE	SERVICE
80016	Automated multichannel test; 13-16 clinical chemistry tests

CPT NOTES

- The following list contains those tests that can be and are frequently done as groups and combinations ("profiles") on automated multichannel equipment. For any combination of tests among those listed immediately below, use the appropriate number 80002–80019. Groups of the tests listed here are distinguished from multiple tests performed individually for immediate or "stat" reporting. (For handling of specimen, see 99000 and 99001.)

Alanine aminotransferase (ALT, SGPT)
Albumin
Aspartate aminotransferase (AST, SGOT)
Bilirubin, direct
Bilirubin, total
Calcium
Carbon dioxide content
Chloride
Cholesterol
Creatinine
Glucose
Lactate dehydrogenase (LD)
Phosphatase, alkaline
Phosphorus (inorganic phosphate)
Potassium
Protein, total
Sodium
Urea Nitrogen (BUN)
Uric acid

ICD–9–CM

173.3	M-Neoplasm, Skin of face NEC
241.0	Nontoxic uninodular goiter
386.0x	Meniere's disease
386.1x	Peripheral vertigo
477.9	Allergic rhinitis NOS
780.4	Dizziness and giddiness
780.7	Malaise and fatigue
784.49	Voice disturbance NEC

CPT CODE	SERVICE
80018	Automated multichannel test; 17-18 clinical chemistry tests

CPT NOTES

- The following list contains those tests that can be and are frequently done as groups and combinations ("profiles") on automated multichannel equipment. For any combination of tests among those listed immediately below, use the appropriate number 80002–80019. Groups of the tests listed here are distinguished from multiple tests performed individually for immediate or "stat" reporting. (For handling of specimen, see 99000 and 99001.)

Alanine aminotransferase (ALT, SGPT)
Albumin
Aspartate aminotransferase (AST, SGOT)
Bilirubin, direct
Bilirubin, total
Calcium
Carbon dioxide content
Chloride
Cholesterol
Creatinine
Glucose
Lactate dehydrogenase (LD)
Phosphatase, alkaline
Phosphorus (inorganic phosphate)
Potassium
Protein, total
Sodium
Urea Nitrogen (BUN)
Uric acid

ICD–9–CM

173.3	M Neoplasm, Skin of face NEC
241.0	Nontoxic uninodular goiter
386.0x	Meniere's disease
386.1x	Peripheral vertigo
477.9	Allergic rhinitis NOS
780.4	Dizziness and giddiness
780.7	Malaise and fatigue
784.49	Voice disturbance NEC

CPT CODE **SERVICE**

80019 Automated multichannel test; 19 or more clinical chemistry tests

CPT NOTES

- The following list contains those tests that can be and are frequently done as groups and combinations ("profiles") on automated multichannel equipment. For any combination of tests among those listed immediately below, use the appropriate number 80002–80019. Groups of the tests listed here are distinguished from multiple tests performed individually for immediate or "stat" reporting. (For handling of specimen, see 99000 and 99001.)

  Alanine aminotransferase (ALT, SGPT)
  Albumin
  Aspartate aminotransferase (AST, SGOT)
  Bilirubin, direct
  Bilirubin, total
  Calcium
  Carbon dioxide content
  Chloride
  Cholesterol
  Creatinine
  Glucose
  Lactate dehydrogenase (LD)
  Phosphatase, alkaline
  Phosphorus (inorganic phosphate)
  Potassium
  Protein, total
  Sodium
  Urea Nitrogen (BUN)
  Uric acid

ICD–9–CM

173.3	M-Neoplasm, Skin of face NEC
241.0	Nontoxic uninodular goiter
386.0x	Meniere's disease
386.1x	Peripheral vertigo
477.9	Allergic rhinitis NOS
780.4	Dizziness and giddiness
780.7	Malaise and fatigue
784.49	Voice disturbance NEC

CPT CODE	SERVICE	ICD–9–CM
80091	Thyroid panel This panel must include the following tests: Thyroxine, total (84436) Triodothyroine (T-3), resin uptake (84479)	240.9 Goiter NOS 241.0 Nontoxic uninodular goiter 242.8x Thyrotoxicosis 243 Congenital hypothyroidism 245.1 Subacute thyroiditis 246.9 Disorder of thyroid NOS

CPT NOTES

- This panel was developed for coding purposes only and should not be interpreted as a clinical parameter. The tests listed with the panel identify the defined components of the panel. These panel components are not intended to limit the performance of other tests. If one performs tests in addition to those specifically indicated for this particular panel, those tests should be reported separately in addition to the panel code.

CPT CODE	SERVICE	ICD–9–CM
80092	Thyroid panel; with thyroid stimulating hormone (TSH) This panel must include the following tests: Thyroxine, total (84436) Thyroid stimulating hormone (TSH) (84443) Triodothyroine (T-3), resin uptake (84479)	240.9 Goiter NOS 241.0 Nontoxic uninodular goiter 242.8x Thyrotoxicosis 243 Congenital hypothyroidism 245.1 Subacute thyroiditis 246.9 Disorder of thyroid NOS

CPT NOTES

- This panel was developed for coding purposes only and should not be interpreted as a clinical parameter. The tests listed with the panel identify the defined components of the panel. These panel components are not intended to limit the performance of other tests. If one performs tests in addition to those specifically indicated for this particular panel, those tests should be reported separately in addition to the panel code.

CPT CODE	SERVICE	ICD–9–CM
82784	Gammaglobulin; IgA, IgD, IgG, IgM, each	381.3 Chronic nonsuppurative otitis media 473.9 Chronic sinusitis NOS 477.9 Allergic rhinitis NOS 490 Bronchitis NOS

CPT NOTES

- The material for examination may be from any source. Examination is quantitative unless specified. (For automated, multichannel tests, see 80002-80019.)
- Clinical information derived from the results of laboratory data that is mathematically calculated (e.g., free thyroxine index (T7)) is considered part of the test procedure and therefore is not a separately reportable service.
- For allergen specific IgE, see 86003, 86005.
- Gamma-glutamyltransferase (GGT), see 82977.

CPT CODE	SERVICE	ICD–9–CM
82785	Gammaglobulin; IgE	472.0 Chronic rhinitis 473.9 Chronic sinusitis NOS 477.0 Allergic rhinitis d/t pollen 477.8 Allergic rhinitis NEC 477.9 Allergic rhinitis NOS

CPT NOTES

- The material for examination may be from any source. Examination is quantitative unless specified. (For automated, multichannel tests, see 80002-80019.)
- Clinical information derived from the results of laboratory data that is mathematically calculated (e.g., free thyroxine index (T7)) is considered part of the test procedure and therefore is not a separately reportable service.
- For allergen specific IgE, see 86003, 86005.
- Gamma-glutamyltransferase (GGT), see 82977.

CPT CODE	SERVICE	ICD–9–CM	
84436	Thyroxine; total	240.9	Goiter NOS
		241.0	Nontoxic uninodular goiter
		242.8x	Thyrotoxicosis
		243	Congenital hypothyroidism
		245.1	Subacute thyroiditis
		246.9	Disorder of thyroid NOS
		780.4	Dizziness and giddiness
		780.7	Malaise and fatigue
		784.2	Swelling in head/neck

CPT NOTES

- The material for examination may be from any source. Examination is quantitative unless specified. (For list of automated, multichannel tests, see 80002-80019.)
- Clinical information derived from the results of laboratory data that is mathematically calculated (e.g., free thyroxine index (T7)) is considered part of the test procedure and therefore is not a separately reportable service.
- This code is intended for use with molecular diagnostic techniques for analysis of nucleic acids. The service is coded by procedure rather than analyte. Code separately for each procedure used in an analysis. For example, a procedure requiring isolation of DNA, restriction endonuclease digestion, electrophoresis, and nucleic acid probe amplification would be coded 83890, 83892, 83894, and 83898.
- For microbial identification, see 87178, 87179.

CPT CODE	SERVICE	ICD–9–CM	
84439	Thyroxine; free	240.9	Goiter NOS
		241.0	Nontoxic uninodular goiter
		242.8x	Thyrotoxicosis
		243	Congenital hypothyroidism
		245.1	Subacute thyroiditis
		246.9	Disorder of thyroid NOS
		780.4	Dizziness and giddiness
		780.7	Malaise and fatigue
		784.2	Swelling in head/neck

CPT NOTES

- The material for examination may be from any source. Examination is quantitative unless specified. (For list of automated, multichannel tests, see 80002-80019.)
- Clinical information derived from the results of laboratory data that is mathematically calculated (e.g., free thyroxine index (T7)) is considered part of the test procedure and therefore is not a separately reportable service.
- This code is intended for use with molecular diagnostic techniques for analysis of nucleic acids. The service is coded by procedure rather than analyte. Code separately for each procedure used in an analysis. For example, a procedure requiring isolation of DNA, restriction endonuclease digestion, electrophoresis, and nucleic acid probe amplification would be coded 83890, 83892, 83894, and 83898.
- For microbial identification, see 87178, 87179.

CPT CODE	SERVICE	ICD–9–CM	
84443	Thyroid stimulating hormone (TSH)	240.9	Goiter NOS
		241.0	Nontoxic uninodular goiter
		242.8x	Thyrotoxicosis
		243	Congenital hypothyroidism
		245.1	Subacute thyroiditis
		246.9	Disorder of thyroid NOS
		780.4	Dizziness and giddiness
		780.7	Malaise and fatigue
		784.2	Swelling in head/neck

CPT NOTES

- The material for examination may be from any source. Examination is quantitative unless specified. (For list of automated, multichannel tests, see 80002-80019.)
- Clinical information derived from the results of laboratory data that is mathematically calculated (e.g., free thyroxine index (T7)) is considered part of the test procedure and therefore is not a separately reportable service.
- This code is intended for use with molecular diagnostic techniques for analysis of nucleic acids. The service is coded by procedure rather than analyte. Code separately for each procedure used in an analysis. For example, a procedure requiring isolation of DNA, restriction endonuclease digestion, electrophoresis, and nucleic acid probe amplification would be coded 83890, 83892, 83894, and 83898.
- For microbial identification, see 87178, 87179.

CPT CODE	SERVICE	ICD–9–CM	
84479	Triidothyronine (T-3); resin uptake	240.9	Goiter NOS
		241.0	Nontoxic uninodular goiter
		242.8x	Thyrotoxicosis
		243	Congenital hypothyroidism
		245.1	Subacute thyroiditis
		246.9	Disorder of thyroid NOS
		780.4	Dizziness and giddiness
		780.7	Malaise and fatigue
		784.2	Swelling in head/neck

CPT NOTES

- The material for examination may be from any source. Examination is quantitative unless specified. (For list of automated, multichannel tests, see 80002-80019.)
- Clinical information derived from the results of laboratory data that is mathematically calculated (e.g., free thyroxine index (T7)) is considered part of the test procedure and therefore is not a separately reportable service.
- This code is intended for use with molecular diagnostic techniques for analysis of nucleic acids. The service is coded by procedure rather than analyte. Code separately for each procedure used in an analysis. For example, a procedure requiring isolation of DNA, restriction endonuclease digestion, electrophoresis, and nucleic acid probe amplification would be coded 83890, 83892, 83894, and 83898.
- For microbial identification, see 87178, 87179.

CPT CODE	SERVICE
84480	Triiodothyronine (T-3); total (TT-3)

CPT NOTES

- The material for examination may be from any source. Examination is quantitative unless specified. (For list of automated, multichannel tests, see 80002-80019.)
- Clinical information derived from the results of laboratory data that is mathematically calculated (e.g., free thyroxine index (T7)) is considered part of the test procedure and therefore is not a separately reportable service.
- This code is intended for use with molecular diagnostic techniques for analysis of nucleic acids. The service is coded by procedure rather than analyte. Code separately for each procedure used in an analysis. For example, a procedure requiring isolation of DNA, restriction endonuclease digestion, electrophoresis, and nucleic acid probe amplification would be coded 83890, 83892, 83894, and 83898.
- For microbial identification, see 87178, 87179.

ICD–9–CM

240.9	Goiter NOS
241.0	Nontoxic uninodular goiter
242.8x	Thyrotoxicosis
243	Congenital hypothyroidism
245.1	Subacute thyroiditis
246.9	Disorder of thyroid NOS
780.4	Dizziness and giddiness
780.7	Malaise and fatigue
784.2	Swelling in head/neck

CPT CODE SERVICE	ICD–9–CM
85002 Bleeding time **CPT NOTES** ♦ For blood banking procedures, see **Transfusion Medicine.** ♦ Agglutinins, see **Immunology**. ♦ Antiplasmin, see 85410. ♦ Antithrombin III, see 85300, 85301.	470 Deviated nasal septum 473.9 Chronic sinusitis NOS 784.7 Epistaxis
85595 Platelet; automated count **CPT NOTES** ♦ For blood banking procedures, see **Transfusion Medicine.** ♦ Agglutinins, see **Immunology**. ♦ Antiplasmin, see 85410. ♦ Antithrombin III, see 85300, 85301.	287.3 Primary thrombocytopenia 784.7 Epistaxis
85610 Prothrombin time **CPT NOTES** ♦ For blood banking procedures, see **Transfusion Medicine.** ♦ Agglutinins, see **Immunology**. ♦ Antiplasmin, see 85410. ♦ Antithrombin III, see 85300, 85301.	463 Acute tonsillitis 474x Chronic tonsil/adenoid disease 475 Peritonsillar abscess
85651 Sedimentation rate, erythrocyte; non-automated **CPT NOTES** ♦ For blood banking procedures, see **Transfusion Medicine.** ♦ Agglutinins, see **Immunology**. ♦ Antiplasmin, see 85410. ♦ Antithrombin III, see 85300, 85301.	243 Congenital hypothyroidism 245.9 Thyroiditis NOS 780.4 Dizziness and giddiness 780.7 Malaise and fatigue

CPT CODE / SERVICE	ICD-9-CM
86003 Allergen specific IgE, quantitative, each panel of up to 12 allergens **CPT NOTES** ♦ Acetylcholine receptor antibody, see 86255, 86256. ♦ Actinomyces, antibodies to, see 86602. ♦ Adrenal cortex antibodies, see 86255, 86256. ♦ For total quantitative IgE, use 82785.	477.0 Allergic rhinitis d/t pollen 477.8 Allergic rhinitis NEC 477.9 Allergic rhinitis NOS
86161 Complement; functional activity, each component **CPT NOTES** ♦ Acetylcholine receptor antibody, see 86255, 86256. ♦ Actinomyces, antibodies to, see 86602. ♦ Adrenal cortex antibodies, see 86255, 86256.	477.9 Allergic rhinitis NOS
86317 Immunoassay for infectious agent antibody, quantitative, not elsewhere specified **CPT NOTES** ♦ Acetylcholine receptor antibody, see 86255, 86256. ♦ Actinomyces, antibodies to, see 86602. ♦ Adrenal cortex antibodies, see 86255, 86256. ♦ For immunoassay techniques for antigens, see 83516, 83518, 83519, 83520, 86313, 86315. ♦ For particle agglutination procedures, see 86403.	461.9 Acute sinusitis NOS 462 Acute pharyngitis 477.9 Allergic rhinitis NOS
86329 Immunodiffusion; not elsewhere specified **CPT NOTES** ♦ Acetylcholine receptor antibody, see 86255, 86256. ♦ Actinomyces, antibodies to, see 86602. ♦ Adrenal cortex antibodies, see 86255, 86256.	461.9 Acute sinusitis NOS 462 Acute pharyngitis 477.9 Allergic rhinitis NOS

CPT CODE	SERVICE	ICD-9-CM
▲ **86403**	Particle agglutination; screen, each antibody	461.9 Acute sinusitis NOS 462 Acute pharyngitis 477.9 Allergic rhinitis NOS

CPT NOTES

- Acetylcholine receptor antibody, see 86255, 86256.
- Actinomyces, antibodies to, see 86602.
- Adrenal cortex antibodies, see 86255, 86256.
- Pregnancy test, see 84702, 84703.
- Rapid plasma reagin test (RPR), see 86592, 86593.

REIMBURSEMENT INFORMATION

General

- Description changed in 1995 CPT.

86580 Skin test; tuberculosis, intradermal

380.1x Infective otitis externa
382.0x Acute suppurative otitis media
388.60 Otorrhea NOS
784.2 Swelling in head/neck

CPT NOTES

- Acetylcholine receptor antibody, see 86255, 86256.
- Actinomyces, antibodies to, see 86602.
- Adrenal cortex antibodies, see 86255, 86256.
- For skin test for allergy, see 95010-95199.
- Smooth muscle antibody, see 86255, 86256.
- Sporothrix, antibodies to, see code for specific method.

CPT CODE	SERVICE
86781	Antibody; Treponema Pallidum, confirmatory test (eg, FTA-abs)

ICD–9–CM	
389.1	Sensorineural hearing loss
780.4	Dizziness and giddiness

CPT NOTES

- Acetylcholine receptor antibody, see 86255, 86256.
- Actinomyces, antibodies to, see 86602.
- Adrenal cortex antibodies, see 86255, 86256.
- Qualitative or semiquantitative immunoassay performed by multiple step methods. For immunoassay by single step method (e.g., reagent strips), use code 86318. Procedures for identification of antibodies should be coded as precisely as possible.

  For example, an antibody to a virus could be coded with increasing specificity for virus, family, genus, species, or type. In some cases, further precision may be added to codes by specifying the class of immunoglobulin being detected. When multiple tests are done to detect antibodies to organisms classified more precisely than the specificity allowed by available codes, it is appropriate to code each as a separate service. For example, a test for antibody to an enterovirus is coded as 86658. Coxsackie viruses are enteroviruses, but there are no codes for the individual species of enterovirus. If assays are performed for antibodies to Coxsackie A and B species, each assay should be separately coded. Similarly, if multiple assays are performed for antibodies of different immunoglobulin classes, each assay should be coded separately.

CPT CODE	SERVICE	ICD–9–CM	
87060	Culture, bacterial, definitive; throat or nose **CPT NOTES** ♦ Microbiology codes include bacteriology, mycology, parasitology, and virology. ♦ For urine, see 87086-87088.	380.1x 382.0x 382.9 460 461x 462 463 464.0 465.9 472.0 472.2 473.2 473.9 477.0 477.8 477.9 478.1 490 491.0 529.0 786.2	Infective otitis externa Acute suppurative otitis media Otitis media NOS Acute nasopharyngitis Acute sinusitis Acute pharyngitis Acute tonsillitis Acute laryngitis Acute upper respiratory infect NOS Chronic rhinitis Chronic nasopharyngitis Chronic ethmoidal sinusitis Chronic sinusitis NOS Allergic rhinitis d/t pollen Allergic rhinitis NEC Allergic rhinitis NOS Nasal and sinus disease NEC Bronchitis NOS Simple chronic bronchitis Glossitis Cough
87072	Culture or direct bacterial identification method, each organism, by commercial kit, any source except urine **CPT NOTES** ♦ Microbiology codes include bacteriology, mycology, parasitology, and virology. ♦ For urine, see 87087.	034.0 462 465.9	Streptococcal sore throat Acute pharyngitis Acute upper respiratory infect NOS
87081	Culture, bacterial, screening only, for single organisms **CPT NOTES** ♦ Microbiology codes include bacteriology, mycology, parasitology, and virology.	034.0 462 465.9	Streptococcal sore throat Acute pharyngitis Acute upper respiratory infect NOS
87082	Culture, presumptive, pathogenic organisms, screening only, by commercial kit (specify type); for single organisms **CPT NOTES** ♦ Microbiology codes include bacteriology, mycology, parasitology, and virology. ♦ For urine colony count, see 87086.	034.0 462 465.9	Streptococcal sore throat Acute pharyngitis Acute upper respiratory infect NOS

CPT CODE	SERVICE	ICD-9-CM	
87181	Sensitivity studies, antibiotic; agar diffusion method, per antibiotic **CPT NOTES** ♦ Microbiology codes include bacteriology, mycology, parasitology, and virology.	460 461x 462 464.0 465.9 472.0 472.2 473x 477.9 490	Acute nasopharyngitis Acute sinusitis Acute pharyngitis Acute laryngitis Acute upper respiratory infect NOS Chronic rhinitis Chronic nasopharyngitis Chronic sinusitis Allergic rhinitis NOS Bronchitis NOS
87184	Sensitivity studies, antibiotic; disc method, per plate (12 or less discs) **CPT NOTES** ♦ Microbiology codes include bacteriology, mycology, parasitology, and virology.	460 461x 462 464.0 465.9 472.0 472.2 473x 477.9 490	Acute nasopharyngitis Acute sinusitis Acute pharyngitis Acute laryngitis Acute upper respiratory infect NOS Chronic rhinitis Chronic nasopharyngitis Chronic sinusitis Allergic rhinitis NOS Bronchitis NOS
87186	Sensitivity studies, antibiotic; microtiter, minimum inhibitory concentration (MIC), any number of antibiotics **CPT NOTES** ♦ Microbiology codes include bacteriology, mycology, parasitology, and virology.	460 461x 462 464.0 465.9 472x 473x 477.9 490	Acute nasopharyngitis Acute sinusitis Acute pharyngitis Acute laryngitis Acute upper respiratory infect NOS Chronic pharyngitis/nasopharyngitis Chronic sinusitis Allergic rhinitis NOS Bronchitis NOS

CPT CODE	SERVICE	ICD–9–CM	

87205 Smear, primary source, with interpretation; routine stain for bacteria, fungi, or cell types

ICD–9–CM	
461x	Acute sinusitis
462	Acute pharyngitis

CPT NOTES

- Microbiology codes include bacteriology, mycology, parasitology, and virology.
- For concentration, see 87015; complete examination, see 87177.
- For complex special stains, see 88312, 88313.
- For fat, meat, fibers, nasal eosinophils, and starch, see miscellaneous section.

88160 Cytopathology, smears, any other source; screening and interpretation

ICD–9–CM	
245.9	Thyroiditis NOS
252.9	Parathyroid gland disorder NOS
288.3	Eosinophilia
461x	Acute sinusitis
462	Acute pharyngitis
464.0	Acute laryngitis
784.2	Swelling in head/neck
786.2	Cough
786.9	Respiratory system, chest sympt NEC

CPT NOTES

- For obtaining specimen, see percutaneous needle biopsy under individual organ in **Surgery**.
- For aerosol collection of sputum, see 89350.
- For special stains, see 88312-88314.

88161 Cytopathology, smears, any other source; preparation, screening and interpretation

ICD–9–CM	
245.9	Thyroiditis NOS
252.9	Parathyroid gland disorder NOS
461x	Acute sinusitis
462	Acute pharyngitis
464.0	Acute laryngitis
784.2	Swelling in head/neck
786.2	Cough
786.9	Respiratory system, chest sympt NEC

CPT NOTES

- For obtaining specimen, see percutaneous needle biopsy under individual organ in **Surgery**.
- For aerosol collection of sputum, see 89350.
- For special stains, see 88312-88314.

CPT CODE	SERVICE
88170	Fine needle aspiration with or without preparation of smears; superficial tissue (eg, thyroid, breast, prostate)

CPT NOTES

- For percutaneous needle biopsy, see 60100 for thyroid, 19100 for breast, 55700 for prostate.

ICD–9–CM

142.0	M-Neoplasm, Parotid gland
145.9	M-Neoplasm, Mouth NOS
147.8	M-Neoplasm, Nasopharynx NEC
161.9	M-Neoplasm, Larynx NOS
173.2	M-Neoplasm, Skin of ear
193	M-Neoplasm, Thyroid gland
195.0	M-Neoplasm, Head/face/neck
196.0	M-Neoplasm, Lymph head/neck/face
202.81	Lymphoma NEC, head/neck
210.2	B-Neoplasm, Major salivary glands
235.0	UB-Neoplasm, Major salivary glands
240.9	Goiter NOS
241.0	Nontoxic uninodular goiter
245.9	Thyroiditis NOS
252.9	Parathyroid gland disorder NOS
527.1	Salivary gland hypertrophy
527.2	Sialoadenitis
683	Acute lymphadenitis
784.2	Swelling in head/neck
785.6	Enlargement of lymph nodes

SURGICAL PATHOLOGY
88300–88399

Services 88300 through 88309 include accession, examination, and reporting. They do not include the services designated in codes 88311 through 88365 and 88399, which are coded in addition when provided.

The unit of service for codes 88300 through 88309 is the specimen. A specimen is defined as tissue or tissues that is (are) submitted for individual and separate attention, requiring individual examination and pathologic diagnosis. Two or more such specimens from the same patient (e.g., separately identified endoscopic biopsies, skin lesions, etc.) are each appropriately assigned an individual code reflective of its proper level of service.

Service code 88300 is used for any specimen that in the opinion of the examining pathologist can be accurately diagnosed without microscopic examination. Service code 88302 is used when gross and microscopic examination is performed on a specimen to confirm identification and the absence of disease. Service codes 88304 through 88309 describe all other specimens requiring gross and microscopic examination, and represent additional ascending levels of physician work. Levels 88302 through 88309 are specifically defined by the assigned specimens.

Any unlisted specimen should be assigned to the code which most closely reflects the physician work involved when compared to other specimens assigned to that code.

See your CPT for the list of assigned specimens.

CPT CODE **SERVICE** | **ICD-9-CM**

88304 LEVEL III - Surgical pathology, gross and microscopic examination

160x	M-Neoplasm, Ear/Sinus/Nasal cavity
463	Acute tonsillitis
478.1	Nasal and sinus disease NEC
709.9	Skin disorder NOS

REIMBURSEMENT INFORMATION

General

- See notes on page 369.

88305 LEVEL IV - Surgical pathology, gross and microscopic examination

173.9	M-Neoplasm, Skin NOS
210.5	B-Neoplasm, Tonsil

REIMBURSEMENT INFORMATION

General

- See notes on page 369.

88331 Pathology consultation during surgery; with frozen section(s), single specimen

141x	Malignant neoplasm of tongue
142x	Malignant neoplasm, salivary glands
146x	Malignant neoplasm, Oropharynx
147x	Malignant neoplasm, Nasopharynx
148x	Malignant neoplasm, Hypopharynx
149x	M-Neoplasm, Lip/Oral cavity/Pharynx
150.0	M-Neoplasm, Cervical esophagus
160x	M-Neoplasm, Ear/Sinus/Nasal cavity
161x	Malignant neoplasm, Larynx
173.2	M-Neoplasm, Skin of ear
173.3	M-Neoplasm, Skin of face NEC
195.0	M-Neoplasm, Head/face/neck
V58.0	Radiotherapy encounter

REIMBURSEMENT INFORMATION

General

- See notes on page 369.

89190 Nasal smear for eosinophils

CPT NOTES

- Occult blood, feces, see 82270.
- Paternity tests, see 86910.

470	Deviated nasal septum
472.0	Chronic rhinitis
473.9	Chronic sinusitis NOS
477.0	Allergic rhinitis d/t pollen
477.8	Allergic rhinitis NEC
477.9	Allergic rhinitis NOS

MEDICINE

CPT CODE	SERVICE	ICD–9–CM
90724	Immunization, active; influenza virus vaccine	V07.8 Prophylactic measures NEC

CPT NOTES

- Immunizations are usually given in conjunction with a medical service. When an immunization is the only service performed, a minimal service may be listed in addition to the injection. Immunization procedures include the supply of materials.
- For allergy testing, see 95004 et seq.
- For skin testing of bacterial, viral, fungal extracts, see 86485–86586.
- For therapeutic or diagnostic injections, see 90782–90799.

REIMBURSEMENT INFORMATION

Medicare

- Follow–up Days — global concept does not apply
- Assistant Surgeon — not paid
- Supply Charges — not allowed
- Outpatient Limit — does not apply

92502 Otolaryngologic examination under general anesthesia

CPT NOTES

- Diagnostic or treatment procedures usually included in a comprehensive otorhinolaryngologic evaluation or office visit, are reported as an integrated medical service, using appropriate descriptors from the 99201 series. Itemization of component procedures (e.g., otoscopy, rhinoscopy, tuning fork test) does not apply.

  Special otorhinolaryngologic services are those diagnostic and treatment services not usually included in a comprehensive otorhinolaryngologic evaluation or office visit. These services are reported separately, using descriptors from the 92500 series.

  All services include medical diagnostic evaluation. Technical procedures (which may or may not be performed by the physician personally) are often part of the service, but should not be mistaken to constitute the service itself.
- For laryngoscopy with stroboscopy, use 31579.

ICD–9–CM	
380.10	Infective otitis externa NOS
380.11	Acute infection of pinna
380.12	Acute swimmers' ear
381.00	Acute nonsup otitis media NOS
381.10	Chron serous otitis media simp/NOS
382.00	Acute suppurative otitis media NOS
382.2	Chronic atticoantral suppurative OM
382.3	Chronic suppurativ otitis media NOS
382.4	Suppurative otitis media NOS
383.0x	Acute mastoiditis
383.1	Chronic mastoiditis
385.10	Adhesive middle ear disease NOS
385.30	Cholesteatoma NOS
385.83	Old foreign body of middle ear
388.60	Otorrhea NOS
388.70	Otalgia NOS
389.9	Hearing loss NOS
474.10	Hypertrophy of tonsils/adenoids
474.11	Hypertrophy of tonsils
474.12	Hypertrophy of adenoids
959.0	Face and neck injury NOS

REIMBURSEMENT INFORMATION

Medicare

- Follow–up Days — 0
- Assistant Surgeon — by report
- Supply Charges — not allowed
- Outpatient Limit — does not apply
- Minor Surgery Rules Apply

CPT CODE	SERVICE
92504	Binocular microscopy (separate diagnostic procedure)

CPT NOTES

- Diagnostic or treatment procedures usually included in a comprehensive otorhinolaryngologic evaluation or office visit, are reported as an integrated medical service, using appropriate descriptors from the 99201 series. Itemization of component procedures (e.g., otoscopy, rhinoscopy, tuning fork test) does not apply.

  Special otorhinolaryngologic services are those diagnostic and treatment services not usually included in a comprehensive otorhinolaryngologic evaluation or office visit. These services are reported separately, using descriptors from the 92500 series.

  All services include medical diagnostic evaluation. Technical procedures (which may or may not be performed by the physician personally) are often part of the service, but should not be mistaken to constitute the service itself.
- For laryngoscopy with stroboscopy, use 31579.

ICD–9–CM

053.71	Otitis externa d/t herpes zoster
112.82	Candidal otitis externa
230.0	CA in situ, Oral cavity/pharynx
315.39	Speech/language develop disord NEC
380.01	Acute perichondritis of pinna
380.02	Chronic perichondritis of pinna
380.10	Infective otitis externa NOS
380.11	Acute infection of pinna
380.12	Acute swimmers' ear
380.14	Malignant otitis externa
380.16	Chron infective otitis externa NEC
380.21	Cholesteatoma of external ear
380.22	Acute otitis externa NEC
380.23	Chronic otitis externa NEC
381.00	Acute nonsup otitis media NOS
381.10	Chron serous otitis media simp/NOS
381.19	Chronic serous otitis media NEC
381.20	Chron mucoid otitis media simp/NOS
381.29	Chronic mucoid otitis media NEC
381.4	Chron nonsup otitis media NOS
381.81	Dysfunction of Eustachian tube
382.00	Acute suppurative otitis media NOS
382.01	Ac suppur otitis media w/drum rupt
382.3	Chronic suppurativ otitis media NOS
382.4	Suppurative otitis media NOS
383.00	Acute mastoiditis w/o complications
383.01	Subperiosteal mastoid abscess
383.02	Acute mastoiditis w/complic NEC
383.1	Chronic mastoiditis
383.32	Postmastoidectomy cholesteatoma
383.9	Mastoiditis NOS
384.00	Acute myringitis NOS
384.01	Bullous myringitis
384.2x	Perforation tympanic membrane
385.3x	Cholesteatoma
385.82	Cholesterin granuloma
388.60	Otorrhea NOS
388.70	Otalgia NOS
389.00	Conductive hearing loss NOS
389.2	Mixed hearing loss
389.8	Hearing loss NEC
389.9	Hearing loss NOS
474.11	Hypertrophy of tonsils
474.9	Chronic tonsil/adenoid disease NOS
478.4	Polyp of vocal cord/larynx

REIMBURSEMENT INFORMATION

Medicare

- Follow–up Days — global concept does not apply
- Assistant Surgeon — by report
- Supply Charges — not allowed
- Outpatient Limit — applies

CPT CODE	SERVICE	ICD–9–CM
92506	Medical evaluation speech, language and/or hearing problems	315.31 Developmental language disorder 315.39 Speech/language develop disord NEC 381.81 Dysfunction of Eustachian tube 382.00 Acute suppurative otitis media NOS 389.00 Conductive hearing loss NOS 389.10 Sensorineural hearing loss NOS 389.11 Sensory hearing loss 474.10 Hypertrophy of tonsils/adenoids 478.5 Vocal cord disease NEC 750.0 Tongue tie 784.40 Voice disturbance NOS 784.49 Voice disturbance NEC 784.69 Symbolic dysfunction NEC V20.2 Routine child health exam

CPT NOTES

- Diagnostic or treatment procedures usually included in a comprehensive otorhinolaryngologic evaluation or office visit, are reported as an integrated medical service, using appropriate descriptors from the 99201 series. Itemization of component procedures (e.g., otoscopy, rhinoscopy, tuning fork test) does not apply.

  Special otorhinolaryngologic services are those diagnostic and treatment services not usually included in a comprehensive otorhinolaryngologic evaluation or office visit. These services are reported separately, using descriptors from the 92500 series.

  All services include medical diagnostic evaluation. Technical procedures (which may or may not be performed by the physician personally) are often part of the service, but should not be mistaken to constitute the service itself.
- For laryngoscopy with stroboscopy, use 31579.

REIMBURSEMENT INFORMATION

Medicare

- Follow–up Days — global concept does not apply
- Assistant Surgeon — by report
- Supply Charges — not allowed
- Outpatient Limit — applies

CPT CODE	SERVICE	ICD–9–CM
92507	Speech, language or hearing therapy, with continuing medical supervision; individual	145.3 M-Neoplasm, Soft palate 231.0 CA in situ, Larynx 315.31 Developmental language disorder 315.39 Speech/language develop disord NEC 381.00 Acute nonsup otitis media NOS 388.30 Tinnitus NOS 389.8 Hearing loss NEC 437.0 Cerebral atherosclerosis 464.0 Acute laryngitis 476.0 Chronic laryngitis 478.30 Vocal cord/larynx paralysis NOS 478.4 Polyp of vocal cord/larynx 478.5 Vocal cord disease NEC 780.4 Dizziness and giddiness 784.49 Voice disturbance NEC 784.5 Speech disturbance NEC 787.2 Dysphagia

CPT NOTES

- Diagnostic or treatment procedures usually included in a comprehensive otorhinolaryngologic evaluation or office visit, are reported as an integrated medical service, using appropriate descriptors from the 99201 series. Itemization of component procedures (e.g., otoscopy, rhinoscopy, tuning fork test) does not apply.

  Special otorhinolaryngologic services are those diagnostic and treatment services not usually included in a comprehensive otorhinolaryngologic evaluation or office visit. These services are reported separately, using descriptors from the 92500 series.

  All services include medical diagnostic evaluation. Technical procedures (which may or may not be performed by the physician personally) are often part of the service, but should not be mistaken to constitute the service itself.
- For laryngoscopy with stroboscopy, use 31579.

REIMBURSEMENT INFORMATION

Medicare

- Follow–up Days — global concept does not apply
- Assistant Surgeon — by report
- Supply Charges — not allowed
- Outpatient Limit — applies

CPT CODE	SERVICE
92508	Speech, language or hearing therapy, with continuing medical supervision; group

CPT NOTES

- Diagnostic or treatment procedures usually included in a comprehensive otorhinolaryngologic evaluation or office visit, are reported as an integrated medical service, using appropriate descriptors from the 99201 series. Itemization of component procedures (e.g., otoscopy, rhinoscopy, tuning fork test) does not apply.

  Special otorhinolaryngologic services are those diagnostic and treatment services not usually included in a comprehensive otorhinolaryngologic evaluation or office visit. These services are reported separately, using descriptors from the 92500 series.

  All services include medical diagnostic evaluation. Technical procedures (which may or may not be performed by the physician personally) are often part of the service, but should not be mistaken to constitute the service itself.
- For laryngoscopy with stroboscopy, use 31579.

ICD–9–CM

145.3	M-Neoplasm, Soft palate
231.0	CA in situ, Larynx
315.31	Developmental language disorder
315.39	Speech/language develop disord NEC
381.00	Acute nonsup otitis media NOS
388.30	Tinnitus NOS
389.8	Hearing loss NEC
437.0	Cerebral atherosclerosis
464.0	Acute laryngitis
476.0	Chronic laryngitis
478.30	Vocal cord/larynx paralysis NOS
478.4	Polyp of vocal cord/larynx
478.5	Vocal cord disease NEC
780.4	Dizziness and giddiness
784.49	Voice disturbance NEC
784.5	Speech disturbance NEC
787.2	Dysphagia

REIMBURSEMENT INFORMATION

Medicare

- Follow–up Days — global concept does not apply
- Assistant Surgeon — by report
- Supply Charges — not allowed
- Outpatient Limit — does not apply

CPT CODE	SERVICE
92511	Nasopharyngoscopy with endoscope (separate procedure)

CPT NOTES

- Diagnostic or treatment procedures usually included in a comprehensive otorhinolaryngologic evaluation or office visit, are reported as an integrated medical service, using appropriate descriptors from the 99201 series. Itemization of component procedures (e.g., otoscopy, rhinoscopy, tuning fork test) does not apply.

  Special otorhinolaryngologic services are those diagnostic and treatment services not usually included in a comprehensive otorhinolaryngologic evaluation or office visit. These services are reported separately, using descriptors from the 92500 series.

  All services include medical diagnostic evaluation. Technical procedures (which may or may not be performed by the physician personally) are often part of the service, but should not be mistaken to constitute the service itself.
- For laryngoscopy with stroboscopy, use 31579.

ICD–9–CM

141.0	M-Neoplasm, Tongue base
148.9	M-Neoplasm, Hypopharynx NOS
161.0	M-Neoplasm, Glottis
161.1	M-Neoplasm, Supraglottis
210.1	B-Neoplasm, Tongue
212.0	B-Neoplasm, Nasal cavity/sinus
212.1	B-Neoplasm, Larynx
230.0	CA in situ, Oral cavity/pharynx
235.1	UB-Neoplasm, Oral cavity/pharynx
460	Acute nasopharyngitis
461.0	Acute maxillary sinusitis
464.0	Acute laryngitis
464.21	Acute laryngotracheitis w/obstruct
470	Deviated nasal septum
471.9	Nasal polyp NOS
476.0	Chronic laryngitis
478.29	Disease of pharynx NEC
478.30	Vocal cord/larynx paralysis NOS
478.32	Vocal cord paralysis, unilat, total
478.33	Vocal cord paralysis, bilat, part
478.34	Vocal cord paralysis, bilat, total
478.4	Polyp of vocal cord/larynx
478.5	Vocal cord disease NEC
478.6	Edema of larynx
527.6	Salivary gland mucocele
529.1	Geographic tongue
529.8	Tongue disorder NEC
786.1	Stridor
802.0	Nasal bone Fx, closed

REIMBURSEMENT INFORMATION

General

- Separate procedure rules apply.

Medicare

- Follow–up Days — 0
- Assistant Surgeon — by report
- Supply Charges — not allowed
- Outpatient Limit — applies
- Minor Surgery Rules Apply

CPT CODE	SERVICE	ICD–9–CM

92512 Nasal function studies, eg, rhinomanometry

470 Deviated nasal septum
472.0 Chronic rhinitis
473.9 Chronic sinusitis NOS
478.1 Nasal and sinus disease NEC
750.29 Pharyngeal anomaly NEC
780.50 Sleep disturbance NOS
786.09 Respiratory abnormality NEC
802.0 Nasal bone Fx, closed

CPT NOTES

- Diagnostic or treatment procedures usually included in a comprehensive otorhinolaryngologic evaluation or office visit, are reported as an integrated medical service, using appropriate descriptors from the 99201 series. Itemization of component procedures (e.g., otoscopy, rhinoscopy, tuning fork test) does not apply.

  Special otorhinolaryngologic services are those diagnostic and treatment services not usually included in a comprehensive otorhinolaryngologic evaluation or office visit. These services are reported separately, using descriptors from the 92500 series.

  All services include medical diagnostic evaluation. Technical procedures (which may or may not be performed by the physician personally) are often part of the service, but should not be mistaken to constitute the service itself.
- For laryngoscopy with stroboscopy, use 31579.

REIMBURSEMENT INFORMATION

<u>Medicare</u>

- Follow–up Days — global concept does not apply
- Assistant Surgeon — by report
- Supply Charges — not allowed
- Outpatient Limit — does not apply

92516 Facial nerve function studies

053.71 Otitis externa d/t herpes zoster
351.0 Bell's palsy
767.5 Facial nerve injury at birth

CPT NOTES

- Diagnostic or treatment procedures usually included in a comprehensive otorhinolaryngologic evaluation or office visit, are reported as an integrated medical service, using appropriate descriptors from the 99201 series. Itemization of component procedures (e.g., otoscopy, rhinoscopy, tuning fork test) does not apply.

  Special otorhinolaryngologic services are those diagnostic and treatment services not usually included in a comprehensive otorhinolaryngologic evaluation or office visit. These services are reported separately, using descriptors from the 92500 series.

  All services include medical diagnostic evaluation. Technical procedures (which may or may not be performed by the physician personally) are often part of the service, but should not be mistaken to constitute the service itself.
- For laryngoscopy with stroboscopy, use 31579.

REIMBURSEMENT INFORMATION

<u>Medicare</u>

- Follow–up Days — global concept does not apply
- Assistant Surgeon — by report
- Supply Charges — not allowed
- Outpatient Limit — applies

CPT CODE **SERVICE**

92520 Laryngeal function studies

CPT NOTES

- Diagnostic or treatment procedures usually included in a comprehensive otorhinolaryngologic evaluation or office visit, are reported as an integrated medical service, using appropriate descriptors from the 99201 series. Itemization of component procedures (e.g., otoscopy, rhinoscopy, tuning fork test) does not apply.

  Special otorhinolaryngologic services are those diagnostic and treatment services not usually included in a comprehensive otorhinolaryngologic evaluation or office visit. These services are reported separately, using descriptors from the 92500 series.

  All services include medical diagnostic evaluation. Technical procedures (which may or may not be performed by the physician personally) are often part of the service, but should not be mistaken to constitute the service itself.
- For laryngoscopy with stroboscopy, use 31579.

ICD–9–CM

464.0	Acute laryngitis
464.10	Acute tracheitis, no obstruction
464.20	Acute laryngotracheitis no obstruct
464.30	Acute epiglottitis, no obstruction
464.4	Croup
476.0	Chronic laryngitis
476.1	Chronic laryngotracheitis
478.30	Vocal cord/larynx paralysis NOS
478.31	Vocal cord paralysis, unilat, part
478.32	Vocal cord paralysis, unilat, total
478.33	Vocal cord paralysis, bilat, part
478.34	Vocal cord paralysis, bilat, total
478.5	Vocal cord disease NEC
478.6	Edema of larynx
478.70	Disease of larynx NOS
478.71	Laryngeal cellulitis
478.74	Stenosis of larynx
478.75	Laryngeal spasm
478.79	Disease of larynx NEC
784.40	Voice disturbance NOS
784.41	Aphonia
784.49	Voice disturbance NEC

REIMBURSEMENT INFORMATION

<u>Medicare</u>

- Follow–up Days — global concept does not apply
- Assistant Surgeon — by report
- Supply Charges — not allowed
- Outpatient Limit — does not apply

CPT CODE **SERVICE**

92531 Spontaneous nystagmus, including gaze

CPT NOTES

- Diagnostic or treatment procedures usually included in a comprehensive otorhinolaryngologic evaluation or office visit, are reported as an integrated medical service, using appropriate descriptors from the 99201 series. Itemization of component procedures (e.g., otoscopy, rhinoscopy, tuning fork test) does not apply.

  Special otorhinolaryngologic services are those diagnostic and treatment services not usually included in a comprehensive otorhinolaryngologic evaluation or office visit. These services are reported separately, using descriptors from the 92500 series.

  All services include medical diagnostic evaluation. Technical procedures (which may or may not be performed by the physician personally) are often part of the service, but should not be mistaken to constitute the service itself.
- For laryngoscopy with stroboscopy, use 31579.

ICD–9–CM

386.10	Peripheral vertigo NOS
386.11	Benign paroxysmal position vertigo
386.12	Vestibular neuronitis
386.19	Peripheral vertigo NEC
386.50	Labyrinthine dysfunction NOS
388.10	Noise effects on inner ear NOS
389.10	Sensorineural hearing loss NOS
780.4	Dizziness and giddiness

REIMBURSEMENT INFORMATION

Medicare

- Follow–up Days — global concept does not apply
- Assistant Surgeon — not paid
- Supply Charges — not allowed
- Outpatient Limit — does not apply

92532 Positional nystagmus

CPT NOTES

- Diagnostic or treatment procedures usually included in a comprehensive otorhinolaryngologic evaluation or office visit, are reported as an integrated medical service, using appropriate descriptors from the 99201 series. Itemization of component procedures (e.g., otoscopy, rhinoscopy, tuning fork test) does not apply.

  Special otorhinolaryngologic services are those diagnostic and treatment services not usually included in a comprehensive otorhinolaryngologic evaluation or office visit. These services are reported separately, using descriptors from the 92500 series.

  All services include medical diagnostic evaluation. Technical procedures (which may or may not be performed by the physician personally) are often part of the service, but should not be mistaken to constitute the service itself.
- For laryngoscopy with stroboscopy, use 31579.

386.10	Peripheral vertigo NOS
386.11	Benign paroxysmal position vertigo
386.12	Vestibular neuronitis
386.19	Peripheral vertigo NEC
386.50	Labyrinthine dysfunction NOS
388.10	Noise effects on inner ear NOS
388.31	Subjective tinnitus
389.10	Sensorineural hearing loss NOS
780.4	Dizziness and giddiness

REIMBURSEMENT INFORMATION

Medicare

- Follow–up Days — global concept does not apply
- Assistant Surgeon — not paid
- Supply Charges — not allowed
- Outpatient Limit — does not apply

CPT CODE **SERVICE**

92533 Caloric vestibular test, each irrigation (binaural, bithermal stimulation constitutes four tests)

CPT NOTES

- Diagnostic or treatment procedures usually included in a comprehensive otorhinolaryngologic evaluation or office visit, are reported as an integrated medical service, using appropriate descriptors from the 99201 series. Itemization of component procedures (e.g., otoscopy, rhinoscopy, tuning fork test) does not apply.

  Special otorhinolaryngologic services are those diagnostic and treatment services not usually included in a comprehensive otorhinolaryngologic evaluation or office visit. These services are reported separately, using descriptors from the 92500 series.

  All services include medical diagnostic evaluation. Technical procedures (which may or may not be performed by the physician personally) are often part of the service, but should not be mistaken to constitute the service itself.
- For laryngoscopy with stroboscopy, use 31579.

ICD–9–CM

383.1 Chronic mastoiditis
386.12 Vestibular neuronitis
386.50 Labyrinthine dysfunction NOS
388.31 Subjective tinnitus
780.4 Dizziness and giddiness

REIMBURSEMENT INFORMATION

Medicare

- Follow–up Days — global concept does not apply
- Assistant Surgeon — not paid
- Supply Charges — not allowed
- Outpatient Limit — does not apply

92534 Optokinetic nystagmus

CPT NOTES

- Diagnostic or treatment procedures usually included in a comprehensive otorhinolaryngologic evaluation or office visit, are reported as an integrated medical service, using appropriate descriptors from the 99201 series. Itemization of component procedures (e.g., otoscopy, rhinoscopy, tuning fork test) does not apply.

  Special otorhinolaryngologic services are those diagnostic and treatment services not usually included in a comprehensive otorhinolaryngologic evaluation or office visit. These services are reported separately, using descriptors from the 92500 series.

  All services include medical diagnostic evaluation. Technical procedures (which may or may not be performed by the physician personally) are often part of the service, but should not be mistaken to constitute the service itself.
- For laryngoscopy with stroboscopy, use 31579.

386.10 Peripheral vertigo NOS
386.11 Benign paroxysmal position vertigo
386.12 Vestibular neuronitis
386.19 Peripheral vertigo NEC
386.50 Labyrinthine dysfunction NOS
388.10 Noise effects on inner ear NOS
389.10 Sensorineural hearing loss NOS
780.4 Dizziness and giddiness

REIMBURSEMENT INFORMATION

Medicare

- Follow–up Days — global concept does not apply
- Assistant Surgeon — not paid
- Supply Charges — not allowed
- Outpatient Limit — does not apply

CPT CODE	SERVICE
92541	Spontaneous nystagmus test, including gaze and fixation nystagmus, with recording

CPT NOTES

- Diagnostic or treatment procedures usually included in a comprehensive otorhinolaryngologic evaluation or office visit, are reported as an integrated medical service, using appropriate descriptors from the 99201 series. Itemization of component procedures (e.g., otoscopy, rhinoscopy, tuning fork test) does not apply.

  Special otorhinolaryngologic services are those diagnostic and treatment services not usually included in a comprehensive otorhinolaryngologic evaluation or office visit. These services are reported separately, using descriptors from the 92500 series.

  All services include medical diagnostic evaluation. Technical procedures (which may or may not be performed by the physician personally) are often part of the service, but should not be mistaken to constitute the service itself.
- For laryngoscopy with stroboscopy, use 31579.
- For unlisted vestibular tests, see 92599.

ICD–9–CM

225.0	B-Neoplasm, Brain
382.2	Chronic atticoantral suppurative OM
386.00	Meniere's disease NOS
386.01	Meniere's disease cochleovestibular
386.10	Peripheral vertigo NOS
386.11	Benign paroxysmal position vertigo
386.12	Vestibular neuronitis
386.2	Central origin vertigo
386.30	Labyrinthitis NOS
386.40	Labyrinthine fistula NOS
386.50	Labyrinthine dysfunction NOS
386.9	Vertiginous syndromes NOS
388.10	Noise effects on inner ear NOS
388.30	Tinnitus NOS
388.31	Subjective tinnitus
388.5	Acoustic nerve disorders
389.10	Sensorineural hearing loss NOS
389.2	Mixed hearing loss
389.8	Hearing loss NEC
780.4	Dizziness and giddiness

REIMBURSEMENT INFORMATION

Medicare

- Follow–up Days — global concept does not apply
- Assistant Surgeon — by report
- Supply Charges — not allowed
- Outpatient Limit — does not apply

CPT CODE **SERVICE**

92542 Positional nystagmus test, minimum of 4 positions, with recording

CPT NOTES

- Diagnostic or treatment procedures usually included in a comprehensive otorhinolaryngologic evaluation or office visit, are reported as an integrated medical service, using appropriate descriptors from the 99201 series. Itemization of component procedures (e.g., otoscopy, rhinoscopy, tuning fork test) does not apply.

  Special otorhinolaryngologic services are those diagnostic and treatment services not usually included in a comprehensive otorhinolaryngologic evaluation or office visit. These services are reported separately, using descriptors from the 92500 series.

  All services include medical diagnostic evaluation. Technical procedures (which may or may not be performed by the physician personally) are often part of the service, but should not be mistaken to constitute the service itself.
- For laryngoscopy with stroboscopy, use 31579.
- For unlisted vestibular tests, see 92599.

ICD–9–CM

225.0	B-Neoplasm, Brain
386.00	Meniere's disease NOS
386.01	Meniere's disease cochleovestibular
386.10	Peripheral vertigo NOS
386.11	Benign paroxysmal position vertigo
386.12	Vestibular neuronitis
386.2	Central origin vertigo
386.30	Labyrinthitis NOS
386.31	Serous labyrinthitis
386.40	Labyrinthine fistula NOS
386.50	Labyrinthine dysfunction NOS
386.9	Vertiginous syndromes NOS
388.30	Tinnitus NOS
388.31	Subjective tinnitus
388.5	Acoustic nerve disorders
389.10	Sensorineural hearing loss NOS
389.14	Central hearing loss
389.8	Hearing loss NEC
780.4	Dizziness and giddiness

REIMBURSEMENT INFORMATION

Medicare

- Follow–up Days — global concept does not apply
- Assistant Surgeon — by report
- Supply Charges — not allowed
- Outpatient Limit — does not apply

CPT CODE	SERVICE
92543	Caloric vestibular test, each irrigation (binaural, bithermal stimulation constitutes four tests), with recording

CPT NOTES

- Diagnostic or treatment procedures usually included in a comprehensive otorhinolaryngologic evaluation or office visit, are reported as an integrated medical service, using appropriate descriptors from the 99201 series. Itemization of component procedures (e.g., otoscopy, rhinoscopy, tuning fork test) does not apply.

  Special otorhinolaryngologic services are those diagnostic and treatment services not usually included in a comprehensive otorhinolaryngologic evaluation or office visit. These services are reported separately, using descriptors from the 92500 series.

  All services include medical diagnostic evaluation. Technical procedures (which may or may not be performed by the physician personally) are often part of the service, but should not be mistaken to constitute the service itself.
- For laryngoscopy with stroboscopy, use 31579.
- For unlisted vestibular tests, see 92599.

ICD–9–CM

225.0	Benign neoplasm, brain
386.00	Meniere's disease NOS
386.01	Meniere's disease cochleovestibular
386.10	Peripheral vertigo NOS
386.11	Benign paroxysmal position vertigo
386.12	Vestibular neuronitis
386.2	Central origin vertigo
386.30	Labyrinthitis NOS
386.40	Labyrinthine fistula NOS
386.50	Labyrinthine dysfunction NOS
386.9	Vertiginous syndromes NOS
388.30	Tinnitus NOS
388.31	Subjective tinnitus
388.5	Acoustic nerve disorders
389.10	Sensorineural hearing loss NOS
389.14	Central hearing loss
389.8	Hearing loss NEC
780.4	Dizziness and giddiness

REIMBURSEMENT INFORMATION

Medicare

- Follow–up Days — global concept does not apply
- Assistant Surgeon — by report
- Supply Charges — not allowed
- Outpatient Limit — does not apply

92544	Optokinetic nystagmus test, bidirectional, foveal or peripheral stimulation, with recording

CPT NOTES

- Diagnostic or treatment procedures usually included in a comprehensive otorhinolaryngologic evaluation or office visit, are reported as an integrated medical service, using appropriate descriptors from the 99201 series. Itemization of component procedures (e.g., otoscopy, rhinoscopy, tuning fork test) does not apply.

  Special otorhinolaryngologic services are those diagnostic and treatment services not usually included in a comprehensive otorhinolaryngologic evaluation or office visit. These services are reported separately, using descriptors from the 92500 series.

  All services include medical diagnostic evaluation. Technical procedures (which may or may not be performed by the physician personally) are often part of the service, but should not be mistaken to constitute the service itself.
- For laryngoscopy with stroboscopy, use 31579.
- For unlisted vestibular tests, see 92599.

386.00	Meniere's disease NOS
386.01	Meniere's disease cochleovestibular
386.10	Peripheral vertigo NOS
386.11	Benign paroxysmal position vertigo
386.12	Vestibular neuronitis
386.2	Central origin vertigo
386.30	Labyrinthitis NOS
386.40	Labyrinthine fistula NOS
386.50	Labyrinthine dysfunction NOS
386.9	Vertiginous syndromes NOS
388.30	Tinnitus NOS
388.5	Acoustic nerve disorders
389.10	Sensorineural hearing loss NOS
389.14	Central hearing loss
389.2	Mixed hearing loss
389.8	Hearing loss NEC
780.4	Dizziness and giddiness

REIMBURSEMENT INFORMATION

Medicare

- Follow–up Days — global concept does not apply
- Assistant Surgeon — by report
- Supply Charges — not allowed
- Outpatient Limit — does not apply

CPT CODE	SERVICE	ICD–9–CM

92545 Oscillating tracking test, with recording

CPT NOTES

- Diagnostic or treatment procedures usually included in a comprehensive otorhinolaryngologic evaluation or office visit, are reported as an integrated medical service, using appropriate descriptors from the 99201 series. Itemization of component procedures (e.g., otoscopy, rhinoscopy, tuning fork test) does not apply.

  Special otorhinolaryngologic services are those diagnostic and treatment services not usually included in a comprehensive otorhinolaryngologic evaluation or office visit. These services are reported separately, using descriptors from the 92500 series.

  All services include medical diagnostic evaluation. Technical procedures (which may or may not be performed by the physician personally) are often part of the service, but should not be mistaken to constitute the service itself.
- For laryngoscopy with stroboscopy, use 31579.
- For unlisted vestibular tests, see 92599.

ICD–9–CM

386.00 Meniere's disease NOS
386.01 Meniere's disease cochleovestibular
386.10 Peripheral vertigo NOS
386.11 Benign paroxysmal position vertigo
386.12 Vestibular neuronitis
386.2 Central origin vertigo
386.30 Labyrinthitis NOS
386.40 Labyrinthine fistula NOS
386.50 Labyrinthine dysfunction NOS
386.9 Vertiginous syndromes NOS
388.30 Tinnitus NOS
388.5 Acoustic nerve disorders
389.10 Sensorineural hearing loss NOS
389.14 Central hearing loss
389.2 Mixed hearing loss
780.4 Dizziness and giddiness

REIMBURSEMENT INFORMATION

Medicare

- Follow–up Days — global concept does not apply
- Assistant Surgeon — by report
- Supply Charges — not allowed
- Outpatient Limit — does not apply

92546 Torsion swing test, with recording

CPT NOTES

- Diagnostic or treatment procedures usually included in a comprehensive otorhinolaryngologic evaluation or office visit, are reported as an integrated medical service, using appropriate descriptors from the 99201 series. Itemization of component procedures (e.g., otoscopy, rhinoscopy, tuning fork test) does not apply.

  Special otorhinolaryngologic services are those diagnostic and treatment services not usually included in a comprehensive otorhinolaryngologic evaluation or office visit. These services are reported separately, using descriptors from the 92500 series.

  All services include medical diagnostic evaluation. Technical procedures (which may or may not be performed by the physician personally) are often part of the service, but should not be mistaken to constitute the service itself.
- For laryngoscopy with stroboscopy, use 31579.
- For unlisted vestibular tests, see 92599.

387.0 Otosclerosis, oval window, nonoblit
388.30 Tinnitus NOS
780.4 Dizziness and giddiness

REIMBURSEMENT INFORMATION

Medicare

- Follow–up Days — global concept does not apply
- Assistant Surgeon — by report
- Supply Charges — not allowed
- Outpatient Limit — does not apply

CPT CODE	SERVICE
92547	Use of vertical electrodes in any or all of above tests counts as one additional test

CPT NOTES

- Diagnostic or treatment procedures usually included in a comprehensive otorhinolaryngologic evaluation or office visit, are reported as an integrated medical service, using appropriate descriptors from the 99201 series. Itemization of component procedures (e.g., otoscopy, rhinoscopy, tuning fork test) does not apply.

  Special otorhinolaryngologic services are those diagnostic and treatment services not usually included in a comprehensive otorhinolaryngologic evaluation or office visit. These services are reported separately, using descriptors from the 92500 series.

  All services include medical diagnostic evaluation. Technical procedures (which may or may not be performed by the physician personally) are often part of the service, but should not be mistaken to constitute the service itself.
- For laryngoscopy with stroboscopy, use 31579.
- For unlisted vestibular tests, see 92599.

ICD–9–CM

386.01	Meniere's disease cochleovestibular
386.10	Peripheral vertigo NOS
386.11	Benign paroxysmal position vertigo
386.12	Vestibular neuronitis
386.2	Central origin vertigo
386.40	Labyrinthine fistula NOS
386.50	Labyrinthine dysfunction NOS
386.9	Vertiginous syndromes NOS
388.30	Tinnitus NOS
388.5	Acoustic nerve disorders
389.2	Mixed hearing loss
780.4	Dizziness and giddiness

REIMBURSEMENT INFORMATION

Medicare

- Follow–up Days — global concept does not apply
- Assistant Surgeon — by report
- Supply Charges — not allowed
- Outpatient Limit — does not apply

CPT CODE **SERVICE**

92551 Screening test, pure tone, air only

CPT NOTES

- Diagnostic or treatment procedures usually included in a comprehensive otorhinolaryngologic evaluation or office visit, are reported as an integrated medical service, using appropriate descriptors from the 99201 series. Itemization of component procedures (e.g., otoscopy, rhinoscopy, tuning fork test) does not apply.

  Special otorhinolaryngologic services are those diagnostic and treatment services not usually included in a comprehensive otorhinolaryngologic evaluation or office visit. These services are reported separately, using descriptors from the 92500 series.

  All services include medical diagnostic evaluation. Technical procedures (which may or may not be performed by the physician personally) are often part of the service, but should not be mistaken to constitute the service itself.
- For laryngoscopy with stroboscopy, use 31579.
- For evaluation of speech, language and/or hearing problems through observation and assessment of performance, see 92506.
- This audiometric test implies the use of calibrated electronic equipment. Other hearing tests (such as whispered voice, tuning fork) are considered part of the general otorhinolaryngologic services and are not reported separately. All descriptors refer to testing both ears. Use the modifier '–52' or 09952, if a test is applied to one ear instead of to two ears. All descriptors (except 92559), apply to testing of individuals; for testing of groups, use 92559 and specify test(s) used.

ICD–9–CM

381.00	Acute nonsup otitis media NOS
381.05	Acute allergic mucoid otitis media
381.06	Ac allergic sanguinous otitis media
381.3	Chronic nonsuppurative otitis media
381.4	Chron nonsup otitis media NOS
381.60	Obstruction of Eustachian tube NOS
385.23	Dislocation of ear ossicles
386.00	Meniere's disease NOS
386.30	Labyrinthitis NOS
388.01	Presbyacusis
388.2	Sudden hearing loss NOS
388.30	Tinnitus NOS
388.40	Abnormal auditory perception NOS
388.70	Otalgia NOS
389.00	Conductive hearing loss NOS
389.10	Sensorineural hearing loss NOS
389.11	Sensory hearing loss
389.12	Neural hearing loss
389.14	Central hearing loss
389.8	Hearing loss NEC
389.9	Hearing loss NOS
784.5	Speech disturbance NEC
V72.1	Examination of ears/hearing

REIMBURSEMENT INFORMATION

Medicare

- Follow–up Days — global concept does not apply
- Assistant Surgeon — not paid
- Supply Charges — not allowed
- Outpatient Limit — does not apply

CPT CODE	SERVICE
92552	Pure tone audiometry (threshold); air only

CPT NOTES

- Diagnostic or treatment procedures usually included in a comprehensive otorhinolaryngologic evaluation or office visit, are reported as an integrated medical service, using appropriate descriptors from the 99201 series. Itemization of component procedures (e.g., otoscopy, rhinoscopy, tuning fork test) does not apply.

  Special otorhinolaryngologic services are those diagnostic and treatment services not usually included in a comprehensive otorhinolaryngologic evaluation or office visit. These services are reported separately, using descriptors from the 92500 series.

  All services include medical diagnostic evaluation. Technical procedures (which may or may not be performed by the physician personally) are often part of the service, but should not be mistaken to constitute the service itself.
- For laryngoscopy with stroboscopy, use 31579.
- For evaluation of speech, language and/or hearing problems through observation and assessment of performance, see 92506.
- This audiometric test implies the use of calibrated electronic equipment. Other hearing tests (such as whispered voice, tuning fork) are considered part of the general otorhinolaryngologic services and are not reported separately. All descriptors refer to testing both ears. Use the modifier '–52' or 09952, if a test is applied to one ear instead of to two ears. All descriptors (except 92559), apply to testing of individuals; for testing of groups, use 92559 and specify test(s) used.

ICD–9–CM

112.82	Candidal otitis externa
315.31	Developmental language disorder
380.32	Acquired deformity auricle/pinna
380.50	Acquired stenosis ear canal NOS
381.04	Acute allergic serous otitis media
381.4	Chron nonsup otitis media NOS
381.81	Dysfunction of Eustachian tube
382.3	Chronic suppurativ otitis media NOS
383.1	Chronic mastoiditis
384.00	Acute myringitis NOS
384.01	Bullous myringitis
384.20	Perforation tympanic membrane NOS
384.21	Cent perforate tympanic membrane
384.82	Atrophic nonflaccid tymp membrane
385.82	Cholesterin granuloma
386.00	Meniere's disease NOS
386.10	Peripheral vertigo NOS
386.12	Vestibular neuronitis
386.19	Peripheral vertigo NEC
387.0	Otosclerosis, oval window, nonoblit
387.9	Otosclerosis NOS
388.32	Objective tinnitus
388.42	Hyperacusis
388.69	Otorrhea NEC
388.70	Otalgia NOS
388.71	Otogenic pain
388.9	Ear disorder NOS
389.00	Conductive hearing loss NOS
389.01	Conductive hearing loss, extern ear
389.02	Conductive hearing loss, tympanic
389.03	Conductive hearing loss, middle ear
389.04	Conductive hearing loss, inner ear
389.08	Conductive hearing loss, comb type
389.10	Sensorineural hearing loss NOS
389.11	Sensory hearing loss
389.12	Neural hearing loss
389.14	Central hearing loss
389.18	Sensorineural hear loss comb type
389.2	Mixed hearing loss
389.8	Hearing loss NEC
389.9	Hearing loss NOS
744.02	Ext ear anomaly NEC, hearing impair
744.47	Preauricular cyst
872.61	Open wound of eardrum
951.5	Injury to acoustic nerve
V41.2	Problems with hearing
V72.1	Examination of ears/hearing

REIMBURSEMENT INFORMATION

Medicare

- Follow–up Days — global concept does not apply
- Assistant Surgeon — by report
- Supply Charges — not allowed
- Outpatient Limit — does not apply
- Major Surgery Rules Apply

CPT CODE	SERVICE
92553	Pure tone audiometry (threshold); air and bone

CPT NOTES

- Diagnostic or treatment procedures usually included in a comprehensive otorhinolaryngologic evaluation or office visit, are reported as an integrated medical service, using appropriate descriptors from the 99201 series. Itemization of component procedures (e.g., otoscopy, rhinoscopy, tuning fork test) does not apply.

  Special otorhinolaryngologic services are those diagnostic and treatment services not usually included in a comprehensive otorhinolaryngologic evaluation or office visit. These services are reported separately, using descriptors from the 92500 series.

  All services include medical diagnostic evaluation. Technical procedures (which may or may not be performed by the physician personally) are often part of the service, but should not be mistaken to constitute the service itself.
- For laryngoscopy with stroboscopy, use 31579.
- For evaluation of speech, language and/or hearing problems through observation and assessment of performance, see 92506.
- This audiometric test implies the use of calibrated electronic equipment. Other hearing tests (such as whispered voice, tuning fork) are considered part of the general otorhinolaryngologic services and are not reported separately. All descriptors refer to testing both ears. Use the modifier '–52' or 09952, if a test is applied to one ear instead of to two ears. All descriptors (except 92559), apply to testing of individuals; for testing of groups, use 92559 and specify test(s) used.

ICD–9–CM

112.82	Candidal otitis externa
380.21	Cholesteatoma of external ear
381.00	Acute nonsup otitis media NOS
381.01	Acute serous otitis media
381.02	Acute mucoid otitis media
381.03	Acute sanguinous otitis media
381.04	Acute allergic serous otitis media
381.05	Acute allergic mucoid otitis media
381.06	Ac allergic sanguinous otitis media
381.10	Chron serous otitis media simp/NOS
381.20	Chron mucoid otitis media simp/NOS
381.81	Dysfunction of Eustachian tube
381.9	Eustachian tube disorder NOS
382.3	Chronic suppurativ otitis media NOS
383.01	Subperiosteal mastoid abscess
383.1	Chronic mastoiditis
384.00	Acute myringitis NOS
384.01	Bullous myringitis
384.20	Perforation tympanic membrane NOS
384.21	Cent perforate tympanic membrane
384.82	Atrophic nonflaccid tymp membrane
385.3x	Cholesteatoma
386.00	Meniere's disease NOS
386.35	Viral labyrinthitis
386.42	Labyrinthine, oval window fistula
387.0	Otosclerosis, oval window, nonoblit
387.9	Otosclerosis NOS
388.10	Noise effects on inner ear NOS
388.12	Noise-induced hearing loss
388.2	Sudden hearing loss NOS
388.30	Tinnitus NOS
388.31	Subjective tinnitus
388.32	Objective tinnitus
388.60	Otorrhea NOS
389.00	Conductive hearing loss NOS
389.03	Conductive hearing loss, middle ear
389.08	Conductive hearing loss, comb type
389.10	Sensorineural hearing loss NOS
389.11	Sensory hearing loss
389.12	Neural hearing loss
389.18	Sensorineural hear loss comb type
389.2	Mixed hearing loss
744.02	Ext ear anomaly NEC, hearing impair
852.40	Traumatic extradural hemorrhage
872.11	Open wound of auricle, complicated
872.61	Open wound of eardrum
951.5	Injury to acoustic nerve
V72.1	Examination of ears/hearing

REIMBURSEMENT INFORMATION

Medicare

- Follow–up Days — global concept does not apply
- Assistant Surgeon — by report
- Supply Charges — not allowed
- Outpatient Limit — does not apply

CPT CODE	SERVICE
92555	Speech audiometry; threshold only

CPT NOTES

- Diagnostic or treatment procedures usually included in a comprehensive otorhinolaryngologic evaluation or office visit, are reported as an integrated medical service, using appropriate descriptors from the 99201 series. Itemization of component procedures (e.g., otoscopy, rhinoscopy, tuning fork test) does not apply.

  Special otorhinolaryngologic services are those diagnostic and treatment services not usually included in a comprehensive otorhinolaryngologic evaluation or office visit. These services are reported separately, using descriptors from the 92500 series.

  All services include medical diagnostic evaluation. Technical procedures (which may or may not be performed by the physician personally) are often part of the service, but should not be mistaken to constitute the service itself.
- For laryngoscopy with stroboscopy, use 31579.
- For evaluation of speech, language and/or hearing problems through observation and assessment of performance, see 92506.
- This audiometric test implies the use of calibrated electronic equipment. Other hearing tests (such as whispered voice, tuning fork) are considered part of the general otorhinolaryngologic services and are not reported separately. All descriptors refer to testing both ears. Use the modifier '–52' or 09952, if a test is applied to one ear instead of to two ears. All descriptors (except 92559), apply to testing of individuals; for testing of groups, use 92559 and specify test(s) used.

ICD–9–CM

380.10	Infective otitis externa NOS
381.00	Acute nonsup otitis media NOS
381.01	Acute serous otitis media
381.04	Acute allergic serous otitis media
381.10	Chron serous otitis media simp/NOS
381.3	Chronic nonsuppurative otitis media
381.4	Chron nonsup otitis media NOS
381.81	Dysfunction of Eustachian tube
382.3	Chronic suppurativ otitis media NOS
382.4	Suppurative otitis media NOS
384.00	Acute myringitis NOS
384.20	Perforation tympanic membrane NOS
384.21	Cent perforate tympanic membrane
384.82	Atrophic nonflaccid tymp membrane
385.10	Adhesive middle ear disease NOS
385.30	Cholesteatoma NOS
386.00	Meniere's disease NOS
386.10	Peripheral vertigo NOS
386.11	Benign paroxysmal position vertigo
386.12	Vestibular neuronitis
386.42	Labyrinthine, oval window fistula
387.9	Otosclerosis NOS
388.31	Subjective tinnitus
388.70	Otalgia NOS
388.71	Otogenic pain
389.00	Conductive hearing loss NOS
389.10	Sensorineural hearing loss NOS
389.2	Mixed hearing loss
389.8	Hearing loss NEC
744.02	Ext ear anomaly NEC, hearing impair
744.47	Preauricular cyst
852.40	Traumatic extradural hemorrhage
951.5	Injury to acoustic nerve
V41.2	Problems with hearing
V72.1	Examination of ears/hearing

REIMBURSEMENT INFORMATION

Medicare

- Follow–up Days — global concept does not apply
- Assistant Surgeon — by report
- Supply Charges — not allowed
- Outpatient Limit — does not apply

CPT CODE **SERVICE**

92556 Speech audiometry; threshold and discrimination

CPT NOTES

- Diagnostic or treatment procedures usually included in a comprehensive otorhinolaryngologic evaluation or office visit, are reported as an integrated medical service, using appropriate descriptors from the 99201 series. Itemization of component procedures (e.g., otoscopy, rhinoscopy, tuning fork test) does not apply.

  Special otorhinolaryngologic services are those diagnostic and treatment services not usually included in a comprehensive otorhinolaryngologic evaluation or office visit. These services are reported separately, using descriptors from the 92500 series.

  All services include medical diagnostic evaluation. Technical procedures (which may or may not be performed by the physician personally) are often part of the service, but should not be mistaken to constitute the service itself.
- For laryngoscopy with stroboscopy, use 31579.
- For evaluation of speech, language and/or hearing problems through observation and assessment of performance, see 92506.
- This audiometric test implies the use of calibrated electronic equipment. Other hearing tests (such as whispered voice, tuning fork) are considered part of the general otorhinolaryngologic services and are not reported separately. All descriptors refer to testing both ears. Use the modifier '–52' or 09952, if a test is applied to one ear instead of to two ears. All descriptors (except 92559), apply to testing of individuals; for testing of groups, use 92559 and specify test(s) used.

ICD–9–CM

053.71	Otitis externa d/t herpes zoster
112.82	Candidal otitis externa
380.15	Chronic mycotic otitis externa
380.22	Acute otitis externa NEC
380.4	Impacted cerumen
381.04	Acute allergic serous otitis media
381.10	Chron serous otitis media simp/NOS
381.81	Dysfunction of Eustachian tube
381.9	Eustachian tube disorder NOS
382.3	Chronic suppurativ otitis media NOS
383.1	Chronic mastoiditis
383.9	Mastoiditis NOS
384.01	Bullous myringitis
384.20	Perforation tympanic membrane NOS
384.82	Atrophic nonflaccid tymp membrane
385.30	Cholesteatoma NOS
385.33	Cholesteatoma, middle ear/mastoid
386.00	Meniere's disease NOS
386.11	Benign paroxysmal position vertigo
386.19	Peripheral vertigo NEC
387.0	Otosclerosis, oval window, nonoblit
387.9	Otosclerosis NOS
388.10	Noise effects on inner ear NOS
388.2	Sudden hearing loss NOS
388.30	Tinnitus NOS
388.31	Subjective tinnitus
388.60	Otorrhea NOS
388.70	Otalgia NOS
389.00	Conductive hearing loss NOS
389.10	Sensorineural hearing loss NOS
389.11	Sensory hearing loss
389.12	Neural hearing loss
389.18	Sensorineural hear loss comb type
389.2	Mixed hearing loss
389.8	Hearing loss NEC
V41.2	Problems with hearing
V72.1	Examination of ears/hearing

REIMBURSEMENT INFORMATION

Medicare

- Follow–up Days — global concept does not apply
- Assistant Surgeon — by report
- Supply Charges — not allowed
- Outpatient Limit — does not apply

CPT CODE	SERVICE
92557	Basic comprehensive audiometry (92553 and 92556 combined), (pure tone, air and bone, and speech, threshold and discrimination)

CPT NOTES

- Diagnostic or treatment procedures usually included in a comprehensive otorhinolaryngologic evaluation or office visit, are reported as an integrated medical service, using appropriate descriptors from the 99201 series. Itemization of component procedures (e.g., otoscopy, rhinoscopy, tuning fork test) does not apply.

  Special otorhinolaryngologic services are those diagnostic and treatment services not usually included in a comprehensive otorhinolaryngologic evaluation or office visit. These services are reported separately, using descriptors from the 92500 series.

  All services include medical diagnostic evaluation. Technical procedures (which may or may not be performed by the physician personally) are often part of the service, but should not be mistaken to constitute the service itself.
- For laryngoscopy with stroboscopy, use 31579.
- For evaluation of speech, language and/or hearing problems through observation and assessment of performance, see 92506.
- This audiometric test implies the use of calibrated electronic equipment. Other hearing tests (such as whispered voice, tuning fork) are considered part of the general otorhinolaryngologic services and are not reported separately. All descriptors refer to testing both ears. Use the modifier '–52' or 09952, if a test is applied to one ear instead of to two ears. All descriptors (except 92559), apply to testing of individuals; for testing of groups, use 92559 and specify test(s) used.
- For hearing aid evaluation and selection, see 92590–92595.

ICD–9–CM

380.22	Acute otitis externa NEC
381.01	Acute serous otitis media
381.19	Chronic serous otitis media NEC
383.1	Chronic mastoiditis
384.20	Perforation tympanic membrane NOS
384.23	Marginal perf tympanic membrane NEC
384.82	Atrophic nonflaccid tymp membrane
384.9	Tympanic membrane disorder NOS
385.10	Adhesive middle ear disease NOS
385.30	Cholesteatoma NOS
385.32	Cholesteatoma of middle ear
385.89	Middle Ear/Mastoid disorder NEC
386.01	Meniere's disease cochleovestibular
386.11	Benign paroxysmal position vertigo
386.19	Peripheral vertigo NEC
386.40	Labyrinthine fistula NOS
386.42	Labyrinthine, oval window fistula
386.50	Labyrinthine dysfunction NOS
386.9	Vertiginous syndromes NOS
387.2	Cochlear otosclerosis
388.01	Presbyacusis
388.12	Noise-induced hearing loss
388.2	Sudden hearing loss NOS
388.30	Tinnitus NOS
388.32	Objective tinnitus
388.40	Abnormal auditory perception NOS
388.42	Hyperacusis
388.43	Impairment auditory discrimination
388.5	Acoustic nerve disorders
388.69	Otorrhea NEC
388.9	Ear disorder NOS
389.00	Conductive hearing loss NOS
389.03	Conductive hearing loss, middle ear
389.10	Sensorineural hearing loss NOS
389.11	Sensory hearing loss
389.12	Neural hearing loss
389.18	Sensorineural hear loss comb type
389.2	Mixed hearing loss
389.8	Hearing loss NEC
389.9	Hearing loss NOS
872.11	Open wound of auricle, complicated
872.61	Open wound of eardrum
V72.1	Examination of ears/hearing

REIMBURSEMENT INFORMATION

Medicare

- Follow–up Days — global concept does not apply
- Assistant Surgeon — by report
- Supply Charges — not allowed
- Outpatient Limit — does not apply
- Fragments — 69210, 92552, 92553, 92556

CPT CODE **SERVICE**

92559 Audiometric testing of groups

CPT NOTES

- Diagnostic or treatment procedures usually included in a comprehensive otorhinolaryngologic evaluation or office visit, are reported as an integrated medical service, using appropriate descriptors from the 99201 series. Itemization of component procedures (e.g., otoscopy, rhinoscopy, tuning fork test) does not apply.

  Special otorhinolaryngologic services are those diagnostic and treatment services not usually included in a comprehensive otorhinolaryngologic evaluation or office visit. These services are reported separately, using descriptors from the 92500 series.

  All services include medical diagnostic evaluation. Technical procedures (which may or may not be performed by the physician personally) are often part of the service, but should not be mistaken to constitute the service itself.
- For laryngoscopy with stroboscopy, use 31579.
- For evaluation of speech, language and/or hearing problems through observation and assessment of performance, see 92506.
- This audiometric test implies the use of calibrated electronic equipment. Other hearing tests (such as whispered voice, tuning fork) are considered part of the general otorhinolaryngologic services and are not reported separately. All descriptors refer to testing both ears. Use the modifier '–52' or 09952, if a test is applied to one ear instead of to two ears. All descriptors (except 92559), apply to testing of individuals; for testing of groups, use 92559 and specify test(s) used.

ICD–9–CM

V70.5 Subpopulation health examination
V70.6 Health exam in population survey
V72.1 Examination of ears/hearing

REIMBURSEMENT INFORMATION

Medicare

- Follow–up Days — global concept does not apply
- Assistant Surgeon — not paid
- Supply Charges — not allowed
- Outpatient Limit — does not apply

CPT CODE **SERVICE**

92560 Bekesy audiometry, screening

CPT NOTES

- Diagnostic or treatment procedures usually included in a comprehensive otorhinolaryngologic evaluation or office visit, are reported as an integrated medical service, using appropriate descriptors from the 99201 series. Itemization of component procedures (e.g., otoscopy, rhinoscopy, tuning fork test) does not apply.

  Special otorhinolaryngologic services are those diagnostic and treatment services not usually included in a comprehensive otorhinolaryngologic evaluation or office visit. These services are reported separately, using descriptors from the 92500 series.

  All services include medical diagnostic evaluation. Technical procedures (which may or may not be performed by the physician personally) are often part of the service, but should not be mistaken to constitute the service itself.
- For laryngoscopy with stroboscopy, use 31579.
- For evaluation of speech, language and/or hearing problems through observation and assessment of performance, see 92506.
- This audiometric test implies the use of calibrated electronic equipment. Other hearing tests (such as whispered voice, tuning fork) are considered part of the general otorhinolaryngologic services and are not reported separately. All descriptors refer to testing both ears. Use the modifier '–52' or 09952, if a test is applied to one ear instead of to two ears. All descriptors (except 92559), apply to testing of individuals; for testing of groups, use 92559 and specify test(s) used.

ICD–9–CM

225.0	B Neoplasm, Brain
382.9	Otitis media NOS
388.30	Tinnitus NOS
780.4	Dizziness and giddiness

REIMBURSEMENT INFORMATION

Medicare

- Follow–up Days — global concept does not apply
- Assistant Surgeon — not paid
- Supply Charges — not allowed
- Outpatient Limit — does not apply

CPT CODE **SERVICE**

92561 Bekesy audiometry; diagnostic

CPT NOTES

- Diagnostic or treatment procedures usually included in a comprehensive otorhinolaryngologic evaluation or office visit, are reported as an integrated medical service, using appropriate descriptors from the 99201 series. Itemization of component procedures (e.g., otoscopy, rhinoscopy, tuning fork test) does not apply.

  Special otorhinolaryngologic services are those diagnostic and treatment services not usually included in a comprehensive otorhinolaryngologic evaluation or office visit. These services are reported separately, using descriptors from the 92500 series.

  All services include medical diagnostic evaluation. Technical procedures (which may or may not be performed by the physician personally) are often part of the service, but should not be mistaken to constitute the service itself.
- For laryngoscopy with stroboscopy, use 31579.
- For evaluation of speech, language and/or hearing problems through observation and assessment of performance, see 92506.
- This audiometric test implies the use of calibrated electronic equipment. Other hearing tests (such as whispered voice, tuning fork) are considered part of the general otorhinolaryngologic services and are not reported separately. All descriptors refer to testing both ears. Use the modifier '–52' or 09952, if a test is applied to one ear instead of to two ears. All descriptors (except 92559), apply to testing of individuals; for testing of groups, use 92559 and specify test(s) used.

ICD–9–CM

047.9	Viral meningitis NOS
225.0	B-Neoplasm, Brain
315.39	Speech/language develop disord NEC
381.4	Chron nonsup otitis media NOS
381.81	Dysfunction of Eustachian tube
384.20	Perforation tympanic membrane NOS
389.00	Conductive hearing loss NOS
389.8	Hearing loss NEC
780.4	Dizziness and giddiness

REIMBURSEMENT INFORMATION

Medicare

- Follow–up Days — global concept does not apply
- Assistant Surgeon — by report
- Supply Charges — not allowed
- Outpatient Limit — does not apply

CPT CODE **SERVICE**

92562 Loudness balance test, alternate binaural or monaural

CPT NOTES

- Diagnostic or treatment procedures usually included in a comprehensive otorhinolaryngologic evaluation or office visit, are reported as an integrated medical service, using appropriate descriptors from the 99201 series. Itemization of component procedures (e.g., otoscopy, rhinoscopy, tuning fork test) does not apply.

  Special otorhinolaryngologic services are those diagnostic and treatment services not usually included in a comprehensive otorhinolaryngologic evaluation or office visit. These services are reported separately, using descriptors from the 92500 series.

  All services include medical diagnostic evaluation. Technical procedures (which may or may not be performed by the physician personally) are often part of the service, but should not be mistaken to constitute the service itself.
- For laryngoscopy with stroboscopy, use 31579.
- For evaluation of speech, language and/or hearing problems through observation and assessment of performance, see 92506.
- This audiometric test implies the use of calibrated electronic equipment. Other hearing tests (such as whispered voice, tuning fork) are considered part of the general otorhinolaryngologic services and are not reported separately. All descriptors refer to testing both ears. Use the modifier '–52' or 09952, if a test is applied to one ear instead of to two ears. All descriptors (except 92559), apply to testing of individuals; for testing of groups, use 92559 and specify test(s) used.

ICD–9–CM

389.9 Hearing loss NOS

REIMBURSEMENT INFORMATION

Medicare

- Follow–up Days — global concept does not apply
- Assistant Surgeon — by report
- Supply Charges — not allowed
- Outpatient Limit — does not apply

CPT CODE **SERVICE**

92563 Tone decay test

CPT NOTES

- Diagnostic or treatment procedures usually included in a comprehensive otorhinolaryngologic evaluation or office visit, are reported as an integrated medical service, using appropriate descriptors from the 99201 series. Itemization of component procedures (e.g., otoscopy, rhinoscopy, tuning fork test) does not apply.

  Special otorhinolaryngologic services are those diagnostic and treatment services not usually included in a comprehensive otorhinolaryngologic evaluation or office visit. These services are reported separately, using descriptors from the 92500 series.

  All services include medical diagnostic evaluation. Technical procedures (which may or may not be performed by the physician personally) are often part of the service, but should not be mistaken to constitute the service itself.
- For laryngoscopy with stroboscopy, use 31579.
- For evaluation of speech, language and/or hearing problems through observation and assessment of performance, see 92506.
- This audiometric test implies the use of calibrated electronic equipment. Other hearing tests (such as whispered voice, tuning fork) are considered part of the general otorhinolaryngologic services and are not reported separately. All descriptors refer to testing both ears. Use the modifier '–52' or 09952, if a test is applied to one ear instead of to two ears. All descriptors (except 92559), apply to testing of individuals; for testing of groups, use 92559 and specify test(s) used.

ICD–9–CM

389.8 Hearing loss NEC

REIMBURSEMENT INFORMATION

Medicare

- Follow–up Days — global concept does not apply
- Assistant Surgeon — by report
- Supply Charges — not allowed
- Outpatient Limit — does not apply

CPT CODE	SERVICE	ICD–9–CM
92564	Short increment sensitivity index (SISI)	389.9 Hearing loss NOS

CPT NOTES

- Diagnostic or treatment procedures usually included in a comprehensive otorhinolaryngologic evaluation or office visit, are reported as an integrated medical service, using appropriate descriptors from the 99201 series. Itemization of component procedures (e.g., otoscopy, rhinoscopy, tuning fork test) does not apply.

  Special otorhinolaryngologic services are those diagnostic and treatment services not usually included in a comprehensive otorhinolaryngologic evaluation or office visit. These services are reported separately, using descriptors from the 92500 series.

  All services include medical diagnostic evaluation. Technical procedures (which may or may not be performed by the physician personally) are often part of the service, but should not be mistaken to constitute the service itself.
- For laryngoscopy with stroboscopy, use 31579.
- For evaluation of speech, language and/or hearing problems through observation and assessment of performance, see 92506.
- This audiometric test implies the use of calibrated electronic equipment. Other hearing tests (such as whispered voice, tuning fork) are considered part of the general otorhinolaryngologic services and are not reported separately. All descriptors refer to testing both ears. Use the modifier '–52' or 09952, if a test is applied to one ear instead of to two ears. All descriptors (except 92559), apply to testing of individuals; for testing of groups, use 92559 and specify test(s) used.

REIMBURSEMENT INFORMATION

Medicare

- Follow–up Days — global concept does not apply
- Assistant Surgeon — by report
- Supply Charges — not allowed
- Outpatient Limit — does not apply

CPT CODE **SERVICE**

92565 Stenger test, pure tone

CPT NOTES

- Diagnostic or treatment procedures usually included in a comprehensive otorhinolaryngologic evaluation or office visit, are reported as an integrated medical service, using appropriate descriptors from the 99201 series. Itemization of component procedures (e.g., otoscopy, rhinoscopy, tuning fork test) does not apply.

  Special otorhinolaryngologic services are those diagnostic and treatment services not usually included in a comprehensive otorhinolaryngologic evaluation or office visit. These services are reported separately, using descriptors from the 92500 series.

  All services include medical diagnostic evaluation. Technical procedures (which may or may not be performed by the physician personally) are often part of the service, but should not be mistaken to constitute the service itself.
- For laryngoscopy with stroboscopy, use 31579.
- For evaluation of speech, language and/or hearing problems through observation and assessment of performance, see 92506.
- This audiometric test implies the use of calibrated electronic equipment. Other hearing tests (such as whispered voice, tuning fork) are considered part of the general otorhinolaryngologic services and are not reported separately. All descriptors refer to testing both ears. Use the modifier '–52' or 09952, if a test is applied to one ear instead of to two ears. All descriptors (except 92559), apply to testing of individuals; for testing of groups, use 92559 and specify test(s) used.

ICD–9–CM

386.55 Loss labyrinthine reactivity unilat

REIMBURSEMENT INFORMATION

Medicare

- Follow–up Days — global concept does not apply
- Assistant Surgeon — by report
- Supply Charges — not allowed
- Outpatient Limit — does not apply

CPT CODE	SERVICE
[illegible]	Tympanometry (impedance testing)

CPT NOTES

- Diagnostic or treatment procedures usually included in a comprehensive otorhinolaryngologic evaluation or office visit, are reported as an integrated medical service, using appropriate descriptors from the 99201 series. Itemization of component procedures (e.g., otoscopy, rhinoscopy, tuning fork test) does not apply.

  Special otorhinolaryngologic services are those diagnostic and treatment services not usually included in a comprehensive otorhinolaryngologic evaluation or office visit. These services are reported separately, using descriptors from the 92500 series.

  All services include medical diagnostic evaluation. Technical procedures (which may or may not be performed by the physician personally) are often part of the service, but should not be mistaken to constitute the service itself.
- For laryngoscopy with stroboscopy, use 31579.
- For evaluation of speech, language and/or hearing problems through observation and assessment of performance, see 92506.
- This audiometric test implies the use of calibrated electronic equipment. Other hearing tests (such as whispered voice, tuning fork) are considered part of the general otorhinolaryngologic services and are not reported separately. All descriptors refer to testing both ears. Use the modifier '–52' or 09952, if a test is applied to one ear instead of to two ears. All descriptors (except 92559), apply to testing of individuals; for testing of groups, use 92559 and specify test(s) used.

ICD–9–CM

[illegible]	Speech/language develop disorder NEC
380.32	Acquired deformity auricle/pinna
380.50	Acquired stenosis ear canal NOS
381.0x	Acute otitis media
381.10	Chron serous otitis media simp/NOS
381.19	Chronic serous otitis media NEC
381.3	Chronic nonsuppurative otitis media
381.4	Chron nonsup otitis media NOS
381.81	Dysfunction of Eustachian tube
381.9	Eustachian tube disorder NOS
382.00	Acute suppurative otitis media NOS
382.3	Chronic suppurativ otitis media NOS
384.0x	Acute myringitis
384.1	Chronic myringitis
384.82	Atrophic nonflaccid tymp membrane
384.9	Tympanic membrane disorder NOS
385.10	Adhesive middle ear disease NOS
385.2x	Other acquired abnormality ossicles
385.30	Cholesteatoma NOS
385.89	Middle Ear/Mastoid disorder NEC
387.9	Otosclerosis NOS
388.01	Presbyacusis
388.1x	Noise effects on inner ear
388.3x	Tinnitus
388.42	Hyperacusis
388.43	Impairment auditory discrimination
388.60	Otorrhea NOS
388.69	Otorrhea NEC
388.7x	Otalgia
389.08	Conductive hearing loss, comb type
389.10	Sensorineural hearing loss NOS
389.11	Sensory hearing loss
389.12	Neural hearing loss
389.18	Sensorineural hear loss comb type
389.2	Mixed hearing loss
744.02	Ext ear anomaly NEC, hearing impair
852.40	Traumatic extradural hemorrhage
951.5	Injury to acoustic nerve
V41.2	Problems with hearing
V72.1	Examination of ears/hearing

REIMBURSEMENT INFORMATION

Medicare

- Follow–up Days — global concept does not apply
- Assistant Surgeon — by report
- Supply Charges — not allowed
- Outpatient Limit — does not apply

CPT CODE **SERVICE**

92568 Acoustic reflex testing

CPT NOTES

- Diagnostic or treatment procedures usually included in a comprehensive otorhinolaryngologic evaluation or office visit, are reported as an integrated medical service, using appropriate descriptors from the 99201 series. Itemization of component procedures (e.g., otoscopy, rhinoscopy, tuning fork test) does not apply.

  Special otorhinolaryngologic services are those diagnostic and treatment services not usually included in a comprehensive otorhinolaryngologic evaluation or office visit. These services are reported separately, using descriptors from the 92500 series.

  All services include medical diagnostic evaluation. Technical procedures (which may or may not be performed by the physician personally) are often part of the service, but should not be mistaken to constitute the service itself.
- For laryngoscopy with stroboscopy, use 31579.
- For evaluation of speech, language and/or hearing problems through observation and assessment of performance, see 92506.
- This audiometric test implies the use of calibrated electronic equipment. Other hearing tests (such as whispered voice, tuning fork) are considered part of the general otorhinolaryngologic services and are not reported separately. All descriptors refer to testing both ears. Use the modifier '–52' or 09952, if a test is applied to one ear instead of to two ears. All descriptors (except 92559), apply to testing of individuals; for testing of groups, use 92559 and specify test(s) used.

ICD–9–CM

053.71	Otitis externa d/t herpes zoster
191.6	M-Neoplasm, Cerebellum NOS
225.0	B-Neoplasm, Brain
225.1	B-Neoplasm, Cranial nerve
315.39	Speech/language develop disord NEC
351.0	Bell's palsy
380.11	Acute infection of pinna
380.14	Malignant otitis externa
380.16	Chron infective otitis externa NEC
380.22	Acute otitis externa NEC
381.01	Acute serous otitis media
381.10	Chron serous otitis media simp/NOS
381.20	Chron mucoid otitis media simp/NOS
381.4	Chron nonsup otitis media NOS
381.81	Dysfunction of Eustachian tube
381.9	Eustachian tube disorder NOS
382.3	Chronic suppurativ otitis media NOS
384.20	Perforation tympanic membrane NOS
386.00	Meniere's disease NOS
386.01	Meniere's disease cochleovestibular
386.50	Labyrinthine dysfunction NOS
387.9	Otosclerosis NOS
388.01	Presbyacusis
388.1x	Noise effects on inner ear
388.30	Tinnitus NOS
388.31	Subjective tinnitus
388.42	Hyperacusis
388.70	Otalgia NOS
388.9	Ear disorder NOS
389.00	Conductive hearing loss NOS
389.08	Conductive hearing loss, comb type
389.1x	Sensorineural hearing loss
389.2	Mixed hearing loss
389.8	Hearing loss NEC
389.9	Hearing loss NOS
473.8	Chronic sinusitis NEC
767.5	Facial nerve injury at birth
V72.1	Examination of ears/hearing

REIMBURSEMENT INFORMATION

Medicare

- Follow–up Days — global concept does not apply
- Assistant Surgeon — by report
- Supply Charges — not allowed
- Outpatient Limit — does not apply

CPT CODE	SERVICE
92569	Acoustic reflex decay test

CPT NOTES

- Diagnostic or treatment procedures usually included in a comprehensive otorhinolaryngologic evaluation or office visit, are reported as an integrated medical service, using appropriate descriptors from the 99201 series. Itemization of component procedures (e.g., otoscopy, rhinoscopy, tuning fork test) does not apply.

  Special otorhinolaryngologic services are those diagnostic and treatment services not usually included in a comprehensive otorhinolaryngologic evaluation or office visit. These services are reported separately, using descriptors from the 92500 series.

  All services include medical diagnostic evaluation. Technical procedures (which may or may not be performed by the physician personally) are often part of the service, but should not be mistaken to constitute the service itself.
- For laryngoscopy with stroboscopy, use 31579.
- For evaluation of speech, language and/or hearing problems through observation and assessment of performance, see 92506.
- This audiometric test implies the use of calibrated electronic equipment. Other hearing tests (such as whispered voice, tuning fork) are considered part of the general otorhinolaryngologic services and are not reported separately. All descriptors refer to testing both ears. Use the modifier '–52' or 09952, if a test is applied to one ear instead of to two ears. All descriptors (except 92559), apply to testing of individuals; for testing of groups, use 92559 and specify test(s) used.

ICD–9–CM

053.71	Otitis externa d/t herpes zoster
225.1	B-Neoplasm, Cranial nerve
386.00	Meniere's disease NOS
386.11	Benign paroxysmal position vertigo
387.0	Otosclerosis, oval window, nonoblit
388.12	Noise-induced hearing loss
388.2	Sudden hearing loss NOS
388.30	Tinnitus NOS
388.31	Subjective tinnitus
388.42	Hyperacusis
388.70	Otalgia NOS
389.00	Conductive hearing loss NOS
389.10	Sensorineural hearing loss NOS
389.2	Mixed hearing loss
389.8	Hearing loss NEC
389.9	Hearing loss NOS
V72.1	Examination of ears/hearing

REIMBURSEMENT INFORMATION

Medicare

- Follow–up Days — global concept does not apply
- Assistant Surgeon — by report
- Supply Charges — not allowed
- Outpatient Limit — does not apply

CPT CODE **SERVICE**

92571 Filtered speech test

CPT NOTES

- Diagnostic or treatment procedures usually included in a comprehensive otorhinolaryngologic evaluation or office visit, are reported as an integrated medical service, using appropriate descriptors from the 99201 series. Itemization of component procedures (e.g., otoscopy, rhinoscopy, tuning fork test) does not apply.

  Special otorhinolaryngologic services are those diagnostic and treatment services not usually included in a comprehensive otorhinolaryngologic evaluation or office visit. These services are reported separately, using descriptors from the 92500 series.

  All services include medical diagnostic evaluation. Technical procedures (which may or may not be performed by the physician personally) are often part of the service, but should not be mistaken to constitute the service itself.
- For laryngoscopy with stroboscopy, use 31579.
- For evaluation of speech, language and/or hearing problems through observation and assessment of performance, see 92506.
- This audiometric test implies the use of calibrated electronic equipment. Other hearing tests (such as whispered voice, tuning fork) are considered part of the general otorhinolaryngologic services and are not reported separately. All descriptors refer to testing both ears. Use the modifier '–52' or 09952, if a test is applied to one ear instead of to two ears. All descriptors (except 92559), apply to testing of individuals; for testing of groups, use 92559 and specify test(s) used.

ICD–9–CM

053.71	Otitis externa d/t herpes zoster
112.82	Candidal otitis externa
225.1	B-Neoplasm, Cranial nerve
380.10	Infective otitis externa NOS
380.4	Impacted cerumen
381.10	Chron serous otitis media simp/NOS
381.4	Chron nonsup otitis media NOS
381.81	Dysfunction of Eustachian tube
382.3	Chronic suppurativ otitis media NOS
382.9	Otitis media NOS
384.20	Perforation tympanic membrane NOS
386.00	Meniere's disease NOS
386.11	Benign paroxysmal position vertigo
387.0	Otosclerosis, oval window, nonoblit
388.12	Noise-induced hearing loss
388.2	Sudden hearing loss NOS
388.30	Tinnitus NOS
388.31	Subjective tinnitus
388.42	Hyperacusis
388.70	Otalgia NOS
389.00	Conductive hearing loss NOS
389.10	Sensorineural hearing loss NOS
389.2	Mixed hearing loss
389.8	Hearing loss NEC
389.9	Hearing loss NOS
V72.1	Examination of ears/hearing

REIMBURSEMENT INFORMATION

Medicare

- Follow–up Days — global concept does not apply
- Assistant Surgeon — by report
- Supply Charges — not allowed
- Outpatient Limit — does not apply

CPT CODE **SERVICE**

92572 Staggered spondaic word test

CPT NOTES

- Diagnostic or treatment procedures usually included in a comprehensive otorhinolaryngologic evaluation or office visit, are reported as an integrated medical service, using appropriate descriptors from the 99201 series. Itemization of component procedures (e.g., otoscopy, rhinoscopy, tuning fork test) does not apply.

  Special otorhinolaryngologic services are those diagnostic and treatment services not usually included in a comprehensive otorhinolaryngologic evaluation or office visit. These services are reported separately, using descriptors from the 92500 series.

  All services include medical diagnostic evaluation. Technical procedures (which may or may not be performed by the physician personally) are often part of the service, but should not be mistaken to constitute the service itself.
- For laryngoscopy with stroboscopy, use 31579.
- For evaluation of speech, language and/or hearing problems through observation and assessment of performance, see 92506.
- This audiometric test implies the use of calibrated electronic equipment. Other hearing tests (such as whispered voice, tuning fork) are considered part of the general otorhinolaryngologic services and are not reported separately. All descriptors refer to testing both ears. Use the modifier '–52' or 09952, if a test is applied to one ear instead of to two ears. All descriptors (except 92559), apply to testing of individuals; for testing of groups, use 92559 and specify test(s) used.

ICD–9–CM

389.9 Hearing loss NOS

REIMBURSEMENT INFORMATION

Medicare

- Follow–up Days — global concept does not apply
- Assistant Surgeon — by report
- Supply Charges — not allowed
- Outpatient Limit — does not apply

CPT CODE **SERVICE**

92573 Lombard test

CPT NOTES

- Diagnostic or treatment procedures usually included in a comprehensive otorhinolaryngologic evaluation or office visit, are reported as an integrated medical service, using appropriate descriptors from the 99201 series. Itemization of component procedures (e.g., otoscopy, rhinoscopy, tuning fork test) does not apply.

  Special otorhinolaryngologic services are those diagnostic and treatment services not usually included in a comprehensive otorhinolaryngologic evaluation or office visit. These services are reported separately, using descriptors from the 92500 series.

  All services include medical diagnostic evaluation. Technical procedures (which may or may not be performed by the physician personally) are often part of the service, but should not be mistaken to constitute the service itself.
- For laryngoscopy with stroboscopy, use 31579.
- For evaluation of speech, language and/or hearing problems through observation and assessment of performance, see 92506.
- This audiometric test implies the use of calibrated electronic equipment. Other hearing tests (such as whispered voice, tuning fork) are considered part of the general otorhinolaryngologic services and are not reported separately. All descriptors refer to testing both ears. Use the modifier '–52' or 09952, if a test is applied to one ear instead of to two ears. All descriptors (except 92559), apply to testing of individuals; for testing of groups, use 92559 and specify test(s) used.

ICD–9–CM

300.11 Conversion disorder

REIMBURSEMENT INFORMATION

Medicare

- Follow–up Days — global concept does not apply
- Assistant Surgeon — by report
- Supply Charges — not allowed
- Outpatient Limit — does not apply

CPT CODE	SERVICE
92574	Swinging story test

CPT NOTES

- Diagnostic or treatment procedures usually included in a comprehensive otorhinolaryngologic evaluation or office visit, are reported as an integrated medical service, using appropriate descriptors from the 99201 series. Itemization of component procedures (e.g., otoscopy, rhinoscopy, tuning fork test) does not apply.

  Special otorhinolaryngologic services are those diagnostic and treatment services not usually included in a comprehensive otorhinolaryngologic evaluation or office visit. These services are reported separately, using descriptors from the 92500 series.

  All services include medical diagnostic evaluation. Technical procedures (which may or may not be performed by the physician personally) are often part of the service, but should not be mistaken to constitute the service itself.
- For laryngoscopy with stroboscopy, use 31579.
- For evaluation of speech, language and/or hearing problems through observation and assessment of performance, see 92506.
- This audiometric test implies the use of calibrated electronic equipment. Other hearing tests (such as whispered voice, tuning fork) are considered part of the general otorhinolaryngologic services and are not reported separately. All descriptors refer to testing both ears. Use the modifier '–52' or 09952, if a test is applied to one ear instead of to two ears. All descriptors (except 92559), apply to testing of individuals; for testing of groups, use 92559 and specify test(s) used.

ICD–9–CM	
389.9	Hearing loss NOS

REIMBURSEMENT INFORMATION

Medicare

- Follow–up Days — global concept does not apply
- Assistant Surgeon — by report
- Supply Charges — not allowed
- Outpatient Limit — does not apply

CPT CODE	SERVICE
92575	Sensorineural acuity level test

CPT NOTES

- Diagnostic or treatment procedures usually included in a comprehensive otorhinolaryngologic evaluation or office visit, are reported as an integrated medical service, using appropriate descriptors from the 99201 series. Itemization of component procedures (e.g., otoscopy, rhinoscopy, tuning fork test) does not apply.

  Special otorhinolaryngologic services are those diagnostic and treatment services not usually included in a comprehensive otorhinolaryngologic evaluation or office visit. These services are reported separately, using descriptors from the 92500 series.

  All services include medical diagnostic evaluation. Technical procedures (which may or may not be performed by the physician personally) are often part of the service, but should not be mistaken to constitute the service itself.
- For laryngoscopy with stroboscopy, use 31579.
- For evaluation of speech, language and/or hearing problems through observation and assessment of performance, see 92506.
- This audiometric test implies the use of calibrated electronic equipment. Other hearing tests (such as whispered voice, tuning fork) are considered part of the general otorhinolaryngologic services and are not reported separately. All descriptors refer to testing both ears. Use the modifier ' 52' or 09952, if a test is applied to one ear instead of to two ears. All descriptors (except 92559), apply to testing of individuals; for testing of groups, use 92559 and specify test(s) used.

ICD-9-CM

389.10	Sensorineural hearing loss NOS
389.11	Sensory hearing loss
389.12	Neural hearing loss
389.14	Central hearing loss
389.18	Sensorineural hear loss comb type
389.8	Hearing loss NEC
389.9	Hearing loss NOS

REIMBURSEMENT INFORMATION

Medicare

- Follow-up Days — global concept does not apply
- Assistant Surgeon — by report
- Supply Charges — not allowed
- Outpatient Limit — does not apply

CPT CODE	SERVICE
92576	Synthetic sentence identification test

ICD–9–CM

389.9 Hearing loss NOS

CPT NOTES

- Diagnostic or treatment procedures usually included in a comprehensive otorhinolaryngologic evaluation or office visit, are reported as an integrated medical service, using appropriate descriptors from the 99201 series. Itemization of component procedures (e.g., otoscopy, rhinoscopy, tuning fork test) does not apply.

  Special otorhinolaryngologic services are those diagnostic and treatment services not usually included in a comprehensive otorhinolaryngologic evaluation or office visit. These services are reported separately, using descriptors from the 92500 series.

  All services include medical diagnostic evaluation. Technical procedures (which may or may not be performed by the physician personally) are often part of the service, but should not be mistaken to constitute the service itself.
- For laryngoscopy with stroboscopy, use 31579.
- For evaluation of speech, language and/or hearing problems through observation and assessment of performance, see 92506.
- This audiometric test implies the use of calibrated electronic equipment. Other hearing tests (such as whispered voice, tuning fork) are considered part of the general otorhinolaryngologic services and are not reported separately. All descriptors refer to testing both ears. Use the modifier '–52' or 09952, if a test is applied to one ear instead of to two ears. All descriptors (except 92559), apply to testing of individuals; for testing of groups, use 92559 and specify test(s) used.

REIMBURSEMENT INFORMATION

Medicare

- Follow–up Days — global concept does not apply
- Assistant Surgeon — by report
- Supply Charges — not allowed
- Outpatient Limit — does not apply

CPT CODE **SERVICE**

92577 Stenger test, speech

CPT NOTES

- Diagnostic or treatment procedures usually included in a comprehensive otorhinolaryngologic evaluation or office visit, are reported as an integrated medical service, using appropriate descriptors from the 99201 series. Itemization of component procedures (e.g., otoscopy, rhinoscopy, tuning fork test) does not apply.

  Special otorhinolaryngologic services are those diagnostic and treatment services not usually included in a comprehensive otorhinolaryngologic evaluation or office visit. These services are reported separately, using descriptors from the 92500 series.

  All services include medical diagnostic evaluation. Technical procedures (which may or may not be performed by the physician personally) are often part of the service, but should not be mistaken to constitute the service itself.
- For laryngoscopy with stroboscopy, use 31579.
- For evaluation of speech, language and/or hearing problems through observation and assessment of performance, see 92506.
- This audiometric test implies the use of calibrated electronic equipment. Other hearing tests (such as whispered voice, tuning fork) are considered part of the general otorhinolaryngologic services and are not reported separately. All descriptors refer to testing both ears. Use the modifier '–52' or 09952, if a test is applied to one ear instead of to two ears. All descriptors (except 92559), apply to testing of individuals; for testing of groups, use 92559 and specify test(s) used.

ICD–9–CM

389.9 Hearing loss NOS

REIMBURSEMENT INFORMATION

Medicare

- Follow–up Days — global concept does not apply
- Assistant Surgeon — by report
- Supply Charges — not allowed
- Outpatient Limit — does not apply

CPT CODE	SERVICE	ICD-9-CM
92578	Delayed auditory feedback test	389.9 Hearing loss NOS

CPT NOTES

- Diagnostic or treatment procedures usually included in a comprehensive otorhinolaryngologic evaluation or office visit, are reported as an integrated medical service, using appropriate descriptors from the 99201 series. Itemization of component procedures (e.g., otoscopy, rhinoscopy, tuning fork test) does not apply.

  Special otorhinolaryngologic services are those diagnostic and treatment services not usually included in a comprehensive otorhinolaryngologic evaluation or office visit. These services are reported separately, using descriptors from the 92500 series.

  All services include medical diagnostic evaluation. Technical procedures (which may or may not be performed by the physician personally) are often part of the service, but should not be mistaken to constitute the service itself.
- For laryngoscopy with stroboscopy, use 31579.
- For evaluation of speech, language and/or hearing problems through observation and assessment of performance, see 92506.
- This audiometric test implies the use of calibrated electronic equipment. Other hearing tests (such as whispered voice, tuning fork) are considered part of the general otorhinolaryngologic services and are not reported separately. All descriptors refer to testing both ears. Use the modifier '–52' or 09952, if a test is applied to one ear instead of to two ears. All descriptors (except 92559), apply to testing of individuals; for testing of groups, use 92559 and specify test(s) used.

REIMBURSEMENT INFORMATION

Medicare

- Follow–up Days — global concept does not apply
- Assistant Surgeon — by report
- Supply Charges — not allowed
- Outpatient Limit — does not apply

CPT CODE **SERVICE**

92580 Electrodermal audiometry

CPT NOTES

- Diagnostic or treatment procedures usually included in a comprehensive otorhinolaryngologic evaluation or office visit, are reported as an integrated medical service, using appropriate descriptors from the 99201 series. Itemization of component procedures (e.g., otoscopy, rhinoscopy, tuning fork test) does not apply.

  Special otorhinolaryngologic services are those diagnostic and treatment services not usually included in a comprehensive otorhinolaryngologic evaluation or office visit. These services are reported separately, using descriptors from the 92500 series.

  All services include medical diagnostic evaluation. Technical procedures (which may or may not be performed by the physician personally) are often part of the service, but should not be mistaken to constitute the service itself.
- For laryngoscopy with stroboscopy, use 31579.
- For evaluation of speech, language and/or hearing problems through observation and assessment of performance, see 92506.
- This audiometric test implies the use of calibrated electronic equipment. Other hearing tests (such as whispered voice, tuning fork) are considered part of the general otorhinolaryngologic services and are not reported separately. All descriptors refer to testing both ears. Use the modifier '–52' or 09952, if a test is applied to one ear instead of to two ears. All descriptors (except 92559), apply to testing of individuals; for testing of groups, use 92559 and specify test(s) used.

ICD–9–CM

389.9 Hearing loss NOS

REIMBURSEMENT INFORMATION

Medicare

- Follow–up Days — global concept does not apply
- Assistant Surgeon — by report
- Supply Charges — not allowed
- Outpatient Limit — does not apply

CPT CODE	SERVICE
92582	Conditioning play audiometry

CPT NOTES

- Diagnostic or treatment procedures usually included in a comprehensive otorhinolaryngologic evaluation or office visit, are reported as an integrated medical service, using appropriate descriptors from the 99201 series. Itemization of component procedures (e.g., otoscopy, rhinoscopy, tuning fork test) does not apply.

  Special otorhinolaryngologic services are those diagnostic and treatment services not usually included in a comprehensive otorhinolaryngologic evaluation or office visit. These services are reported separately, using descriptors from the 92500 series.

  All services include medical diagnostic evaluation. Technical procedures (which may or may not be performed by the physician personally) are often part of the service, but should not be mistaken to constitute the service itself.
- For laryngoscopy with stroboscopy, use 31579.
- For evaluation of speech, language and/or hearing problems through observation and assessment of performance, see 92506.
- This audiometric test implies the use of calibrated electronic equipment. Other hearing tests (such as whispered voice, tuning fork) are considered part of the general otorhinolaryngologic services and are not reported separately. All descriptors refer to testing both ears. Use the modifier '–52' or 09952, if a test is applied to one ear instead of to two ears. All descriptors (except 92559), apply to testing of individuals; for testing of groups, use 92559 and specify test(s) used.

ICD–9–CM

315.39	Speech/language develop disord NEC
320.2	Streptococcal meningitis
380.10	Infective otitis externa NOS
381.10	Chron serous otitis media simp/NOS
381.3	Chronic nonsuppurative otitis media
381.4	Chron nonsup otitis media NOS
381.81	Dysfunction of Eustachian tube
382.00	Acute suppurative otitis media NOS
382.3	Chronic suppurativ otitis media NOS
382.9	Otitis media NOS
384.20	Perforation tympanic membrane NOS
389.00	Conductive hearing loss NOS
389.10	Sensorineural hearing loss NOS
389.8	Hearing loss NEC
V41.2	Problems with hearing
V72.1	Examination of ears/hearing

REIMBURSEMENT INFORMATION

Medicare

- Follow–up Days — global concept does not apply
- Assistant Surgeon — by report
- Supply Charges — not allowed
- Outpatient Limit — does not apply

CPT CODE	SERVICE
92583	Select picture audiometry

CPT NOTES

- Diagnostic or treatment procedures usually included in a comprehensive otorhinolaryngologic evaluation or office visit, are reported as an integrated medical service, using appropriate descriptors from the 99201 series. Itemization of component procedures (e.g., otoscopy, rhinoscopy, tuning fork test) does not apply.

  Special otorhinolaryngologic services are those diagnostic and treatment services not usually included in a comprehensive otorhinolaryngologic evaluation or office visit. These services are reported separately, using descriptors from the 92500 series.

  All services include medical diagnostic evaluation. Technical procedures (which may or may not be performed by the physician personally) are often part of the service, but should not be mistaken to constitute the service itself.
- For laryngoscopy with stroboscopy, use 31579.
- For evaluation of speech, language and/or hearing problems through observation and assessment of performance, see 92506.
- This audiometric test implies the use of calibrated electronic equipment. Other hearing tests (such as whispered voice, tuning fork) are considered part of the general otorhinolaryngologic services and are not reported separately. All descriptors refer to testing both ears. Use the modifier '–52' or 09952, if a test is applied to one ear instead of to two ears. All descriptors (except 92559), apply to testing of individuals; for testing of groups, use 92559 and specify test(s) used.

ICD–9–CM

V41.2 Problems with hearing

REIMBURSEMENT INFORMATION

Medicare

- Follow–up Days — global concept does not apply
- Assistant Surgeon — by report
- Supply Charges — not allowed
- Outpatient Limit — does not apply

CPT CODE **SERVICE**

92584 Electrocochleography

CPT NOTES

- Diagnostic or treatment procedures usually included in a comprehensive otorhinolaryngologic evaluation or office visit, are reported as an integrated medical service, using appropriate descriptors from the 99201 series. Itemization of component procedures (e.g., otoscopy, rhinoscopy, tuning fork test) does not apply.

  Special otorhinolaryngologic services are those diagnostic and treatment services not usually included in a comprehensive otorhinolaryngologic evaluation or office visit. These services are reported separately, using descriptors from the 92500 series.

  All services include medical diagnostic evaluation. Technical procedures (which may or may not be performed by the physician personally) are often part of the service, but should not be mistaken to constitute the service itself.
- For laryngoscopy with stroboscopy, use 31579.
- For evaluation of speech, language and/or hearing problems through observation and assessment of performance, see 92506.
- This audiometric test implies the use of calibrated electronic equipment. Other hearing tests (such as whispered voice, tuning fork) are considered part of the general otorhinolaryngologic services and are not reported separately. All descriptors refer to testing both ears. Use the modifier '–52' or 09952, if a test is applied to one ear instead of to two ears. All descriptors (except 92559), apply to testing of individuals; for testing of groups, use 92559 and specify test(s) used.

ICD–9–CM

368.10	Subjective visual disturbance NOS
386.00	Meniere's disease NOS
386.01	Meniere's disease cochleovestibular
386.10	Peripheral vertigo NOS
386.11	Benign paroxysmal position vertigo
386.2	Central origin vertigo
386.40	Labyrinthine fistula NOS
386.50	Labyrinthine dysfunction NOS
386.9	Vertiginous syndromes NOS
388.5	Acoustic nerve disorders
389.10	Sensorineural hearing loss NOS
780.4	Dizziness and giddiness

REIMBURSEMENT INFORMATION

Medicare

- Follow–up Days — global concept does not apply
- Assistant Surgeon — by report
- Supply Charges — not allowed
- Outpatient Limit — does not apply

CPT CODE **SERVICE**

92585 Brainstem evoked response recording (evoked response (EEG) audiometry)

CPT NOTES

- Diagnostic or treatment procedures usually included in a comprehensive otorhinolaryngologic evaluation or office visit, are reported as an integrated medical service, using appropriate descriptors from the 99201 series. Itemization of component procedures (e.g., otoscopy, rhinoscopy, tuning fork test) does not apply.

  Special otorhinolaryngologic services are those diagnostic and treatment services not usually included in a comprehensive otorhinolaryngologic evaluation or office visit. These services are reported separately, using descriptors from the 92500 series.

  All services include medical diagnostic evaluation. Technical procedures (which may or may not be performed by the physician personally) are often part of the service, but should not be mistaken to constitute the service itself.
- For laryngoscopy with stroboscopy, use 31579.
- For evaluation of speech, language and/or hearing problems through observation and assessment of performance, see 92506.
- This audiometric test implies the use of calibrated electronic equipment. Other hearing tests (such as whispered voice, tuning fork) are considered part of the general otorhinolaryngologic services and are not reported separately. All descriptors refer to testing both ears. Use the modifier '–52' or 09952, if a test is applied to one ear instead of to two ears. All descriptors (except 92559), apply to testing of individuals; for testing of groups, use 92559 and specify test(s) used.

ICD–9–CM

192.0	M-Neoplasm, Cranial nerves
198.4	M2-Neoplasm, Nervous system NEC
225.0	B-Neoplasm, Brain
225.1	B-Neoplasm, Cranial nerve
237.9	UB-Neoplasm, Nervous system NEC
307.81	Tension headache
315.39	Speech/language develop disord NEC
346.1	Common migraine
346.9	Migraine NOS
351.0	Bell's palsy
381.9	Eustachian tube disorder NOS
386.00	Meniere's disease NOS
386.01	Meniere's disease cochleovestibular
386.10	Peripheral vertigo NOS
386.11	Benign paroxysmal position vertigo
386.12	Vestibular neuronitis
386.2	Central origin vertigo
386.30	Labyrinthitis NOS
386.40	Labyrinthine fistula NOS
386.50	Labyrinthine dysfunction NOS
386.9	Vertiginous syndromes NOS
388.30	Tinnitus NOS
388.32	Objective tinnitus
388.5	Acoustic nerve disorders
388.70	Otalgia NOS
388.8	Ear disorders NEC
389.00	Conductive hearing loss NOS
389.01	Conductive hearing loss, extern ear
389.02	Conductive hearing loss, tympanic
389.03	Conductive hearing loss, middle ear
389.04	Conductive hearing loss, inner ear
389.08	Conductive hearing loss, comb type
389.10	Sensorineural hearing loss NOS
389.11	Sensory hearing loss
389.12	Neural hearing loss
389.14	Central hearing loss
389.18	Sensorineural hear loss comb type
389.2	Mixed hearing loss
389.8	Hearing loss NEC
389.9	Hearing loss NOS
780.4	Dizziness and giddiness
781.3	Lack of coordination
784.0	Headache

REIMBURSEMENT INFORMATION

Medicare

- Follow–up Days — global concept does not apply
- Assistant Surgeon — by report
- Supply Charges — not allowed
- Outpatient Limit — does not apply

CPT CODE **SERVICE**

● 92587 Evoked otoacoustic emissions; limited (single stimulus level, either transient or distortion products)

CPT NOTES

- Diagnostic or treatment procedures usually included in a comprehensive otorhinolaryngologic evaluation or office visit, are reported as an integrated medical service, using appropriate descriptors from the 99201 series. Itemization of component procedures (e.g., otoscopy, rhinoscopy, tuning fork test) does not apply.

  Special otorhinolaryngologic services are those diagnostic and treatment services not usually included in a comprehensive otorhinolaryngologic evaluation or office visit. These services are reported separately, using descriptors from the 92500 series.

  All services include medical diagnostic evaluation. Technical procedures (which may or may not be performed by the physician personally) are often part of the service, but should not be mistaken to constitute the service itself.
- For laryngoscopy with stroboscopy, use 31579.
- For evaluation of speech, language and/or hearing problems through observation and assessment of performance, see 92506.
- This audiometric test implies the use of calibrated electronic equipment. Other hearing tests (such as whispered voice, tuning fork) are considered part of the general otorhinolaryngologic services and are not reported separately. All descriptors refer to testing both ears. Use the modifier '–52' or 09952, if a test is applied to one ear instead of to two ears. All descriptors (except 92559), apply to testing of individuals; for testing of groups, use 92559 and specify test(s) used.

ICD–9–CM

225.1	B Neoplasm, Cranial nerve
315.39	Speech/language develop disord NEC
322.9	Meningitis NOS
340	Multiple sclerosis
388.2	Sudden hearing loss NOS
389.10	Sensorineural hearing loss NOS
765.10	Preterm infant NEC, weight NOS
765.11	Preterm infant NEC, 500 gram

REIMBURSEMENT INFORMATION

General

- New procedure, 1995 CPT.

Medicare

- Follow–up Days — global concept does not apply
- Assistant Surgeon — by report
- Supply Charges — not allowed
- Outpatient Limit — does not apply

CPT CODE	SERVICE
● **92588**	Evoked otoacoustic emissions; comprehensive or diagnostic evaluation (comparison of transient and distortion product otoacoustic emissions at multiple levels and frequencies)

CPT NOTES

- Diagnostic or treatment procedures usually included in a comprehensive otorhinolaryngologic evaluation or office visit, are reported as an integrated medical service, using appropriate descriptors from the 99201 series. Itemization of component procedures (e.g., otoscopy, rhinoscopy, tuning fork test) does not apply.

  Special otorhinolaryngologic services are those diagnostic and treatment services not usually included in a comprehensive otorhinolaryngologic evaluation or office visit. These services are reported separately, using descriptors from the 92500 series.

  All services include medical diagnostic evaluation. Technical procedures (which may or may not be performed by the physician personally) are often part of the service, but should not be mistaken to constitute the service itself.
- For laryngoscopy with stroboscopy, use 31579.
- For evaluation of speech, language and/or hearing problems through observation and assessment of performance, see 92506.
- This audiometric test implies the use of calibrated electronic equipment. Other hearing tests (such as whispered voice, tuning fork) are considered part of the general otorhinolaryngologic services and are not reported separately. All descriptors refer to testing both ears. Use the modifier '–52' or 09952, if a test is applied to one ear instead of to two ears. All descriptors (except 92559), apply to testing of individuals; for testing of groups, use 92559 and specify test(s) used.

ICD–9–CM

225.1	B-Neoplasm, Cranial nerve
315.39	Speech/language develop disord NEC
322.9	Meningitis NOS
340	Multiple sclerosis
388.2	Sudden hearing loss NOS
389.10	Sensorineural hearing loss NOS
765.10	Preterm infant NEC, weight NOS
765.11	Preterm infant NEC, 500 gram

REIMBURSEMENT INFORMATION

General

- New procedure, 1995 CPT.

Medicare

- Follow–up Days — global concept does not apply
- Assistant Surgeon — by report
- Supply Charges — not allowed
- Outpatient Limit — does not apply

CPT CODE **SERVICE**

92589 Central auditory function test(s) (specify)

CPT NOTES

- Diagnostic or treatment procedures usually included in a comprehensive otorhinolaryngologic evaluation or office visit, are reported as an integrated medical service, using appropriate descriptors from the 99201 series. Itemization of component procedures (e.g., otoscopy, rhinoscopy, tuning fork test) does not apply.

  Special otorhinolaryngologic services are those diagnostic and treatment services not usually included in a comprehensive otorhinolaryngologic evaluation or office visit. These services are reported separately, using descriptors from the 92500 series.

  All services include medical diagnostic evaluation. Technical procedures (which may or may not be performed by the physician personally) are often part of the service, but should not be mistaken to constitute the service itself.
- For laryngoscopy with stroboscopy, use 31579.
- For evaluation of speech, language and/or hearing problems through observation and assessment of performance, see 92506.
- This audiometric test implies the use of calibrated electronic equipment. Other hearing tests (such as whispered voice, tuning fork) are considered part of the general otorhinolaryngologic services and are not reported separately. All descriptors refer to testing both ears. Use the modifier '–52' or 09952, if a test is applied to one ear instead of to two ears. All descriptors (except 92559), apply to testing of individuals; for testing of groups, use 92559 and specify test(s) used.

ICD–9–CM

389.9 Hearing loss NOS

REIMBURSEMENT INFORMATION

Medicare

- Follow–up Days — global concept does not apply
- Assistant Surgeon — by report
- Supply Charges — not allowed
- Outpatient Limit — does not apply

CPT CODE **SERVICE**

92590 Hearing aid examination and selection; monaural

CPT NOTES

- Diagnostic or treatment procedures usually included in a comprehensive otorhinolaryngologic evaluation or office visit, are reported as an integrated medical service, using appropriate descriptors from the 99201 series. Itemization of component procedures (e.g., otoscopy, rhinoscopy, tuning fork test) does not apply.

  Special otorhinolaryngologic services are those diagnostic and treatment services not usually included in a comprehensive otorhinolaryngologic evaluation or office visit. These services are reported separately, using descriptors from the 92500 series.

  All services include medical diagnostic evaluation. Technical procedures (which may or may not be performed by the physician personally) are often part of the service, but should not be mistaken to constitute the service itself.
- For laryngoscopy with stroboscopy, use 31579.
- For evaluation of speech, language and/or hearing problems through observation and assessment of performance, see 92506.
- This audiometric test implies the use of calibrated electronic equipment. Other hearing tests (such as whispered voice, tuning fork) are considered part of the general otorhinolaryngologic services and are not reported separately. All descriptors refer to testing both ears. Use the modifier '–52' or 09952, if a test is applied to one ear instead of to two ears. All descriptors (except 92559), apply to testing of individuals; for testing of groups, use 92559 and specify test(s) used.

ICD–9–CM

388.5 Acoustic nerve disorders
389.10 Sensorineural hearing loss NOS

REIMBURSEMENT INFORMATION

Medicare

- Follow–up Days — global concept does not apply
- Assistant Surgeon — not paid
- Supply Charges — not allowed
- Outpatient Limit — does not apply

CPT CODE **SERVICE**

92591 Hearing aid examination and selection, binaural

CPT NOTES

- Diagnostic or treatment procedures usually included in a comprehensive otorhinolaryngologic evaluation or office visit, are reported as an integrated medical service, using appropriate descriptors from the 99201 series. Itemization of component procedures (e.g., otoscopy, rhinoscopy, tuning fork test) does not apply.

  Special otorhinolaryngologic services are those diagnostic and treatment services not usually included in a comprehensive otorhinolaryngologic evaluation or office visit. These services are reported separately, using descriptors from the 92500 series.

  All services include medical diagnostic evaluation. Technical procedures (which may or may not be performed by the physician personally) are often part of the service, but should not be mistaken to constitute the service itself.
- For laryngoscopy with stroboscopy, use 31579.
- For evaluation of speech, language and/or hearing problems through observation and assessment of performance, see 92506.
- This audiometric test implies the use of calibrated electronic equipment. Other hearing tests (such as whispered voice, tuning fork) are considered part of the general otorhinolaryngologic services and are not reported separately. All descriptors refer to testing both ears. Use the modifier '–52' or 09952, if a test is applied to one ear instead of to two ears. All descriptors (except 92559), apply to testing of individuals; for testing of groups, use 92559 and specify test(s) used.

ICD–9–CM

388.5 Acoustic nerve disorders
389.18 Sensorineural hear loss comb type

REIMBURSEMENT INFORMATION

Medicare

- Follow–up Days — global concept does not apply
- Assistant Surgeon — not paid
- Supply Charges — not allowed
- Outpatient Limit — does not apply

CPT CODE **SERVICE**

92592 Hearing aid check; monaural

CPT NOTES

- Diagnostic or treatment procedures usually included in a comprehensive otorhinolaryngologic evaluation or office visit, are reported as an integrated medical service, using appropriate descriptors from the 99201 series. Itemization of component procedures (e.g., otoscopy, rhinoscopy, tuning fork test) does not apply.

  Special otorhinolaryngologic services are those diagnostic and treatment services not usually included in a comprehensive otorhinolaryngologic evaluation or office visit. These services are reported separately, using descriptors from the 92500 series.

  All services include medical diagnostic evaluation. Technical procedures (which may or may not be performed by the physician personally) are often part of the service, but should not be mistaken to constitute the service itself.
- For laryngoscopy with stroboscopy, use 31579.
- For evaluation of speech, language and/or hearing problems through observation and assessment of performance, see 92506.
- This audiometric test implies the use of calibrated electronic equipment. Other hearing tests (such as whispered voice, tuning fork) are considered part of the general otorhinolaryngologic services and are not reported separately. All descriptors refer to testing both ears. Use the modifier '–52' or 09952, if a test is applied to one ear instead of to two ears. All descriptors (except 92559), apply to testing of individuals; for testing of groups, use 92559 and specify test(s) used.

ICD–9–CM

389.10 Sensorineural hearing loss NOS
V41.2 Problems with hearing

REIMBURSEMENT INFORMATION

Medicare

- Follow–up Days — global concept does not apply
- Assistant Surgeon — not paid
- Supply Charges — not allowed
- Outpatient Limit — does not apply

CPT CODE **SERVICE**

92593 Hearing aid check; binaural

CPT NOTES

- Diagnostic or treatment procedures usually included in a comprehensive otorhinolaryngologic evaluation or office visit, are reported as an integrated medical service, using appropriate descriptors from the 99201 series. Itemization of component procedures (e.g., otoscopy, rhinoscopy, tuning fork test) does not apply.

  Special otorhinolaryngologic services are those diagnostic and treatment services not usually included in a comprehensive otorhinolaryngologic evaluation or office visit. These services are reported separately, using descriptors from the 92500 series.

  All services include medical diagnostic evaluation. Technical procedures (which may or may not be performed by the physician personally) are often part of the service, but should not be mistaken to constitute the service itself.
- For laryngoscopy with stroboscopy, use 31579.
- For evaluation of speech, language and/or hearing problems through observation and assessment of performance, see 92506.
- This audiometric test implies the use of calibrated electronic equipment. Other hearing tests (such as whispered voice, tuning fork) are considered part of the general otorhinolaryngologic services and are not reported separately. All descriptors refer to testing both ears. Use the modifier '–52' or 09952, if a test is applied to one ear instead of to two ears. All descriptors (except 92559), apply to testing of individuals; for testing of groups, use 92559 and specify test(s) used.

ICD–9–CM

V41.2 Problems with hearing

REIMBURSEMENT INFORMATION

Medicare

- Follow–up Days — global concept does not apply
- Assistant Surgeon — not paid
- Supply Charges — not allowed
- Outpatient Limit — does not apply

CPT CODE **SERVICE**

92594 Electroacoustic evaluation for hearing aid; monaural

CPT NOTES

- Diagnostic or treatment procedures usually included in a comprehensive otorhinolaryngologic evaluation or office visit, are reported as an integrated medical service, using appropriate descriptors from the 99201 series. Itemization of component procedures (e.g., otoscopy, rhinoscopy, tuning fork test) does not apply.

  Special otorhinolaryngologic services are those diagnostic and treatment services not usually included in a comprehensive otorhinolaryngologic evaluation or office visit. These services are reported separately, using descriptors from the 92500 series.

  All services include medical diagnostic evaluation. Technical procedures (which may or may not be performed by the physician personally) are often part of the service, but should not be mistaken to constitute the service itself.
- For laryngoscopy with stroboscopy, use 31579.
- For evaluation of speech, language and/or hearing problems through observation and assessment of performance, see 92506.
- This audiometric test implies the use of calibrated electronic equipment. Other hearing tests (such as whispered voice, tuning fork) are considered part of the general otorhinolaryngologic services and are not reported separately. All descriptors refer to testing both ears. Use the modifier '–52' or 09952, if a test is applied to one ear instead of to two ears. All descriptors (except 92559), apply to testing of individuals; for testing of groups, use 92559 and specify test(s) used.

ICD–9–CM

388.5 Acoustic nerve disorders

REIMBURSEMENT INFORMATION

Medicare

- Follow–up Days — global concept does not apply
- Assistant Surgeon — not paid
- Supply Charges — not allowed
- Outpatient Limit — does not apply

CPT CODE **SERVICE**

92595 Electroacoustic evaluation for hearing aid; binaural

CPT NOTES

- Diagnostic or treatment procedures usually included in a comprehensive otorhinolaryngologic evaluation or office visit, are reported as an integrated medical service, using appropriate descriptors from the 99201 series. Itemization of component procedures (e.g., otoscopy, rhinoscopy, tuning fork test) does not apply.

  Special otorhinolaryngologic services are those diagnostic and treatment services not usually included in a comprehensive otorhinolaryngologic evaluation or office visit. These services are reported separately, using descriptors from the 92500 series.

  All services include medical diagnostic evaluation. Technical procedures (which may or may not be performed by the physician personally) are often part of the service, but should not be mistaken to constitute the service itself.
- For laryngoscopy with stroboscopy, use 31579.
- For evaluation of speech, language and/or hearing problems through observation and assessment of performance, see 92506.
- This audiometric test implies the use of calibrated electronic equipment. Other hearing tests (such as whispered voice, tuning fork) are considered part of the general otorhinolaryngologic services and are not reported separately. All descriptors refer to testing both ears. Use the modifier '–52' or 09952, if a test is applied to one ear instead of to two ears. All descriptors (except 92559), apply to testing of individuals; for testing of groups, use 92559 and specify test(s) used.

ICD–9–CM

388.5 Acoustic nerve disorders

REIMBURSEMENT INFORMATION

Medicare

- Follow–up Days — global concept does not apply
- Assistant Surgeon — not paid
- Supply Charges — not allowed
- Outpatient Limit — does not apply

CPT CODE **SERVICE**

92596 Ear protector attenuation measurements

CPT NOTES

- Diagnostic or treatment procedures usually included in a comprehensive otorhinolaryngologic evaluation or office visit, are reported as an integrated medical service, using appropriate descriptors from the 99201 series. Itemization of component procedures (e.g., otoscopy, rhinoscopy, tuning fork test) does not apply.

  Special otorhinolaryngologic services are those diagnostic and treatment services not usually included in a comprehensive otorhinolaryngologic evaluation or office visit. These services are reported separately, using descriptors from the 92500 series.

  All services include medical diagnostic evaluation. Technical procedures (which may or may not be performed by the physician personally) are often part of the service, but should not be mistaken to constitute the service itself.
- For laryngoscopy with stroboscopy, use 31579.
- For evaluation of speech, language and/or hearing problems through observation and assessment of performance, see 92506.
- This audiometric test implies the use of calibrated electronic equipment. Other hearing tests (such as whispered voice, tuning fork) are considered part of the general otorhinolaryngologic services and are not reported separately. All descriptors refer to testing both ears. Use the modifier '–52' or 09952, if a test is applied to one ear instead of to two ears. All descriptors (except 92559), apply to testing of individuals; for testing of groups, use 92559 and specify test(s) used.

ICD–9–CM

389.12 Neural hearing loss

REIMBURSEMENT INFORMATION

Medicare

- Follow–up Days — global concept does not apply
- Assistant Surgeon — by report
- Supply Charges — not allowed
- Outpatient Limit — does not apply

CPT CODE **SERVICE**

92599 Unlisted otorhinolaryngological service or procedure

CPT NOTES

- Diagnostic or treatment procedures usually included in a comprehensive otorhinolaryngologic evaluation or office visit, are reported as an integrated medical service, using appropriate descriptors from the 99201 series. Itemization of component procedures (e.g., otoscopy, rhinoscopy, tuning fork test) does not apply.

  Special otorhinolaryngologic services are those diagnostic and treatment services not usually included in a comprehensive otorhinolaryngologic evaluation or office visit. These services are reported separately, using descriptors from the 92500 series.

  All services include medical diagnostic evaluation. Technical procedures (which may or may not be performed by the physician personally) are often part of the service, but should not be mistaken to constitute the service itself.
- For laryngoscopy with stroboscopy, use 31579.

ICD-9-CM

381.00	Acute nonsup otitis media NOS
381.10	Chron serous otitis media simp/NOS
381.81	Dysfunction of Eustachian tube
382.00	Acute suppurative otitis media NOS
386.30	Labyrinthitis NOS
388.30	Tinnitus NOS
388.31	Subjective tinnitus
388.60	Otorrhea NOS
389.10	Sensorineural hearing loss NOS
389.8	Hearing loss NEC
461.0	Acute maxillary sinusitis
466.0	Acute bronchitis
784.49	Voice disturbance NEC

REIMBURSEMENT INFORMATION

Medicare

- Follow–up Days — global concept does not apply
- Assistant Surgeon — by report
- Supply Charges — not allowed
- Outpatient Limit — does not apply
- Major Surgery Rules Apply

94010 Spirometry, including graphic record, total and timed vital capacity, expiratory flow rate measurement(s), and/or maximal voluntary ventilation

CPT NOTES

- Includes laboratory procedure(s) and interpretation of test results. If a separate identifiable Evaluation and Management service is performed, the appropriate E/M service codes should be reported in addition to this code.

135	Sarcoidosis
490	Bronchitis NOS
491.20	Obstr chron bronchitis w/o exacerb
491.21	Obstr chron bronchitis w/exacerb
492.8	Emphysema NEC
493.00	Extrinsic asthma w/o stat asthmat
493.01	Extrinsic asthma w/stat asthmaticus
493.10	Intrinsic asthma w/o stat asthmat
493.90	Asthma NOS w/o status asthmaticus
496	Chronic airway obstruction NEC
501	Asbestosis
518.81	Respiratory failure
518.82	Other pulmonary insufficiency
786.09	Respiratory abnormality NEC
786.2	Cough

REIMBURSEMENT INFORMATION

Medicare

- Follow–up Days — global concept does not apply
- Assistant Surgeon — by report
- Supply Charges — not allowed
- Outpatient Limit — does not apply
- Fragments — 94160, 94200

CPT CODE	SERVICE	ICD–9–CM
94060	Bronchospasm evaluation: spirometry as in 94010, before and after bronchodilator (aerosol or parenteral) or exercise **CPT NOTES** ♦ Includes laboratory procedure(s) and interpretation of test results. If a separate identifiable Evaluation and Management service is performed, the appropriate E/M service codes should be reported in addition to this code.	135 Sarcoidosis 491.20 Obstr chron bronchitis w/o exacerb 491.21 Obstr chron bronchitis w/exacerb 493.00 Extrinsic asthma w/o stat asthmat 493.01 Extrinsic asthma w/stat asthmaticus 493.10 Intrinsic asthma w/o stat asthmat 493.90 Asthma NOS w/o status asthmaticus 496 Chronic airway obstruction NEC 501 Asbestosis 518.81 Respiratory failure 518.82 Other pulmonary insufficiency 530.6 Acquired esophageal diverticulum 780.53 Hypersomnia w/sleep apnea 786.09 Respiratory abnormality NEC 786.2 Cough **REIMBURSEMENT INFORMATION** <u>Medicare</u> ♦ Follow–up Days — global concept does not apply ♦ Assistant Surgeon — by report ♦ Supply Charges — not allowed ♦ Outpatient Limit — does not apply
94375	Respiratory flow volume loop **CPT NOTES** ♦ Includes laboratory procedure(s) and interpretation of test results. If a separate identifiable Evaluation and Management service is performed, the appropriate E/M service codes should be reported in addition to this code.	135 Sarcoidosis 491.20 Obstr chron bronchitis w/o exacerb 491.21 Obstr chron bronchitis w/exacerb 493.00 Extrinsic asthma w/o stat asthmat 493.01 Extrinsic asthma w/stat asthmaticus 493.10 Intrinsic asthma w/o stat asthmat 493.90 Asthma NOS w/o status asthmaticus 496 Chronic airway obstruction NEC 501 Asbestosis 518.81 Respiratory failure 518.82 Other pulmonary insufficiency 530.6 Acquired esophageal diverticulum 780.53 Hypersomnia w/sleep apnea 786.09 Respiratory abnormality NEC 786.2 Cough **REIMBURSEMENT INFORMATION** <u>Medicare</u> ♦ Follow–up Days — global concept does not apply ♦ Assistant Surgeon — by report ♦ Supply Charges — not allowed ♦ Outpatient Limit — does not apply

CPT CODE **SERVICE**

94040 Nonpressurized inhalation treatment for acute airway obstruction

CPT NOTES

- Includes laboratory procedure(s) and interpretation of test results. If a separate identifiable Evaluation and Management service is performed, the appropriate E/M service codes should be reported in addition to this code.

ICD–9–CM

464.31	Acute epiglottitis w/obstruction
464.4	Croup
466.0	Acute bronchitis
486	Pneumonia, organism NOS
490	Bronchitis NOS
491.20	Obstr chron bronchitis w/o exacerb
491.21	Obstr chron bronchitis w/exacerb
493.00	Extrinsic asthma w/o stat asthmat
493.01	Extrinsic asthma w/stat asthmaticus
493.10	Intrinsic asthma w/o stat asthmat
493.90	Asthma NOS w/o status asthmaticus
496	Chronic airway obstruction NEC
501	Asbestosis
518.82	Other pulmonary insufficiency
519.1	Trachea/bronchus disease NEC
519.8	Respiratory system disease NEC
786.09	Respiratory abnormality NEC
786.2	Cough
995.0	Anaphylactic shock NEC

REIMBURSEMENT INFORMATION

Medicare

- Follow–up Days — global concept does not apply
- Assistant Surgeon — by report
- Supply Charges — not allowed
- Outpatient Limit — does not apply

CPT CODE **SERVICE**

94664 Aerosol or vapor inhalations for sputum mobilization, bronchodilation, or sputum induction for diagnostic purposes; initial demonstration and/or evaluation

CPT NOTES

- Includes laboratory procedure(s) and interpretation of test results. If a separate identifiable Evaluation and Management service is performed, the appropriate E/M service codes should be reported in addition to this code.

ICD–9–CM

464.31	Acute epiglottitis w/obstruction
464.4	Croup
466.0	Acute bronchitis
486	Pneumonia, organism NOS
490	Bronchitis NOS
491.20	Obstr chron bronchitis w/o exacerb
491.21	Obstr chron bronchitis w/exacerb
493.00	Extrinsic asthma w/o stat asthmat
493.01	Extrinsic asthma w/stat asthmaticus
493.10	Intrinsic asthma w/o stat asthmat
493.90	Asthma NOS w/o status asthmaticus
496	Chronic airway obstruction NEC
501	Asbestosis
518.82	Other pulmonary insufficiency
519.1	Trachea/bronchus disease NEC
519.8	Respiratory system disease NEC
786.09	Respiratory abnormality NEC
786.2	Cough
995.0	Anaphylactic shock NEC

REIMBURSEMENT INFORMATION

Medicare

- Follow–up Days — global concept does not apply
- Assistant Surgeon — by report
- Supply Charges — not allowed
- Outpatient Limit — does not apply

CPT CODE	SERVICE
95004	Percutaneous tests (scratch, puncture, prick) with allergenic extracts, immediate type reaction, specify number of tests

CPT NOTES

Definitions

- ***Allergy sensitivity tests***: the performance and evaluation of selective cutaneous and mucous membrane tests in correlation with the history, physical examination, and other observations of the patient. The number of tests performed should be judicious and dependent upon the history, physical findings, and clinical judgment. All patients should not necessarily receive the same tests nor the same number of sensitivity tests.
- ***Immunotherapy (desensitization, hyposensitization)***: the parenteral administration of allergenic extracts as antigens at periodic intervals, usually on an increasing dosage scale to a dosage which is maintained as maintenance therapy. Indications for immunotherapy are determined by appropriate diagnostic procedures coordinated with clinical judgment and knowledge of the natural history of allergic diseases.
- ***Other therapy***: for medical conferences on the use of mechanical and electronic devices (precipitators, air conditioners, air filters, humidifiers, dehumidifiers), climatotherapy, physical therapy, occupational and recreational therapy, see Evaluation and Management section.

ICD–9–CM

346.9	Migraine NOS
372.05	Acute atopic conjunctivitis
372.14	Chronic allergic conjunctivitis NEC
381.00	Acute nonsup otitis media NOS
381.01	Acute serous otitis media
381.10	Chron serous otitis media simp/NOS
381.4	Chron nonsup otitis media NOS
381.81	Dysfunction of Eustachian tube
382.9	Otitis media NOS
461.9	Acute sinusitis NOS
466.0	Acute bronchitis
471.0	Polyp of nasal cavity
472.0	Chronic rhinitis
473.8	Chronic sinusitis NEC
473.9	Chronic sinusitis NOS
477.0	Allergic rhinitis d/t pollen
477.8	Allergic rhinitis NEC
477.9	Allergic rhinitis NOS
478.1	Nasal and sinus disease NEC
490	Bronchitis NOS
493.00	Extrinsic asthma w/o stat asthmat
493.90	Asthma NOS w/o status asthmaticus
496	Chronic airway obstruction NEC
519.1	Trachea/bronchus disease NEC
691.8	Other atopic dermatitis
692.5	Topical food dermatitis
692.9	Dermatitis NOS
693.1	Dermatitis d/t food ingestion
693.9	Dermatitis d/t internal agent NOS
698.2	Prurigo
698.9	Pruritic disorder NOS
708.0	Allergic urticaria
708.9	Urticaria NOS
780.53	Hypersomnia w/sleep apnea
784.0	Headache
786.09	Respiratory abnormality NEC
786.2	Cough
787.3	Flatulence/eructation/gas pain
989.5	Toxic effect of venom
995.0	Anaphylactic shock NEC
995.2	Adverse effect med/biol substnc NOS
995.3	Allergy, unspecified
V72.7	Skin/sensitization tests

REIMBURSEMENT INFORMATION

<u>Medicare</u>

- Follow–up Days — global concept does not apply
- Assistant Surgeon — by report
- Supply Charges — not allowed
- Outpatient Limit — does not apply

CPT CODE **SERVICE**

95010 Percutaneous tests (scratch, puncture, prick) sequential and incremental, with drugs, biologicals or venoms, immediate type reaction, specify number of tests

CPT NOTES

Definitions

- ***Allergy sensitivity tests***: the performance and evaluation of selective cutaneous and mucous membrane tests in correlation with the history, physical examination, and other observations of the patient. The number of tests performed should be judicious and dependent upon the history, physical findings, and clinical judgment. All patients should not necessarily receive the same tests nor the same number of sensitivity tests.
- ***Immunotherapy (desensitization, hyposensitization)***: the parenteral administration of allergenic extracts as antigens at periodic intervals, usually on an increasing dosage scale to a dosage which is maintained as maintenance therapy. Indications for immunotherapy are determined by appropriate diagnostic procedures coordinated with clinical judgment and knowledge of the natural history of allergic diseases.
- ***Other therapy***: for medical conferences on the use of mechanical and electronic devices (precipitators, air conditioners, air filters, humidifiers, dehumidifiers), climatotherapy, physical therapy, occupational and recreational therapy, see Evaluation and Management section.

ICD–9–CM

346.9	Migraine NOS
372.05	Acute atopic conjunctivitis
372.14	Chronic allergic conjunctivitis NEC
381.00	Acute nonsup otitis media NOS
381.01	Acute serous otitis media
381.10	Chron serous otitis media simp/NOS
381.4	Chron nonsup otitis media NOS
381.8	Eustachian tube disorder
382.9	Otitis media NOS
461.9	Acute sinusitis NOS
466.0	Acute bronchitis
471.0	Polyp of nasal cavity
472.0	Chronic rhinitis
473.8	Chronic sinusitis NEC
473.9	Chronic sinusitis NOS
477.0	Allergic rhinitis d/t pollen
477.9	Allergic rhinitis NOS
478.1	Nasal and sinus disease NEC
493.90	Asthma NOS w/o status asthmaticus
496	Chronic airway obstruction NEC
519.1	Trachea/bronchus disease NEC
691.8	Other atopic dermatitis
692.5	Topical food dermatitis
692.9	Dermatitis NOS
693.1	Dermatitis d/t food ingestion
693.9	Dermatitis d/t internal agent NOS
698.2	Prurigo
698.9	Pruritic disorder NOS
708.0	Allergic urticaria
708.9	Urticaria NOS
780.53	Hypersomnia w/sleep apnea
784.0	Headache
786.09	Respiratory abnormality NEC
786.2	Cough
989.5	Toxic effect of venom
995.0	Anaphylactic shock NEC
995.2	Adverse effect med/biol substnc NOS
995.3	Allergy, unspecified

REIMBURSEMENT INFORMATION

Medicare

- Follow–up Days — global concept does not apply
- Assistant Surgeon — by report
- Supply Charges — not allowed
- Outpatient Limit — does not apply

CPT CODE **SERVICE**

[illegible] Intracutaneous (intradermal) tests, sequential and incremental, with drugs, biologicals, or venoms, immediate type reaction, specify number of tests

CPT NOTES

Definitions

- ***Allergy sensitivity tests:*** the performance and evaluation of selective cutaneous and mucous membrane tests in correlation with the history, physical examination, and other observations of the patient. The number of tests performed should be judicious and dependent upon the history, physical findings, and clinical judgment. All patients should not necessarily receive the same tests nor the same number of sensitivity tests.
- ***Immunotherapy (desensitization, hyposensitization)***: the parenteral administration of allergenic extracts as antigens at periodic intervals, usually on an increasing dosage scale to a dosage which is maintained as maintenance therapy. Indications for immunotherapy are determined by appropriate diagnostic procedures coordinated with clinical judgment and knowledge of the natural history of allergic diseases.
- ***Other therapy***: for medical conferences on the use of mechanical and electronic devices (precipitators, air conditioners, air filters, humidifiers, dehumidifiers), climatotherapy, physical therapy, occupational and recreational therapy, see Evaluation and Management section.

ICD–9–CM

[illegible]	Migraine NOS
372.05	Acute atopic conjunctivitis
372.14	Chronic allergic conjunctivitis NEC
381.00	Acute nonsup otitis media NOS
381.01	Acute serous otitis media
381.10	Chron serous otitis media simp/NOS
381.4	Chron nonsup otitis media NOS
381.8	Eustachian tube disorder
382.9	Otitis media NOS
461.9	Acute sinusitis NOS
466.0	Acute bronchitis
471.0	Polyp of nasal cavity
472.0	Chronic rhinitis
473.8	Chronic sinusitis NEC
477.0	Allergic rhinitis d/t pollen
477.8	Allergic rhinitis NEC
477.9	Allergic rhinitis NOS
478.1	Nasal and sinus disease NEC
490	Bronchitis NOS
493.00	Extrinsic asthma w/o stat asthmat
519.1	Trachea/bronchus disease NEC
691.8	Other atopic dermatitis
692.5	Topical food dermatitis
692.9	Dermatitis NOS
693.1	Dermatitis d/t food ingestion
693.9	Dermatitis d/t internal agent NOS
698.2	Prurigo
698.9	Pruritic disorder NOS
708.0	Allergic urticaria
708.9	Urticaria NOS
784.0	Headache
786.09	Respiratory abnormality NEC
786.2	Cough
989.5	Toxic effect of venom
995.0	Anaphylactic shock NEC
995.2	Adverse effect med/biol substnc NOS
995.3	Allergy, unspecified

REIMBURSEMENT INFORMATION

Medicare

- Follow–up Days — global concept does not apply
- Assistant Surgeon — by report
- Supply Charges — not allowed
- Outpatient Limit — does not apply

CPT CODE **SERVICE**

95024 Intracutaneous (intradermal) tests with allergenic extracts, immediate type reaction, specify number of tests

CPT NOTES

Definitions

- ***Allergy sensitivity tests:*** the performance and evaluation of selective cutaneous and mucous membrane tests in correlation with the history, physical examination, and other observations of the patient. The number of tests performed should be judicious and dependent upon the history, physical findings, and clinical judgment. All patients should not necessarily receive the same tests nor the same number of sensitivity tests.
- ***Immunotherapy (desensitization, hyposensitization)***: the parenteral administration of allergenic extracts as antigens at periodic intervals, usually on an increasing dosage scale to a dosage which is maintained as maintenance therapy. Indications for immunotherapy are determined by appropriate diagnostic procedures coordinated with clinical judgment and knowledge of the natural history of allergic diseases.
- ***Other therapy***: for medical conferences on the use of mechanical and electronic devices (precipitators, air conditioners, air filters, humidifiers, dehumidifiers), climatotherapy, physical therapy, occupational and recreational therapy, see Evaluation and Management section.

ICD–9–CM

346.9	Migraine NOS
381.01	Acute serous otitis media
381.10	Chron serous otitis media simp/NOS
382.9	Otitis media NOS
386.01	Meniere's disease cochleovestibular
386.9	Vertiginous syndromes NOS
461.9	Acute sinusitis NOS
466.0	Acute bronchitis
471.0	Polyp of nasal cavity
472.0	Chronic rhinitis
473.9	Chronic sinusitis NOS
477.0	Allergic rhinitis d/t pollen
477.8	Allergic rhinitis NEC
477.9	Allergic rhinitis NOS
478.1	Nasal and sinus disease NEC
490	Bronchitis NOS
493.00	Extrinsic asthma w/o stat asthmat
493.90	Asthma NOS w/o status asthmaticus
518.1	Interstitial emphysema
519.1	Trachea/bronchus disease NEC
691.8	Other atopic dermatitis
692.5	Topical food dermatitis
692.9	Dermatitis NOS
693.1	Dermatitis d/t food ingestion
693.9	Dermatitis d/t internal agent NOS
698.2	Prurigo
698.9	Pruritic disorder NOS
708.0	Allergic urticaria
708.9	Urticaria NOS
784.0	Headache
786.09	Respiratory abnormality NEC
786.2	Cough
989.5	Toxic effect of venom
995.0	Anaphylactic shock NEC
995.2	Adverse effect med/biol substnc NOS
995.3	Allergy, unspecified
V72.7	Skin/sensitization tests

REIMBURSEMENT INFORMATION

Medicare

- Follow–up Days — global concept does not apply
- Assistant Surgeon — by report
- Supply Charges — not allowed
- Outpatient Limit — does not apply

CPT CODE **SERVICE**

95027 Skin end point titration

CPT NOTES

Definitions

- ***Allergy sensitivity tests:*** the performance and evaluation of selective cutaneous and mucous membrane tests in correlation with the history, physical examination, and other observations of the patient. The number of tests performed should be judicious and dependent upon the history, physical findings, and clinical judgment. All patients should not necessarily receive the same tests nor the same number of sensitivity tests.
- ***Immunotherapy (desensitization, hyposensitization)***: the parenteral administration of allergenic extracts as antigens at periodic intervals, usually on an increasing dosage scale to a dosage which is maintained as maintenance therapy. Indications for immunotherapy are determined by appropriate diagnostic procedures coordinated with clinical judgment and knowledge of the natural history of allergic diseases.
- ***Other therapy***: for medical conferences on the use of mechanical and electronic devices (precipitators, air conditioners, air filters, humidifiers, dehumidifiers), climatotherapy, physical therapy, occupational and recreational therapy, see Evaluation and Management section.

ICD–9–CM

346.9	Migraine NOS
381.01	Acute serous otitis media
381.10	Chron serous otitis media simp/NOS
382.9	Otitis media NOS
386.01	Meniere's disease cochleovestibular
386.30	Labyrinthitis NOS
386.9	Vertiginous syndromes NOS
388.30	Tinnitus NOS
388.71	Otogenic pain
471.0	Polyp of nasal cavity
472.0	Chronic rhinitis
473.9	Chronic sinusitis NOS
477.0	Allergic rhinitis d/t pollen
477.8	Allergic rhinitis NEC
477.9	Allergic rhinitis NOS
490	Bronchitis NOS
491.9	Chronic bronchitis NOS
493.00	Extrinsic asthma w/o stat asthmat
493.90	Asthma NOS w/o status asthmaticus
691.8	Other atopic dermatitis
692.5	Topical food dermatitis
692.9	Dermatitis NOS
693.1	Dermatitis d/t food ingestion
693.9	Dermatitis d/t internal agent NOS
698.2	Prurigo
698.9	Pruritic disorder NOS
708.0	Allergic urticaria
708.9	Urticaria NOS
784.0	Headache
786.09	Respiratory abnormality NEC
786.2	Cough
989.5	Toxic effect of venom
995.0	Anaphylactic shock NEC
995.2	Adverse effect med/biol substnc NOS
995.3	Allergy, unspecified

REIMBURSEMENT INFORMATION

Medicare

- Follow–up Days — global concept does not apply
- Assistant Surgeon — by report
- Supply Charges — not allowed
- Outpatient Limit — does not apply

CPT CODE **SERVICE**

95028 Intracutaneous (intradermal) tests with allergenic extracts, delayed type reaction, including reading, specify number of tests

CPT NOTES

Definitions

- ***Allergy sensitivity tests:*** the performance and evaluation of selective cutaneous and mucous membrane tests in correlation with the history, physical examination, and other observations of the patient. The number of tests performed should be judicious and dependent upon the history, physical findings, and clinical judgment. All patients should not necessarily receive the same tests nor the same number of sensitivity tests.
- ***Immunotherapy (desensitization, hyposensitization)***: the parenteral administration of allergenic extracts as antigens at periodic intervals, usually on an increasing dosage scale to a dosage which is maintained as maintenance therapy. Indications for immunotherapy are determined by appropriate diagnostic procedures coordinated with clinical judgment and knowledge of the natural history of allergic diseases.
- ***Other therapy***: for medical conferences on the use of mechanical and electronic devices (precipitators, air conditioners, air filters, humidifiers, dehumidifiers), climatotherapy, physical therapy, occupational and recreational therapy, see Evaluation and Management section.

ICD–9–CM

477.0	Allergic rhinitis d/t pollen
477.8	Allergic rhinitis NEC
493.00	Extrinsic asthma w/o stat asthmat
691.8	Other atopic dermatitis
692.6	Dermatitis due to plants
701.8	Hypertrophic/atrophic skin NEC
780.7	Malaise and fatigue
784.2	Swelling in head/neck

REIMBURSEMENT INFORMATION

Medicare

- Follow–up Days — global concept does not apply
- Assistant Surgeon — by report
- Supply Charges — not allowed
- Outpatient Limit — does not apply

CPT CODE **SERVICE**

95044 Patch or application test(s) (specify number of tests)

CPT NOTES

Definitions

- ***Allergy sensitivity tests:*** the performance and evaluation of selective cutaneous and mucous membrane tests in correlation with the history, physical examination, and other observations of the patient. The number of tests performed should be judicious and dependent upon the history, physical findings, and clinical judgment. All patients should not necessarily receive the same tests nor the same number of sensitivity tests.
- ***Immunotherapy (desensitization, hyposensitization)***: the parenteral administration of allergenic extracts as antigens at periodic intervals, usually on an increasing dosage scale to a dosage which is maintained as maintenance therapy. Indications for immunotherapy are determined by appropriate diagnostic procedures coordinated with clinical judgment and knowledge of the natural history of allergic diseases.
- ***Other therapy***: for medical conferences on the use of mechanical and electronic devices (precipitators, air conditioners, air filters, humidifiers, dehumidifiers), climatotherapy, physical therapy, occupational and recreational therapy, see Evaluation and Management section.

ICD–9–CM

692.3	Topical medicine dermatitis
692.5	Topical food dermatitis
692.6	Dermatitis due to plants
692.81	Cosmetic dermatitis
692.89	Dermatitis NEC
692.9	Dermatitis NOS

REIMBURSEMENT INFORMATION

Medicare

- Follow–up Days — global concept does not apply
- Assistant Surgeon — by report
- Supply Charges — not allowed
- Outpatient Limit — does not apply

CPT CODE **SERVICE**

95052 Photo patch test(s) (specify number of tests)

CPT NOTES

Definitions

- ***Allergy sensitivity tests:*** the performance and evaluation of selective cutaneous and mucous membrane tests in correlation with the history, physical examination, and other observations of the patient. The number of tests performed should be judicious and dependent upon the history, physical findings, and clinical judgment. All patients should not necessarily receive the same tests nor the same number of sensitivity tests.
- ***Immunotherapy (desensitization, hyposensitization)***: the parenteral administration of allergenic extracts as antigens at periodic intervals, usually on an increasing dosage scale to a dosage which is maintained as maintenance therapy. Indications for immunotherapy are determined by appropriate diagnostic procedures coordinated with clinical judgment and knowledge of the natural history of allergic diseases.
- ***Other therapy***: for medical conferences on the use of mechanical and electronic devices (precipitators, air conditioners, air filters, humidifiers, dehumidifiers), climatotherapy, physical therapy, occupational and recreational therapy, see Evaluation and Management section.

ICD–9–CM

370.33 Keratoconjunctivitis sicca
692.3 Topical medicine dermatitis
995.2 Adverse effect med/biol substnc NOS

REIMBURSEMENT INFORMATION

Medicare

- Follow–up Days — global concept does not apply
- Assistant Surgeon — by report
- Supply Charges — not allowed
- Outpatient Limit — does not apply

CPT CODE **SERVICE**

[illegible]

CPT NOTES

Definitions

- ***Allergy sensitivity tests:*** the performance and evaluation of selective cutaneous and mucous membrane tests in correlation with the history, physical examination, and other observations of the patient. The number of tests performed should be judicious and dependent upon the history, physical findings, and clinical judgment. All patients should not necessarily receive the same tests nor the same number of sensitivity tests.
- ***Immunotherapy (desensitization, hyposensitization)***: the parenteral administration of allergenic extracts as antigens at periodic intervals, usually on an increasing dosage scale to a dosage which is maintained as maintenance therapy. Indications for immunotherapy are determined by appropriate diagnostic procedures coordinated with clinical judgment and knowledge of the natural history of allergic diseases.
- ***Other therapy***: for medical conferences on the use of mechanical and electronic devices (precipitators, air conditioners, air filters, humidifiers, dehumidifiers), climatotherapy, physical therapy, occupational and recreational therapy, see Evaluation and Management section.

ICD–9–CM

[illegible]
692.3 Topical medicine dermatitis
692.81 Cosmetic dermatitis
995.2 Adverse effect med/biol substnc NOS

REIMBURSEMENT INFORMATION

Medicare

- Follow–up Days — global concept does not apply
- Assistant Surgeon — by report
- Supply Charges — not allowed
- Outpatient Limit — does not apply

CPT CODE **SERVICE**

95060 Ophthalmic mucous membrane tests

CPT NOTES

Definitions

- ***Allergy sensitivity tests:*** the performance and evaluation of selective cutaneous and mucous membrane tests in correlation with the history, physical examination, and other observations of the patient. The number of tests performed should be judicious and dependent upon the history, physical findings, and clinical judgment. All patients should not necessarily receive the same tests nor the same number of sensitivity tests.
- ***Immunotherapy (desensitization, hyposensitization)***: the parenteral administration of allergenic extracts as antigens at periodic intervals, usually on an increasing dosage scale to a dosage which is maintained as maintenance therapy. Indications for immunotherapy are determined by appropriate diagnostic procedures coordinated with clinical judgment and knowledge of the natural history of allergic diseases.
- ***Other therapy***: for medical conferences on the use of mechanical and electronic devices (precipitators, air conditioners, air filters, humidifiers, dehumidifiers), climatotherapy, physical therapy, occupational and recreational therapy, see Evaluation and Management section.

ICD–9–CM

370.32 Limbar/corneal conjunctivitis
370.33 Keratoconjunctivitis sicca
372.05 Acute atopic conjunctivitis
375.20 Epiphora NOS

REIMBURSEMENT INFORMATION

Medicare

- Follow–up Days — global concept does not apply
- Assistant Surgeon — by report
- Supply Charges — not allowed
- Outpatient Limit — does not apply

CPT CODE **SERVICE**

95065 Direct nasal mucous membrane test

CPT NOTES

Definitions

- ***Allergy sensitivity tests:*** the performance and evaluation of selective cutaneous and mucous membrane tests in correlation with the history, physical examination, and other observations of the patient. The number of tests performed should be judicious and dependent upon the history, physical findings, and clinical judgment. All patients should not necessarily receive the same tests nor the same number of sensitivity tests.
- ***Immunotherapy (desensitization, hyposensitization)***: the parenteral administration of allergenic extracts as antigens at periodic intervals, usually on an increasing dosage scale to a dosage which is maintained as maintenance therapy. Indications for immunotherapy are determined by appropriate diagnostic procedures coordinated with clinical judgment and knowledge of the natural history of allergic diseases.
- ***Other therapy***: for medical conferences on the use of mechanical and electronic devices (precipitators, air conditioners, air filters, humidifiers, dehumidifiers), climatotherapy, physical therapy, occupational and recreational therapy, see Evaluation and Management section.

ICD–9–CM

477.9 Allergic rhinitis NOS
754.0 Congen skull/face/jaw deformity

REIMBURSEMENT INFORMATION

Medicare

- Follow–up Days — global concept does not apply
- Assistant Surgeon — by report
- Supply Charges — not allowed
- Outpatient Limit — does not apply

CPT CODE **SERVICE**

95070 Inhalation bronchial challenge testing (not including necessary pulmonary function tests); with histamine, methacholine, or similar compounds

CPT NOTES

Definitions

- ***Allergy sensitivity tests:*** the performance and evaluation of selective cutaneous and mucous membrane tests in correlation with the history, physical examination, and other observations of the patient. The number of tests performed should be judicious and dependent upon the history, physical findings, and clinical judgment. All patients should not necessarily receive the same tests nor the same number of sensitivity tests.
- ***Immunotherapy (desensitization, hyposensitization)***: the parenteral administration of allergenic extracts as antigens at periodic intervals, usually on an increasing dosage scale to a dosage which is maintained as maintenance therapy. Indications for immunotherapy are determined by appropriate diagnostic procedures coordinated with clinical judgment and knowledge of the natural history of allergic diseases.
- ***Other therapy***: for medical conferences on the use of mechanical and electronic devices (precipitators, air conditioners, air filters, humidifiers, dehumidifiers), climatotherapy, physical therapy, occupational and recreational therapy, see Evaluation and Management section.
- For pulmonary function tests, see 94060, 94070.

ICD–9–CM

491.2	Obstructive chronic bronchitis
493.90	Asthma NOS w/o status asthmaticus
518.82	Other pulmonary insufficiency
519.8	Respiratory system disease NEC
786.09	Respiratory abnormality NEC
786.2	Cough
786.59	Chest pain NEC

REIMBURSEMENT INFORMATION

Medicare

- Follow–up Days — global concept does not apply
- Assistant Surgeon — by report
- Supply Charges — not allowed
- Outpatient Limit — does not apply

CPT CODE **SERVICE**

95071 Inhalation bronchial challenge testing (not including necessary pulmonary function tests); with antigens or gasses, specify

CPT NOTES

Definitions

- ***Allergy sensitivity tests:*** the performance and evaluation of selective cutaneous and mucous membrane tests in correlation with the history, physical examination, and other observations of the patient. The number of tests performed should be judicious and dependent upon the history, physical findings, and clinical judgment. All patients should not necessarily receive the same tests nor the same number of sensitivity tests.
- ***Immunotherapy (desensitization, hyposensitization)***: the parenteral administration of allergenic extracts as antigens at periodic intervals, usually on an increasing dosage scale to a dosage which is maintained as maintenance therapy. Indications for immunotherapy are determined by appropriate diagnostic procedures coordinated with clinical judgment and knowledge of the natural history of allergic diseases.
- ***Other therapy***: for medical conferences on the use of mechanical and electronic devices (precipitators, air conditioners, air filters, humidifiers, dehumidifiers), climatotherapy, physical therapy, occupational and recreational therapy, see Evaluation and Management section.
- For pulmonary function tests, see 94060, 94070.

ICD–9–CM

491.2	Obstructive chronic bronchitis
493.90	Asthma NOS w/o status asthmaticus
518.82	Other pulmonary insufficiency
519.8	Respiratory system disease NEC
786.09	Respiratory abnormality NEC
786.2	Cough
786.59	Chest pain NEC

REIMBURSEMENT INFORMATION

Medicare

- Follow–up Days — global concept does not apply
- Assistant Surgeon — by report
- Supply Charges — not allowed
- Outpatient Limit — does not apply

CPT CODE **SERVICE**

95075 Ingestion challenge test (sequential and incremental ingestion of test items, eg, food, drug or other substance such as metabisulfite)

CPT NOTES

Definitions

- ***Allergy sensitivity tests:*** the performance and evaluation of selective cutaneous and mucous membrane tests in correlation with the history, physical examination, and other observations of the patient. The number of tests performed should be judicious and dependent upon the history, physical findings, and clinical judgment. All patients should not necessarily receive the same tests nor the same number of sensitivity tests.
- ***Immunotherapy (desensitization, hyposensitization)***: the parenteral administration of allergenic extracts as antigens at periodic intervals, usually on an increasing dosage scale to a dosage which is maintained as maintenance therapy. Indications for immunotherapy are determined by appropriate diagnostic procedures coordinated with clinical judgment and knowledge of the natural history of allergic diseases.
- ***Other therapy***: for medical conferences on the use of mechanical and electronic devices (precipitators, air conditioners, air filters, humidifiers, dehumidifiers), climatotherapy, physical therapy, occupational and recreational therapy, see Evaluation and Management section.

ICD–9–CM

477.9	Allergic rhinitis NOS
693.1	Dermatitis d/t food ingestion
989.5	Toxic effect of venom
995.2	Adverse effect med/biol substnc NOS

REIMBURSEMENT INFORMATION

Medicare

- Follow–up Days — global concept does not apply
- Assistant Surgeon — by report
- Supply Charges — not allowed
- Outpatient Limit — does not apply

CPT CODE	SERVICE
95078	Provocative testing (eg, Rinkel test)

CPT NOTES

Definitions

- ***Allergy sensitivity tests:*** the performance and evaluation of selective cutaneous and mucous membrane tests in correlation with the history, physical examination, and other observations of the patient. The number of tests performed should be judicious and dependent upon the history, physical findings, and clinical judgment. All patients should not necessarily receive the same tests nor the same number of sensitivity tests.
- ***Immunotherapy (desensitization, hyposensitization)***: the parenteral administration of allergenic extracts as antigens at periodic intervals, usually on an increasing dosage scale to a dosage which is maintained as maintenance therapy. Indications for immunotherapy are determined by appropriate diagnostic procedures coordinated with clinical judgment and knowledge of the natural history of allergic diseases.
- ***Other therapy***: for medical conferences on the use of mechanical and electronic devices (precipitators, air conditioners, air filters, humidifiers, dehumidifiers), climatotherapy, physical therapy, occupational and recreational therapy, see Evaluation and Management section.
- For allergy laboratory tests, see 86000–86999.
- For intravenous therapy for severe or intractable allergic disease, see 90780, 90781, 90784.

ICD–9–CM	
477.9	Allergic rhinitis NOS
478.1	Nasal and sinus disease NEC
692.9	Dermatitis NOS
786.2	Cough

REIMBURSEMENT INFORMATION

Medicare

- Follow–up Days — global concept does not apply
- Assistant Surgeon — by report
- Supply Charges — not allowed
- Outpatient Limit — does not apply

CPT CODE **SERVICE**

95115 Professional services for allergen immunotherapy not including provision of allergenic extracts; single injection

CPT NOTES

Definitions

- ***Allergy sensitivity tests:*** the performance and evaluation of selective cutaneous and mucous membrane tests in correlation with the history, physical examination, and other observations of the patient. The number of tests performed should be judicious and dependent upon the history, physical findings, and clinical judgment. All patients should not necessarily receive the same tests nor the same number of sensitivity tests.
- ***Immunotherapy (desensitization, hyposensitization)***: the parenteral administration of allergenic extracts as antigens at periodic intervals, usually on an increasing dosage scale to a dosage which is maintained as maintenance therapy. Indications for immunotherapy are determined by appropriate diagnostic procedures coordinated with clinical judgment and knowledge of the natural history of allergic diseases.
- ***Other therapy***: for medical conferences on the use of mechanical and electronic devices (precipitators, air conditioners, air filters, humidifiers, dehumidifiers), climatotherapy, physical therapy, occupational and recreational therapy, see Evaluation and Management section.
- Includes the professional services necessary for allergen immunotherapy. Office visit codes may be used in addition to allergen immunotherapy, if and only if, other identifiable services are provided at that time.

ICD–9–CM

314.01	Attention deficit w/hyperactivity
372.05	Acute atopic conjunctivitis
372.14	Chronic allergic conjunctivitis NEC
381.04	Acute allergic serous otitis media
477.0	Allergic rhinitis d/t pollen
477.8	Allergic rhinitis NEC
477.9	Allergic rhinitis NOS
493.00	Extrinsic asthma w/o stat asthmat
493.90	Asthma NOS w/o status asthmaticus
558.9	Noninfect gastroenteritis NEC
691.8	Other atopic dermatitis
692.6	Dermatitis due to plants
692.9	Dermatitis NOS
698.9	Pruritic disorder NOS
708.0	Allergic urticaria
780.9	General symptoms NEC
995.2	Adverse effect med/biol substnc NOS
995.3	Allergy, unspecified
999.5	Serum reaction NEC
V07.1	Desensitization to allergens
V07.8	Prophylactic measures NEC
V67.9	Follow-up exam NOS
V72.7	Skin/sensitization tests

REIMBURSEMENT INFORMATION

Medicare

- Follow–up Days — global concept does not apply
- Assistant Surgeon — by report
- Supply Charges — not allowed
- Outpatient Limit — does not apply

CPT CODE	SERVICE
95117	Professional services for allergen immunotherapy not including provision of allergenic extracts; multiple injections

CPT NOTES

Definitions

- ***Allergy sensitivity tests:*** the performance and evaluation of selective cutaneous and mucous membrane tests in correlation with the history, physical examination, and other observations of the patient. The number of tests performed should be judicious and dependent upon the history, physical findings, and clinical judgment. All patients should not necessarily receive the same tests nor the same number of sensitivity tests.
- ***Immunotherapy (desensitization, hyposensitization)***: the parenteral administration of allergenic extracts as antigens at periodic intervals, usually on an increasing dosage scale to a dosage which is maintained as maintenance therapy. Indications for immunotherapy are determined by appropriate diagnostic procedures coordinated with clinical judgment and knowledge of the natural history of allergic diseases.
- ***Other therapy***: for medical conferences on the use of mechanical and electronic devices (precipitators, air conditioners, air filters, humidifiers, dehumidifiers), climatotherapy, physical therapy, occupational and recreational therapy, see Evaluation and Management section.
- Includes the professional services necessary for allergen immunotherapy. Office visit codes may be used in addition to allergen immunotherapy, if and only if, other identifiable services are provided at that time.

ICD–9–CM

314.01	Attention deficit w/hyperactivity
372.05	Acute atopic conjunctivitis
372.14	Chronic allergic conjunctivitis NEC
381.04	Acute allergic serous otitis media
477.0	Allergic rhinitis d/t pollen
477.8	Allergic rhinitis NEC
477.9	Allergic rhinitis NOS
493.00	Extrinsic asthma w/o stat asthmat
493.90	Asthma NOS w/o status asthmaticus
558.9	Noninfect gastroenteritis NEC
691.8	Other atopic dermatitis
692.6	Dermatitis due to plants
692.9	Dermatitis NOS
698.9	Pruritic disorder NOS
708.0	Allergic urticaria
780.9	General symptoms NEC
995.2	Adverse effect med/biol substnc NOS
995.3	Allergy, unspecified
999.5	Serum reaction NEC
V07.1	Desensitization to allergens
V07.8	Prophylactic measures NEC
V67.9	Follow-up exam NOS
V72.7	Skin/sensitization tests

REIMBURSEMENT INFORMATION

Medicare

- Follow–up Days — global concept does not apply
- Assistant Surgeon — by report
- Supply Charges — not allowed
- Outpatient Limit — does not apply

CPT CODE **SERVICE**

95120 Professional services for allergen immunotherapy in prescribing physician's office or institution, including provision of allergenic extract; single injection

CPT NOTES

Definitions

- ***Allergy sensitivity tests:*** the performance and evaluation of selective cutaneous and mucous membrane tests in correlation with the history, physical examination, and other observations of the patient. The number of tests performed should be judicious and dependent upon the history, physical findings, and clinical judgment. All patients should not necessarily receive the same tests nor the same number of sensitivity tests.
- ***Immunotherapy (desensitization, hyposensitization)***: the parenteral administration of allergenic extracts as antigens at periodic intervals, usually on an increasing dosage scale to a dosage which is maintained as maintenance therapy. Indications for immunotherapy are determined by appropriate diagnostic procedures coordinated with clinical judgment and knowledge of the natural history of allergic diseases.
- ***Other therapy***: for medical conferences on the use of mechanical and electronic devices (precipitators, air conditioners, air filters, humidifiers, dehumidifiers), climatotherapy, physical therapy, occupational and recreational therapy, see Evaluation and Management section.
- Includes the professional services necessary for allergen immunotherapy. Office visit codes may be used in addition to allergen immunotherapy, if and only if, other identifiable services are provided at that time.

ICD–9–CM

314.01	Attention deficit w/hyperactivity
346.9	Migraine NOS
372.05	Acute atopic conjunctivitis
372.14	Chronic allergic conjunctivitis NEC
381.04	Acute allergic serous otitis media
466.0	Acute bronchitis
477.0	Allergic rhinitis d/t pollen
477.8	Allergic rhinitis NEC
477.9	Allergic rhinitis NOS
493.00	Extrinsic asthma w/o stat asthmat
493.90	Asthma NOS w/o status asthmaticus
558.9	Noninfect gastroenteritis NEC
691.8	Other atopic dermatitis
692.6	Dermatitis due to plants
692.9	Dermatitis NOS
698.2	Prurigo
698.9	Pruritic disorder NOS
708.0	Allergic urticaria
780.9	General symptoms NEC
995.2	Adverse effect med/biol substnc NOS
995.3	Allergy, unspecified
999.5	Serum reaction NEC
V07.1	Desensitization to allergens
V07.8	Prophylactic measures NEC
V67.9	Follow-up exam NOS
V72.7	Skin/sensitization tests

REIMBURSEMENT INFORMATION

Medicare

- Follow–up Days — global concept does not apply
- Assistant Surgeon — not paid
- Supply Charges — not allowed
- Outpatient Limit — does not apply

CPT CODE **SERVICE**

95125 Professional services for allergen immunotherapy in prescribing physician's office or institution, including provision of allergenic extract; multiple injections (specify number of injections)

CPT NOTES

Definitions

- ***Allergy sensitivity tests:*** the performance and evaluation of selective cutaneous and mucous membrane tests in correlation with the history, physical examination, and other observations of the patient. The number of tests performed should be judicious and dependent upon the history, physical findings, and clinical judgment. All patients should not necessarily receive the same tests nor the same number of sensitivity tests.
- ***Immunotherapy (desensitization, hyposensitization)***: the parenteral administration of allergenic extracts as antigens at periodic intervals, usually on an increasing dosage scale to a dosage which is maintained as maintenance therapy. Indications for immunotherapy are determined by appropriate diagnostic procedures coordinated with clinical judgment and knowledge of the natural history of allergic diseases.
- ***Other therapy***: for medical conferences on the use of mechanical and electronic devices (precipitators, air conditioners, air filters, humidifiers, dehumidifiers), climatotherapy, physical therapy, occupational and recreational therapy, see Evaluation and Management section.
- Includes the professional services necessary for allergen immunotherapy. Office visit codes may be used in addition to allergen immunotherapy, if and only if, other identifiable services are provided at that time.

ICD–9–CM

314.01	Attention deficit w/hyperactivity
346.9	Migraine NOS
372.05	Acute atopic conjunctivitis
372.14	Chronic allergic conjunctivitis NEC
381.04	Acute allergic serous otitis media
466.0	Acute bronchitis
477.0	Allergic rhinitis d/t pollen
477.8	Allergic rhinitis NEC
477.9	Allergic rhinitis NOS
493.00	Extrinsic asthma w/o stat asthmat
493.90	Asthma NOS w/o status asthmaticus
558.9	Noninfect gastroenteritis NEC
691.8	Other atopic dermatitis
692.6	Dermatitis due to plants
692.9	Dermatitis NOS
698.2	Prurigo
698.9	Pruritic disorder NOS
708.0	Allergic urticaria
780.9	General symptoms NEC
995.2	Adverse effect med/biol substnc NOS
995.3	Allergy, unspecified
999.5	Serum reaction NEC
V07.1	Desensitization to allergens
V07.8	Prophylactic measures NEC
V67.9	Follow-up exam NOS
V72.7	Skin/sensitization tests

REIMBURSEMENT INFORMATION

Medicare

- Follow–up Days — global concept does not apply
- Assistant Surgeon — not paid
- Supply Charges — not allowed
- Outpatient Limit — does not apply

CPT CODE **SERVICE**

95130 Professional services for allergen immunotherapy in prescribing physician's office or institution, including provision of allergenic extract; single stinging insect venom

CPT NOTES

Definitions

- ***Allergy sensitivity tests:*** the performance and evaluation of selective cutaneous and mucous membrane tests in correlation with the history, physical examination, and other observations of the patient. The number of tests performed should be judicious and dependent upon the history, physical findings, and clinical judgment. All patients should not necessarily receive the same tests nor the same number of sensitivity tests.
- ***Immunotherapy (desensitization, hyposensitization)***: the parenteral administration of allergenic extracts as antigens at periodic intervals, usually on an increasing dosage scale to a dosage which is maintained as maintenance therapy. Indications for immunotherapy are determined by appropriate diagnostic procedures coordinated with clinical judgment and knowledge of the natural history of allergic diseases.
- ***Other therapy***: for medical conferences on the use of mechanical and electronic devices (precipitators, air conditioners, air filters, humidifiers, dehumidifiers), climatotherapy, physical therapy, occupational and recreational therapy, see Evaluation and Management section.
- Includes the professional services necessary for allergen immunotherapy. Office visit codes may be used in addition to allergen immunotherapy, if and only if, other identifiable services are provided at that time.

ICD–9–CM

708.0 Allergic urticaria
989.5 Toxic effect of venom

REIMBURSEMENT INFORMATION

Medicare

- Follow–up Days — global concept does not apply
- Assistant Surgeon — not paid
- Supply Charges — not allowed
- Outpatient Limit — does not apply

CPT CODE	SERVICE
95131	Professional services for allergen immunotherapy in prescribing physician's office or institution, including provision of allergenic extract; two stinging insect venoms

CPT NOTES

Definitions

- ***Allergy sensitivity tests:*** the performance and evaluation of selective cutaneous and mucous membrane tests in correlation with the history, physical examination, and other observations of the patient. The number of tests performed should be judicious and dependent upon the history, physical findings, and clinical judgment. All patients should not necessarily receive the same tests nor the same number of sensitivity tests.
- ***Immunotherapy (desensitization, hyposensitization)***: the parenteral administration of allergenic extracts as antigens at periodic intervals, usually on an increasing dosage scale to a dosage which is maintained as maintenance therapy. Indications for immunotherapy are determined by appropriate diagnostic procedures coordinated with clinical judgment and knowledge of the natural history of allergic diseases.
- ***Other therapy***: for medical conferences on the use of mechanical and electronic devices (precipitators, air conditioners, air filters, humidifiers, dehumidifiers), climatotherapy, physical therapy, occupational and recreational therapy, see Evaluation and Management section.
- Includes the professional services necessary for allergen immunotherapy. Office visit codes may be used in addition to allergen immunotherapy, if and only if, other identifiable services are provided at that time.

ICD–9–CM

708.0	Allergic urticaria
989.5	Toxic effect of venom

REIMBURSEMENT INFORMATION

Medicare

- Follow–up Days — global concept does not apply
- Assistant Surgeon — not paid
- Supply Charges — not allowed
- Outpatient Limit — does not apply

CPT CODE **SERVICE**

95132 Professional services for allergen immunotherapy in prescribing physician's office or institution, including provision of allergenic extract; three stinging insect venoms

CPT NOTES

Definitions

- ***Allergy sensitivity tests:*** the performance and evaluation of selective cutaneous and mucous membrane tests in correlation with the history, physical examination, and other observations of the patient. The number of tests performed should be judicious and dependent upon the history, physical findings, and clinical judgment. All patients should not necessarily receive the same tests nor the same number of sensitivity tests.
- ***Immunotherapy (desensitization, hyposensitization)***: the parenteral administration of allergenic extracts as antigens at periodic intervals, usually on an increasing dosage scale to a dosage which is maintained as maintenance therapy. Indications for immunotherapy are determined by appropriate diagnostic procedures coordinated with clinical judgment and knowledge of the natural history of allergic diseases.
- ***Other therapy***: for medical conferences on the use of mechanical and electronic devices (precipitators, air conditioners, air filters, humidifiers, dehumidifiers), climatotherapy, physical therapy, occupational and recreational therapy, see Evaluation and Management section.
- Includes the professional services necessary for allergen immunotherapy. Office visit codes may be used in addition to allergen immunotherapy, if and only if, other identifiable services are provided at that time.

ICD–9–CM

708.0 Allergic urticaria
989.5 Toxic effect of venom

REIMBURSEMENT INFORMATION

Medicare

- Follow–up Days — global concept does not apply
- Assistant Surgeon — not paid
- Supply Charges — not allowed
- Outpatient Limit — does not apply

CPT CODE	SERVICE
95133	Professional services for allergen immunotherapy in prescribing physician's office or institution, including provision of allergenic extract; four stinging insect venoms

CPT NOTES

Definitions

- ***Allergy sensitivity tests:*** the performance and evaluation of selective cutaneous and mucous membrane tests in correlation with the history, physical examination, and other observations of the patient. The number of tests performed should be judicious and dependent upon the history, physical findings, and clinical judgment. All patients should not necessarily receive the same tests nor the same number of sensitivity tests.
- ***Immunotherapy (desensitization, hyposensitization)***: the parenteral administration of allergenic extracts as antigens at periodic intervals, usually on an increasing dosage scale to a dosage which is maintained as maintenance therapy. Indications for immunotherapy are determined by appropriate diagnostic procedures coordinated with clinical judgment and knowledge of the natural history of allergic diseases.
- ***Other therapy***: for medical conferences on the use of mechanical and electronic devices (precipitators, air conditioners, air filters, humidifiers, dehumidifiers), climatotherapy, physical therapy, occupational and recreational therapy, see Evaluation and Management section.
- Includes the professional services necessary for allergen immunotherapy. Office visit codes may be used in addition to allergen immunotherapy, if and only if, other identifiable services are provided at that time.

ICD–9–CM

708.0	Allergic urticaria
989.5	Toxic effect of venom

REIMBURSEMENT INFORMATION

Medicare

- Follow–up Days — global concept does not apply
- Assistant Surgeon — not paid
- Supply Charges — not allowed
- Outpatient Limit — does not apply

CPT CODE **SERVICE**

95144 Professional services for the supervision and provision of antigens for allergen immunotherapy, single or multiple antigens, single dose vials (specify number of vials)

CPT NOTES

Definitions

- ***Allergy sensitivity tests:*** the performance and evaluation of selective cutaneous and mucous membrane tests in correlation with the history, physical examination, and other observations of the patient. The number of tests performed should be judicious and dependent upon the history, physical findings, and clinical judgment. All patients should not necessarily receive the same tests nor the same number of sensitivity tests.
- ***Immunotherapy (desensitization, hyposensitization)***: the parenteral administration of allergenic extracts as antigens at periodic intervals, usually on an increasing dosage scale to a dosage which is maintained as maintenance therapy. Indications for immunotherapy are determined by appropriate diagnostic procedures coordinated with clinical judgment and knowledge of the natural history of allergic diseases.
- ***Other therapy***: for medical conferences on the use of mechanical and electronic devices (precipitators, air conditioners, air filters, humidifiers, dehumidifiers), climatotherapy, physical therapy, occupational and recreational therapy, see Evaluation and Management section.
- Includes the professional services necessary for allergen immunotherapy. Office visit codes may be used in addition to allergen immunotherapy, if and only if, other identifiable services are provided at that time.

ICD–9–CM

372.05	Acute atopic conjunctivitis
372.14	Chronic allergic conjunctivitis NEC
381.04	Acute allergic serous otitis media
477.0	Allergic rhinitis d/t pollen
477.8	Allergic rhinitis NEC
477.9	Allergic rhinitis NOS
493.00	Extrinsic asthma w/o stat asthmat
493.90	Asthma NOS w/o status asthmaticus
558.9	Noninfect gastroenteritis NEC
691.8	Other atopic dermatitis
692.6	Dermatitis due to plants
692.9	Dermatitis NOS
698.9	Pruritic disorder NOS
708.0	Allergic urticaria
780.9	General symptoms NEC
995.3	Allergy, unspecified

REIMBURSEMENT INFORMATION

Medicare

- Follow–up Days — global concept does not apply
- Assistant Surgeon — not paid
- Supply Charges — not allowed
- Outpatient Limit — does not apply

CPT CODE **SERVICE**

95145 Professional services for the supervision and provision of antigens for allergen immunotherapy (specify number of doses); single stinging insect venom, multiple dose vials

CPT NOTES

Definitions

- ***Allergy sensitivity tests:*** the performance and evaluation of selective cutaneous and mucous membrane tests in correlation with the history, physical examination, and other observations of the patient. The number of tests performed should be judicious and dependent upon the history, physical findings, and clinical judgment. All patients should not necessarily receive the same tests nor the same number of sensitivity tests.
- ***Immunotherapy (desensitization, hyposensitization)***: the parenteral administration of allergenic extracts as antigens at periodic intervals, usually on an increasing dosage scale to a dosage which is maintained as maintenance therapy. Indications for immunotherapy are determined by appropriate diagnostic procedures coordinated with clinical judgment and knowledge of the natural history of allergic diseases.
- ***Other therapy***: for medical conferences on the use of mechanical and electronic devices (precipitators, air conditioners, air filters, humidifiers, dehumidifiers), climatotherapy, physical therapy, occupational and recreational therapy, see Evaluation and Management section.
- Includes the professional services necessary for allergen immunotherapy. Office visit codes may be used in addition to allergen immunotherapy, if and only if, other identifiable services are provided at that time.

ICD–9–CM

708.0 Allergic urticaria
989.5 Toxic effect of venom

REIMBURSEMENT INFORMATION

Medicare

- Follow–up Days — global concept does not apply
- Assistant Surgeon — not paid
- Supply Charges — not allowed
- Outpatient Limit — does not apply

CPT CODE	SERVICE
95147	Professional services for the supervision and provision of antigens for allergen immunotherapy (specify number of doses); three single stinging insect venoms, multiple does vials

CPT NOTES

Definitions

- ***Allergy sensitivity tests:*** the performance and evaluation of selective cutaneous and mucous membrane tests in correlation with the history, physical examination, and other observations of the patient. The number of tests performed should be judicious and dependent upon the history, physical findings, and clinical judgment. All patients should not necessarily receive the same tests nor the same number of sensitivity tests.
- ***Immunotherapy (desensitization, hyposensitization)***: the parenteral administration of allergenic extracts as antigens at periodic intervals, usually on an increasing dosage scale to a dosage which is maintained as maintenance therapy. Indications for immunotherapy are determined by appropriate diagnostic procedures coordinated with clinical judgment and knowledge of the natural history of allergic diseases.
- ***Other therapy***: for medical conferences on the use of mechanical and electronic devices (precipitators, air conditioners, air filters, humidifiers, dehumidifiers), climatotherapy, physical therapy, occupational and recreational therapy, see Evaluation and Management section.
- Includes the professional services necessary for allergen immunotherapy. Office visit codes may be used in addition to allergen immunotherapy, if and only if, other identifiable services are provided at that time.

ICD–9–CM

708.0	Allergic urticaria
989.5	Toxic effect of venom

REIMBURSEMENT INFORMATION

Medicare

- Follow–up Days — global concept does not apply
- Assistant Surgeon — not paid
- Supply Charges — not allowed
- Outpatient Limit — does not apply

CPT CODE	SERVICE
95148	Professional services for the supervision and provision of antigens for allergen immunotherapy (specify number of doses); four single stinging insect venoms, multiple does vials

CPT NOTES

Definitions

- ***Allergy sensitivity tests:*** the performance and evaluation of selective cutaneous and mucous membrane tests in correlation with the history, physical examination, and other observations of the patient. The number of tests performed should be judicious and dependent upon the history, physical findings, and clinical judgment. All patients should not necessarily receive the same tests nor the same number of sensitivity tests.
- ***Immunotherapy (desensitization, hyposensitization)***: the parenteral administration of allergenic extracts as antigens at periodic intervals, usually on an increasing dosage scale to a dosage which is maintained as maintenance therapy. Indications for immunotherapy are determined by appropriate diagnostic procedures coordinated with clinical judgment and knowledge of the natural history of allergic diseases.
- ***Other therapy***: for medical conferences on the use of mechanical and electronic devices (precipitators, air conditioners, air filters, humidifiers, dehumidifiers), climatotherapy, physical therapy, occupational and recreational therapy, see Evaluation and Management section.
- Includes the professional services necessary for allergen immunotherapy. Office visit codes may be used in addition to allergen immunotherapy, if and only if, other identifiable services are provided at that time.

ICD–9–CM

708.0	Allergic urticaria
989.5	Toxic effect of venom

REIMBURSEMENT INFORMATION

Medicare

- Follow–up Days — global concept does not apply
- Assistant Surgeon — not paid
- Supply Charges — not allowed
- Outpatient Limit — does not apply

CPT CODE **SERVICE**

95149 Professional services for the supervision and provision of antigens for allergen immunotherapy (specify number of doses); five single stinging insect venoms, multiple does vials

CPT NOTES

Definitions

- ***Allergy sensitivity tests:*** the performance and evaluation of selective cutaneous and mucous membrane tests in correlation with the history, physical examination, and other observations of the patient. The number of tests performed should be judicious and dependent upon the history, physical findings, and clinical judgment. All patients should not necessarily receive the same tests nor the same number of sensitivity tests.
- ***Immunotherapy (desensitization, hyposensitization)***: the parenteral administration of allergenic extracts as antigens at periodic intervals, usually on an increasing dosage scale to a dosage which is maintained as maintenance therapy. Indications for immunotherapy are determined by appropriate diagnostic procedures coordinated with clinical judgment and knowledge of the natural history of allergic diseases.
- ***Other therapy***: for medical conferences on the use of mechanical and electronic devices (precipitators, air conditioners, air filters, humidifiers, dehumidifiers), climatotherapy, physical therapy, occupational and recreational therapy, see Evaluation and Management section.
- Includes the professional services necessary for allergen immunotherapy. Office visit codes may be used in addition to allergen immunotherapy, if and only if, other identifiable services are provided at that time.

ICD–9–CM

708.0 Allergic urticaria
989.5 Toxic effect of venom

REIMBURSEMENT INFORMATION

Medicare

- Follow–up Days — global concept does not apply
- Assistant Surgeon — not paid
- Supply Charges — not allowed
- Outpatient Limit — does not apply

CPT CODE	SERVICE
95165	Professional services for the supervision and provision of antigens for allergen immunotherapy; single or multiple antigens, multiple does vial(s), (specify number of doses)

CPT NOTES

Definitions

- ***Allergy sensitivity tests:*** the performance and evaluation of selective cutaneous and mucous membrane tests in correlation with the history, physical examination, and other observations of the patient. The number of tests performed should be judicious and dependent upon the history, physical findings, and clinical judgment. All patients should not necessarily receive the same tests nor the same number of sensitivity tests.
- ***Immunotherapy (desensitization, hyposensitization)***: the parenteral administration of allergenic extracts as antigens at periodic intervals, usually on an increasing dosage scale to a dosage which is maintained as maintenance therapy. Indications for immunotherapy are determined by appropriate diagnostic procedures coordinated with clinical judgment and knowledge of the natural history of allergic diseases.
- ***Other therapy***: for medical conferences on the use of mechanical and electronic devices (precipitators, air conditioners, air filters, humidifiers, dehumidifiers), climatotherapy, physical therapy, occupational and recreational therapy, see Evaluation and Management section.
- Includes the professional services necessary for allergen immunotherapy. Office visit codes may be used in addition to allergen immunotherapy, if and only if, other identifiable services are provided at that time.

ICD–9–CM

346.2	Variants of migraine
372.05	Acute atopic conjunctivitis
372.14	Chronic allergic conjunctivitis NEC
477.0	Allergic rhinitis d/t pollen
477.8	Allergic rhinitis NEC
477.9	Allergic rhinitis NOS
493.00	Extrinsic asthma w/o stat asthmat
493.90	Asthma NOS w/o status asthmaticus
692.6	Dermatitis due to plants
692.9	Dermatitis NOS
693.1	Dermatitis d/t food ingestion
698.9	Pruritic disorder NOS
708.0	Allergic urticaria
780.9	General symptoms NEC
995.2	Adverse effect med/biol substnc NOS
995.3	Allergy, unspecified
999.5	Serum reaction NEC

REIMBURSEMENT INFORMATION

Medicare

- Follow–up Days — global concept does not apply
- Assistant Surgeon — not paid
- Supply Charges — not allowed
- Outpatient Limit — does not apply

CPT CODE	SERVICE
95170	Professional services for the supervision and provision of antigens for allergen immunotherapy; whole body extract of biting insect or other arthropod (specify number of doses)

CPT NOTES

Definitions

- ***Allergy sensitivity tests:*** the performance and evaluation of selective cutaneous and mucous membrane tests in correlation with the history, physical examination, and other observations of the patient. The number of tests performed should be judicious and dependent upon the history, physical findings, and clinical judgment. All patients should not necessarily receive the same tests nor the same number of sensitivity tests.
- ***Immunotherapy (desensitization, hyposensitization)***: the parenteral administration of allergenic extracts as antigens at periodic intervals, usually on an increasing dosage scale to a dosage which is maintained as maintenance therapy. Indications for immunotherapy are determined by appropriate diagnostic procedures coordinated with clinical judgment and knowledge of the natural history of allergic diseases.
- ***Other therapy***: for medical conferences on the use of mechanical and electronic devices (precipitators, air conditioners, air filters, humidifiers, dehumidifiers), climatotherapy, physical therapy, occupational and recreational therapy, see Evaluation and Management section.
- Includes the professional services necessary for allergen immunotherapy. Office visit codes may be used in addition to allergen immunotherapy, if and only if, other identifiable services are provided at that time.

ICD–9–CM

708.0	Allergic urticaria
989.5	Toxic effect of venom

REIMBURSEMENT INFORMATION

Medicare

- Follow–up Days — global concept does not apply
- Assistant Surgeon — not paid
- Supply Charges — not allowed
- Outpatient Limit — does not apply

CPT CODE	SERVICE
95180	Rapid desensitization procedure, each hour (eg, insulin, penicillin, horse serum)

CPT NOTES

Definitions

- ***Allergy sensitivity tests:*** the performance and evaluation of selective cutaneous and mucous membrane tests in correlation with the history, physical examination, and other observations of the patient. The number of tests performed should be judicious and dependent upon the history, physical findings, and clinical judgment. All patients should not necessarily receive the same tests nor the same number of sensitivity tests.
- ***Immunotherapy (desensitization, hyposensitization)***: the parenteral administration of allergenic extracts as antigens at periodic intervals, usually on an increasing dosage scale to a dosage which is maintained as maintenance therapy. Indications for immunotherapy are determined by appropriate diagnostic procedures coordinated with clinical judgment and knowledge of the natural history of allergic diseases.
- ***Other therapy***: for medical conferences on the use of mechanical and electronic devices (precipitators, air conditioners, air filters, humidifiers, dehumidifiers), climatotherapy, physical therapy, occupational and recreational therapy, see Evaluation and Management section.
- Includes the professional services necessary for allergen immunotherapy. Office visit codes may be used in addition to allergen immunotherapy, if and only if, other identifiable services are provided at that time.

ICD–9–CM

693.0	Drug dermatitis NOS
995.2	Adverse effect med/biol substnc NOS

REIMBURSEMENT INFORMATION

<u>Medicare</u>

- Follow–up Days — global concept does not apply
- Assistant Surgeon — by report
- Supply Charges — not allowed
- Outpatient Limit — does not apply

CPT CODE **SERVICE**

95199 Unlisted allergy/clinical immunologic service or procedure

CPT NOTES

Definitions

- ***Allergy sensitivity tests:*** the performance and evaluation of selective cutaneous and mucous membrane tests in correlation with the history, physical examination, and other observations of the patient. The number of tests performed should be judicious and dependent upon the history, physical findings, and clinical judgment. All patients should not necessarily receive the same tests nor the same number of sensitivity tests.
- ***Immunotherapy (desensitization, hyposensitization)***: the parenteral administration of allergenic extracts as antigens at periodic intervals, usually on an increasing dosage scale to a dosage which is maintained as maintenance therapy. Indications for immunotherapy are determined by appropriate diagnostic procedures coordinated with clinical judgment and knowledge of the natural history of allergic diseases.
- ***Other therapy***: for medical conferences on the use of mechanical and electronic devices (precipitators, air conditioners, air filters, humidifiers, dehumidifiers), climatotherapy, physical therapy, occupational and recreational therapy, see Evaluation and Management section.
- Includes the professional services necessary for allergen immunotherapy. Office visit codes may be used in addition to allergen immunotherapy, if and only if, other identifiable services are provided at that time.
- For skin testing of bacterial, viral, fungal extracts, see 95030-95, 86485-86586.
- For special reports on allergy patients, see 99080.
- For testing procedures such as radioallergosorbent testing (RAST), rat mast cell technique (RMCT), mast cell degranulation test (MCDT), lymphocytic transformations test (LTT), leukocyte histamine release (LHR), migration inhibitory factor test (MIF), transfer factor test (TFT), nitroblue tetrazolium dye test (NTD), see Immunology section in Pathology or use 95199.

ICD–9–CM

472.0	Chronic rhinitis
477.0	Allergic rhinitis d/t pollen
477.9	Allergic rhinitis NOS
493.10	Intrinsic asthma w/o stat asthmat
693.1	Dermatitis d/t food ingestion
708.0	Allergic urticaria
708.5	Cholinergic urticaria
708.9	Urticaria NOS
786.2	Cough
919.5	Insect bite NEC, infected

REIMBURSEMENT INFORMATION

Medicare

- Follow–up Days — global concept does not apply
- Assistant Surgeon — by report
- Supply Charges — not allowed
- Outpatient Limit — does not apply

ISBN 0-07-600762-6
90000
9 780076 007622